FUNDAMENTALS OF
Psychoneuroimmunology

We dedicate this book to our families

FUNDAMENTALS OF
Psychoneuroimmunology

CAI SONG
University of British Columbia, Vancouver, Canada

BRIAN E. LEONARD
National University of Ireland, Galway, Ireland

JOHN WILEY & SONS, LTD
Chichester · New York · Weinheim · Brisbane · Singapore · Toronto

Other Wiley Editorial Offices

John Wiley & Sons, Inc., 605 Third Avenue,
New York, NY 10158-0012, USA

WILEY-VCH Verlag GmbH, Pappelallee 3,
D-69469 Weinheim, Germany

Jacaranda Wiley Ltd, 33 Park Road, Milton,
Queensland 4064, Australia

John Wiley & Sons (Asia) Pte Ltd, 2 Clementi Loop #02-01,
Jin Xing Distripark, Singapore 129809

John Wiley & Sons (Canada) Ltd, 22 Worcester Road,
Rexdale, Ontario M9W 1L1, Canada

Library of Congress Cataloging-in-Publication Data

Song, Cai.
  Fundamentals of psychoneuroimmunology / Cai Song, Brian E. Leonard.
    p. ; cm.
  Includes bibliographical references and index.
  ISBN 0-471-98671-2 (cased : alk. paper)
  1. Psychoneuroimmunology.   I. Leonard, B. E.   II. Title.
  [DNLM: 1. Psychoneuroimmunology.   2. Immune System—physiopathology.   3. Mental
  Disorders—immunology. WL 103.7 S698f 2000]
  RC346.5 .S66 2000
  616.8'0479—dc21
                                                                              99-059485

British Library Cataloguing in Publication Data

A catalogue record for this book is available from the British Library

ISBN 0-471-98671-2

Typeset in 10/12pt Palatino by Dorwyn Ltd, Rowlands Castle, Hants
Printed and bound in Great Britain by Biddles Ltd, Guildford and King's Lynn
This book is printed on acid-free paper responsibly manufactured from sustainable forestry,
in which at least two trees are planted for each one used for paper production.

Contents

Preface

The history of medicine is reflected in the conflict between monist and dualist philosophies, a conflict between those who see a unity between the mind and the body and those who distinguish between the purely organic and the purely mental or spiritual. This struggle goes back over 2000 years in Western Europe to the Greek philosophers. In the Hygeian school of Greek medicine, based on the teachings of Hippocrates, health was viewed as a natural state of the body. The body was believed to be endowed with inherent healing powers which, if the individual lives in harmony with these powers, maintains health and helps to restore the body to health in event of disease. Thus a disease was seen as a reflection of weakness of the inherent healing powers of the body and the function of medicine was to assist the patient to restore health and live within the natural law (vis medicatrix naturae). By contrast, the Asclepian school of medicine (based on the physician Asclepius who is said to have performed miracles) arose about 1200 BC, some 600 years before the Hygeian school, and has profoundly influenced modern medicine by focusing on diseases, their causes and cures. Each disease was considered to be the effect of, or response to, a specific cause that affected a specific organ system. Thus for every disease it was postulated that there was a specific drug or procedure that could alleviate or cure it. A successful clinician was therefore one who was able to make a correct diagnosis and prescribe the correct treatment.

Of the many advances in the neurosciences over the past four decades, the realization that the immune and endocrine systems are profoundly affected by the emotional state and, conversely, that these systems can change the emotional state, has helped to refocus the attention of physicians and researchers on the interrelationship between the mind and the body. Thus psychoneuroimmunoendocrinology has become the discipline that after 2500 years has served to unify the Hygeian and Asclepian schools of thought.

While the origin of the concept that the emotional state and mental processes are linked to physical health and disease can be traced back to antiquity, the scientific basis for understanding the mechanisms whereby these processes are communicated was largely due to the research of Hans Selye in the early part of this century. Selye and his collaborators showed how the hypothalamus and the pituitary gland play a critical role in controlling the release of stress hormones, particularly the glucocorticoids, which modulate immune function. Equally it is now known that the products of the immune system can communicate and modulate the functioning of the endocrine system. The hypothalamus provides the anatomical conduit for relaying the responses of the organism to stressful stimuli not only to the endocrine organs but also to the antonomic nervous system which innervates the tissues of the immune system. The stress hormones, and the cells of the immune system which secrete immunotransmitters, thus act as the cellular links between the central neurotransmitters and pysiological and pathalogical processes. Thus an understanding of the neurochemical, immunological, endocrinological, neurobiological and psychological implications of the cross-talk between the endocrine and immune systems offers exciting approaches to the management of numerous pathological conditions. These range from the autoimmune diseases to the numerous neurological and psychiatric diseases in which the harmonious relationship between the immune, endocrine and neurotransmitter systems are disturbed. Perhaps for the first time, the science of psychoneuroimmunology helps to provide a rational basis for psychosomatic medicine which for decades has tended to be marginalized as a subject of limited scientific merit.

The present volume is an attempt by two psychopharmacologists from different neuroscience backgrounds to demonstrate the importance of psychoneuroimmunology to the practising physician and experimental neuroscientist. This is not intended to be a definitive text and we are well aware of the many limitations that inevitably arise when attempting to cover the impact of the immune system on neurological and psychiatric diseases. Hopefully the text is sufficiently concise and stimulating to encourage the reader to probe further into the subject. To assist the reader in this regard, we have included details of monographs and review articles at the end of each chapter that reflect the basic concepts that have been discussed. Our hope is that you, the reader, will look upon this modest contribution as an introduction to the rapidly developing world of psychoneuroimmunology. Your comments and criticisms will be particularly welcomed.

Finally, we express our gratitude to the many colleagues who have contributed to our research and understanding of the subject over the last decade. BL particularly wishes to thank his secretary, Marie Morrissey, for her dedicated assistance in the word-processing part of the text. Special thanks is also due to Deborah Reece and her staff at John Wiley & Sons for their encouragement and assistance in our realization of this project.

Cai Song, Vancouver
Brian E. Leonard, Galway
August 1999

1 Historical Overview of Mind–Body Interrelationships

The belief that stress and the emotional states of an individual can have a major impact on bodily functions, and even be responsible for cancers, coronary disease and gastrointestinal distress, has been widely held since antiquity. For example, nearly 2000 years ago, the Greek physician Galen proposed that melancholic women were particularly prone to cancer of the reproductive organs due to an excess of "black bile", which was believed to cause melancholia. In the first century BC, the Roman poet Virgil postulated that "mind moves matter", while 300 years earlier the philosopher Aristotle advised that "Just as you ought not to attempt to use eyes without head or head without body, so you should not treat body without soul".

In more recent time, the French philosopher and mathematician René Descartes had a major impact on the way diseases were envisaged. Descartes proposed that the complex study of living organisms could best be understood by investigating the individual components that compromise the individual. He postulated that by considering the smaller and smaller components of the living organism, the functions of these components would probably become simpler to understand. This led to scientific reductionism, a philosophical approach which is particularly prevalent today in molecular neurobiology and many aspects of the neurosciences. The reductionist perspective of Descartes resulted in a number of advances and discoveries leading in the eighteenth and nineteenth centuries to an understanding of the importance of microorganisms in causing disease. Indeed by the nineteenth century, body and mind had become completely separated into those areas that belonged to the attention of philosophers and theologicians (mind) and those areas that belonged to the world of the physiologist, anatomist and clinician. However, despite the separation between mind and body in the eyes of the majority of medical scientists in the nineteenth and early twentieth century, some clinical researchers persisted in emphasizing the importance of emotional factors in physical disease. Thus the father of modern medicine, Sir William Osler, believed that it was more important to know what was going on in a patient's head than in his chest to predict the outcome of pulmonary tuberculosis. He also recognized the psychosomatic nature of conditions such as systemic lupus erythematosus. However, a serious attempt to recognize the interrelation-ship between the mental state of a patient and physical illness only came about early in this century when Meyer proposed the concept of psychobiol-ogy, which emphasized the interrelationship between mental and physical events. Other researchers, such as Franz Alexander and Flanders Dunbar, laid the basis of psychosomatic medicine by investigating the relationship between physical illness and stressful life events, personality and emotions.

In the 1930s, during the period in which psychosomatic medicine was becoming accepted, Hans Selye established the importance of the endocrine system, as influenced by different kinds of external and internal stressors, in causing such pathological changes as adrenal cortical hypertrophy, gastric ulcerations and atrophy of the thymus and lymphatic tissues. Only in more recent times has it become established that changes in the immune system that occur in response to stress are directly influenced by the activity of the endocrine system. Undoubtedly due to the impact of the endocrine system in the understanding of physiological and pathological changes, psycho-endocrinology has become well established as an independent discipline. However, only in the last two decades or so has psychoneuroimmunology become well established with the attempt to integrate the behavioural, neu-ronal, endocrine and immune functions. Each of these "systems" has been shown to respond to information supplied by the other, thereby providing an integrated biological network within the organism. Of those interacting systems, however, it is the immune system which is still considered by many investigators to be an autonomous agency of defence, a system of complex cellular interactions that proceeds independently of changes occurring in the rest of the body. This assumption is still currently held by many immunolo-gists, as witnessed by a total absence of any mention of psychoneuro-immunology in some of the recently published standard textbooks on immunology (cf. Elgert, 1996).

And yet there is substantial evidence to show how the immune system impacts on the endocrine and neurotransmitter systems. Many of these aspects will be discussed in later chapters but, as an example, interleukin-1 (IL-1) not only orchestrates many immune responses but also stimulates the release of corticotrophin-releasing factor (CRF) by the hypothalamus. This causes the release of adrenocorticotrophic hormone (ACTH), resulting in enhanced glucocorticoid secretion. These hormones have well-established immunomodulatory effects. Thus regulation of ACTH secretion by IL-1 might represent a feedback loop that demonstrates a meaningful brain–immune system interrelationship. There are numerous other feedback sys-tems that involve different cytokines influencing neurotransmitter release in the hypothalamus. For example, IL-6 and tumour necrosis factor (TNF) alpha stimulate the release of acetylcholine, serotonin, corticotrophin-releasing hormone (CRH) and IL-1 but inhibit the release of gamma-aminobutyric acid (GABA) from the hypothalamus. These cytokines are released from activated monocytes and macrophages, are important factors in immune–endocrine–neurotransmitter interconnections and are illustrated diagramatically in Figure 1.1.

The recent interest in psychoneuroimmunology has undoubtedly been encouraged by the changes in the immune system and behaviour following infection by the human immunodeficiency virus (HIV). More is known about the immunological characteristics of the various stages of AIDS than any other disorder and it is now becoming apparent that several cytokines (for example, the interleukins, interferons (IFNs), and TNF) can act as markers of the progression of the disease. The almost miraculous recoveries of some AIDS patients that have been associated with major changes in lifestyle, stress reducing strategies, etc. have been accompanied by major changes in their immunological status. Stress management strategies are now frequently being incorporated into the treatment of the AIDS patient as a result of such findings.

Considering the short time during which any attention has been given to brain–immune interrelationships, considerable advances in our understanding of the subject have taken place largely due to the pioneering research and enthusiastic support for psychoneuroimmunology by neuroscientists

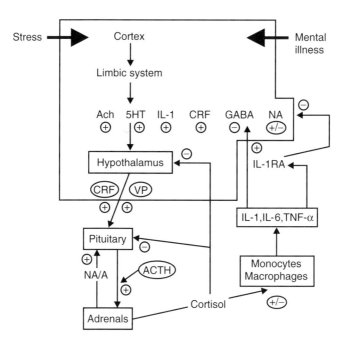

Figure 1.1 Hypothalamic–pituitary–adrenal immune interrelationship. CRF, corticotrophin-releasing factor; VP, vasopressin; ACTH, corticotrophin; IL, interleukin; TNF, tumour necrosis factor; IL-1RA, interleukin-1 receptor antagonist; ACh, acetylcholine; 5-HT, 5-hydroxytryptamine; GABA, gamma-aminobutyric acid; NA, noradrenaline; A, adrenaline.

such as George Solomon and Robert Ader in the Unites States and Robert Dantzer in France. It is now established that primary and secondary lymphoid tissues are sympathetically innervated, which enables the peripheral nervous system to influence immune function. Immune and neurotransmitter receptors occur on lymphocytes and they can respond to the appropriate signals from the endocrine, immune and neurotransmitter systems. Similarly, both experimental and clinical studies have shown that changes in the immune system, caused by infection for example, can profoundly affect the mood state, as anyone who has had an attack of influenza will testify.

Despite the major changes in neuroscience research that have taken place in recent years, there are many major questions that remain to be answered regarding the clinical importance of immune–brain interactions. Many of the difficulties arise from the paucity of information and the action of cytokines and other immune factors on brain function and the need to design research strategies that are consistent with the nature and behaviour of the components of an integrated system. It is evident that the kinetics of the active components of the nervous, immune and endocrine systems differ and raise major difficulties in evaluating the interaction between these systems. Furthermore, an adequate quantitative and qualitative assessment of stress on immune functions has not yet been finalized. These are some of the challenges that face psychoneuroimmunology at present, which is undoubtedly one of the most challenging fields in the neuorosciences. The situation is perhaps best encapsulated by the following quote from the philosopher Arthur Schopenhauer: "All truth passes through three stages. First it is ridiculed. Second it is violently opposed. Third it is accepted as being self-evident." At present, psychoneuroimmunology is between stages one and two. Perhaps the modest contribution that follows this chapter will help to raise its status.

BIBLIOGRAPHY

Ader, R., Felten, D. L. and Cohen, N. (Eds) (1991) *Psychoneuroimmunology*. Academic Press, New York.
Cannon, W. (1932) *The Wisdom of the Body*. Norton, New York.
Dantzer, R. (1989) *The Psychosomatic Delusion*. The Free Press, New York.
Dunbar, F. (1935) *Emotions and Bodily Changes*. Columbia University Press, New York.
Elgert, K. D. (1996) *Immunology: Understanding the Immune System*. Wiley-Liss, New York.
Leonard, B. E. and Miller, K. (Eds) (1995) *Stress, the Immune System and Psychiatry*. John Wiley and Sons, Chichester.
Mire-Sluis, A. and Thorpe, R. (1998) *Cytokines*. Academic Press, New York.
Solomon, G. (1984) Emotions, immunity and disease. In: Cooper, E. L. (Ed.) *Stress, Immunity and Aging*, pp. 1–10. Marcel Dekker, New York.

2 Introduction

The function of the immune system is recognition and defence against foreign substances, in distinguishing what is "self" from "non-self". This function is partly mediated by the central nervous system (CNS) and the endocrine system as the immune system can act as the recipient of afferent signals from these two systems. Thus the CNS receives information from sensory organs, the immune system and the endocrine system, thereby controlling and regulating their responses. Conversely the function of the endocrine system is to receive information from the brain and the immune system and, by secreting different kinds of hormones, to modulate their activities. The three systems are tightly integrated in their functions in order to preserve homeostasis.

STRUCTURE AND FUNCTIONS OF THE IMMUNE SYSTEM

There are two kinds of immunity, innate and acquired. *Innate* immunity includes those aspects occurring in early development that are always present and available to protect the individual from challenges by "foreign" invaders. The protective barriers include the skin, the mucous membrane and the cough reflex, which present effective barriers to environmental agents. Innate immunity also includes substances released from leucocytes, phagocytic cells, macrophages and microglial cells of the central nervous system. Some serum proteins also contribute to the innate immunity. For example, within minutes after injury (exogenous or endogenous tissue damage or infection), the inflammatory process begins and leads to the activation of the liver to secrete a group of serum proteins called *acute phase proteins*. An important member of the acute phase proteins is C-reactive protein. This protein binds to the membrane of certain microorganisms and activates the complement system. This results in a the lysis of the microorganisms and/or the increase of phagocytosis.

Acquired immunity is more specific and comes later. It includes immune organs and cells involved in cellular immunity and humoral (antibody and complement) mediated immunity.

IMMUNE ORGANS

The immune system consists of organs, tissues and cells. Immune organs include the thymus, bone marrow, lymph nodes, spleen and mucosa-associated lymphoid tissue. They have four major functions: (i) to provide an environment for the maturation of the immature cells in the immune system, (ii) to concentrate lymphocytes into organs that drain areas of antigen insult, (iii) to permit the interaction of different classes of lymphocytes and (iv) to provide an efficient vehicle for the dispersal of antibodies and other soluble factors from lymphocytes and other immune cells. There are two types of immune organs, namely the *primary* and *secondary lymphoid organs*. The thymus gland and bone marrow are *primary organs* where antigen-independent differentiation of lymphocytes takes place. The mature lymphocytes produced in the thymus and bone marrow are passed via the blood to the spleen and lymph nodes, which are *secondary lymphoid organs*. The lymphocyte function to encounter antigens and undergo antigen-dependent differentiation in the secondary lymphoid organs.

The bone marrow is the site of B-cell synthesis in mammals and also the origin of all immune cells. The bone marrow provides a microenvironment for B-cell antigen-independent differentiation. Mature B lymphocytes bear antigen-specific receptors and are transported by the circulating blood to the secondary lymphoid organs.

The *thymus gland* is the source of T cells. Progenitor cells from the bone marrow migrate to the thymus gland where they differentiate into T lymphocytes. The thymus grows rapidly during foetal development until puberty, and then undergoes atrophy with ageing. There are two lobes in the thymus, each of which consists of two main parts, the cortex and the medulla. Lymphocytes (thymocytes) of various sizes, most of which are immature, and also epithelial cells are located in the cortex. After maturation, lymphocytes migrate to the medulla where they are able to respond to foreign antigens. Thymus epithelial cells produce *thymic hormones* such as thymulin, thymosin and thymopoietin. These hormones are critical for lymphocyte differentiation and proliferation.

Lymph nodes are small ovoid structures located along the lymphatic routes. They serve to recover materials lost from the blood capillary network together with antigens that have entered into the tissue spaces and return them to the blood. Lymph nodes act primarily as filters for lymph. They (i) provide a site for phagocytosis and antibody production against antigens; (ii) act as a connection between the lymphatic system and the circulatory system; (iii) support the induction, proliferation and differentiation of lymphocytes and (iv) allow the lymphocytes to be recirculated.

The *spleen* is the largest secondary lymphoid organ. It is the major organ in the body in which antibodies are synthesized and from which they are released into the circulation. The spleen is composed of white pulp, rich in lymphoid cells, and red pulp, which contains macrophages, lymphocytes and erythrocytes. White pulp is divided into the peripheral region, central artery and germinal centre. Approximately 50% of spleen cells are B lymphocytes, and 30–40% are T lymphocytes. Following antigenic stimulation,

B cells and plasma cells in the germinal centre synthesize and release antibodies.

IMMUNE CELLS

The immune system is made up of five major kinds of cells (Table 2.1). These are T lymphocytes, B lymphocytes, monocytes, natural killer (NK) cells and granulocytes. These cells originate from the bone marrow, and are called pluripotent haematopoietic stem cells. They have the ability both to self-renew and to differentiate to all blood cell lineages under the influence of different immunotransmitters called *cytokines*. As indicated in Table 2.1, these leucocytes have different functions. During an antigen invasion or an inflammatory response, they may increase or decrease. The activities of immune cells (indicated by lymphocyte proliferation, NK cell cytotoxicity, neutrophil phagocytosis and macrophage activity) are important markers for infection, inflammation and many diseases.

Table 2.1 Five major immune cells and their functions

	T cell	B cell	NK cell	Monocyte/ Macrophage	Granulocyte (Neutrophil)
Antigen receptor	TCR αβ	Ig	?	None	None
Membrane markers	CD3, CD4 or CD8	Ig, CD5, CD9, CD10, CD19, CD20	CD16, CD56	CD11b, CD35, Fc receptor	CD16, CD18
Functions	Cytotoxicity	Ig secretion, antigen presentation	Cytotoxicity ADCC	Phagocytosis, antigen presentation	Phagocytosis
Cytokine secretion	IL-2, IL-3, IL-4, IL-5, IL-6, IFN-γ, TNF	IL-1, IL-6, IL-10, TNF, IFN	IL-1, IFN, TNF, IL-4, IL-8	IL-1, IL-6, IL-10, TNF, IFN, IL-15	IL-1, IL-3, IL-8, TNF
Percentage	18–32%	3–7%	10–19%	3–7%	50–70%

CD, cluster of differentiation antigen; TCR, T-cell receptor for antigen; Ig, immunoglobulin; ADCC, antibody-dependent cell-mediated cytotoxicity; IL, interleukin; IFN, interferon; TNF, tumour necrosis factor; NK, natural killer

ANTIGEN, IMMUNOGENS AND T-CELL IMMUNE RESPONSES

An *antigen* is any agent capable of binding specifically to components of the immune system, such as lymphocytes or antibodies. An *immunogen* is a high molecular weight compound that is chemically complex and can induce an immune response.

The first exposure of an individual to an immunogen is called the *primary response*. A second exposure to the same immunogen results in a *secondary response* which is more rapid in onset and of greater magnitude. There are two kind of immune responses, *cellular immunity* and *humoral immunity*. Cellular immunity is performed by the five different types of leucocyte, as described above. Humoral immunity involves a class of immunoglobins called *anti-bodies*. In cellular immunity, if immune cells cannot communicate with one another, they cannot provide protection. *Major histocompatibility complex* (MHC) is a cluster of genes responsible for molecules that are essential to T-cell function. Class I MHC activate cytotoxic/suppressor T cells (CD8+) and class II present peptide antigens to helper/inducer T cells (CD4+). T cells, B cells and activated monocytes (macrophages) can communicate only when a fragmented antigen is presented with class II MHC region on B cells and macrophages that can interact with appropriate receptors on T cells. Most T cells kill foreign antigens only when the antigen is on cell surfaces and in association with self-MHC-encoded cell-surface molecules. Thus, T-cell recognition of an antigen is a MHC-restricted process. Each T cell bears many identical complex receptors and circulates directly to the site of antigen.

Activated T cells have several subsets each of which performs its function when interacting with an antigen. (i) T-helper cells (T_H) cooperate with B cells to produce antibodies by releasing cytokines. (ii) T-cytotoxic cells (T_C) are able to kill the cells on contact with their target. (iii) T-suppressor cells (T_S) are able to suppress the immune response leading to a downward modulation or an inhibition in reactivity of other effector cells. (iv) T delayed-type hypersensitivity cells (T_{DTH}) release cytokines which induce the migration and activation of monocytes and macrophages, leading to the so-called delayed-type hypersensitivity inflammatory reactions.

ANTIBODY, ANTIGEN AND ANTIBODY REACTION

An antibody molecule is made up of four polypeptide chains which are divided into two identical light chains and two heavy chains (Figure 2.1). An antibody molecule is Y-shaped, with two identical antigen-binding sites at the ends of the arms of the Y. The light and heavy chains contribute to the antigen-binding sites. The stem of the Y is termed the Fc fragment. The Fc region of the antibody is responsible for its biological properties, which include activation of the complement system, placental transfer and binding to cell-surface receptors. The five different classes of immunoglobulins are called IgG, IgA, IgM, IgD and IgE. The function of an antibody is to combine with and inactivate an antigen, thereby preventing toxins and microorganisms from entering cells. The functions of each antibody are listed in Table 2.2.

COMPLEMENT SYSTEM

The complement system consists of a group of serum proteins that act in cooperation with complexed antigen and antibody. The main sources of

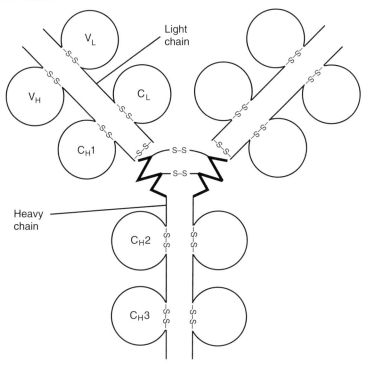

Figure 2.1 Schematic representation of an immunoglobulin molecule (IgG). Antibodies are large proteins shaped to form a Y. The fork in the Y is the hinge region, which connects the arms to the stem and allows them to swing. The stem, or constant (C) region, of the Y serves to link the antibody to other participants in the immune response. V, variable region; H, heavy chain; L, light chain. Reproduced by permission from Benjamini et al. (1996).

complement proteins are the hepatocytes and macrophages. Complements can be activated though two pathways, namely the antigen–antibody complex and the cell walls of some bacteria and yeasts, such as polysaccharides. For example, when a specific antibody binds with an antigen, the complex activates the first component of complement, called C1. Then, the antigen–antibody–C1 complex activates more components in the order C4, C2, C5, C6, C7, C8, C9. This activation can lead to neutralization of virus or the promotion of phagocytosis and lysis of bacteria and other antigenic cells.

CYTOKINES

Activation of immune cells leads to further regulation by soluble molecules called *cytokines*. Cytokines serve as a signal for communications between leucocytes. They are a large group of non-antibody-, non-antigen-special peptides produced by lymphocytes, macrophages, granulocytes and other

Table 2.2   Classified antibodies type and their functions

Name of antibody	Location	Functions
IgG	Blood	Coating microorganism to speed up their uptake by phagocytic cells, and inhibiting B-cell activation
IgA	External secretions	Providing the neonate with a major source of intestinal and respiratory protection against pathogens
IgM	Intravascular spaces	Best agglutinating and complement-acting antibody and the only antibody synthesis by the foetus
IgD	On the surface of lymphocytes	Involved in B-cell maturation, and serving a B-protective function
IgE	Serum	Binding with high affinity to receptors on mast cells and protecting against parasitic infection

cells (Table 2.1). Different cytokines have different biological effects which change the behaviour and function of many leucocytes.

According their source and function, cytokines are divided into inter-leukins, which include lymphokines (produced by lymphocytes) and mono-kines (produced by monocytes), chemokines, interferons, cytotoxic/immunomodulatory and colony-stimulating factors. Table 2.3 lists most cytokines and their functions. In addition to the cytokines, cytokine recep-tors are widely distributed on leucocytes, immune organs and neurons.

AUTOIMMUNITY

Autoimmunity arises as an immune response against the self-constituents, sometimes causing an *autoimmune disease*. Autoimmune diseases may involve either an immune response to a self-antigen changed by infection or drug. The basis of autoimmune disorders is multifactorial. They may result from a de-crease in suppressor cell number or function, enhanced T_H cell activity or inappropriate expression of MHC molecules on non-antigen-presenting cells, hyperactivity of B cells, excessive production of some cytokines, thymic de-fects, genetic factors or hormonal factors. Autoimmune diseases can be classi-fied as either organ-specific or systemic. They can be further divided as diseases mediated by T cells or by antibodies. For instance, Hashimoto's thyroiditis, insulin-dependent diabetes and postvaccinal encephalomyelitis are cell-mediated autoimmune diseases, whereas Graves' disease, systemic lupus erythematosus (SLE), rheumatoid arthritis, autoimmune haemolytic diseases are antibody-mediated autoimmune diseases.

Table 2.3 Cytokines, producers and functions

Cytokine	Abbreviation	Major producers	Functions
Interleukin-1α Interleukin-1β	IL-1α, IL-1β	Monocytes/ macrophages, NK cells, B cells, astrocytes	Stimulates T-cell and B-cell activities, induces IL-2 and receptor expression, increases acute phase proteins, cytocidal activities of NK and macrophages and induces fever
Interleukin-2	IL-2	CD4+ and CD8+ T cells, thymocytes	Stimulates T-cell, thymocyte and B-cell proliferation, induces lymphokine release and enhances NK cell activity
Interleukin-3	IL-3	T cells (Th1 + Th2)	Supports growth of mast cells, multipotential stem cells and progenitors of monocytes and granulocytes
Interleukin-4	IL-4	T cells (Th1)	Co-stimulates B-cell proliferation and antibody production, stimulates T-cell proliferation, activates macrophage activity and mast cell growth factor
Interleukin-5	IL-5	T cells	Co-stimulates B-cell growth and IgA secretion from B cells, induces differentiation of eosinophils
Interleukin-6	IL-6	Monocytes/ macrophages, B cells, T cells	Induces acute phase protein in hepatocytes, stimulates B cell differentiation and IgG secretion, co-stimulates thymocyte proliferation and activates T cells
Interleukin-8	IL-8	Neutrophils, B cells, monocytes, NK cells	Stimulates chemotaxis of neutrophils and T cells and stimulates granulocyte activity
Interleukin-10	IL-10	T cells (CD8+), B cell, monocytes, macrophages	Inhibits cytokine synthesis by Th1 cells and activates macrophages, stimulates T cell growth and differentiation
Interleukin-12	IL-12	Macrophages, neutrophils, mast cells	Induces INF-γ production, augments the NK cytotoxic activity, stimulates differentiation CD4+ T cells to Th1 cells, blocks inflmmatory monokine production
Interferon gamma	INF-γ	T cells, macrophage, NK cells, thymocytes	Induces class II MHC expression on macrophages, inhibits viral replication, activates non-specific tumouricidal and microbicidal activity in macrophages
Tumour necrosis factor alpha	TNF-α	T cells, macrophages, monocytes, NK cells, neutrophils	Cytolysis of tumour cells, induces class I MHC antigen, enhances respiratory burst activity in neutrophils, regulates other immune cell functions
Colony-stimulating factors	GM-CSF	T cells, B cells, NK cells, mast cells	Stimulates the growth of colonies of granulocytes and macrophages from bone marrow precursors, activates macrophage cytocidal activity

IMMUNE–NEUROTRANSMITTER INTERRELATIONSHIPS

The effects of the CNS on functions of the immune system have been extensively studied. These studies revealed that changes in neurotransmitter synthesis, release and metabolism following a brain lesion, stress, psychiatric diseases or neurodegeneration could significantly alter both cellular and humoral immunity. Conversely, a large body of evidence has demonstrated that immunization, inflammatory responses and autoimmune diseases may rapidly influence CNS functions.

BRAIN LESIONS AND IMMUNE FUNCTIONS

Early studies of the influence of the brain on the immune system were performed experimentally in rats or mice. Lesions that affect the immune process are mostly located in the hypothalamus, which suggests that the effect of the lesions may be mediated by alterations of autonomic or endocrine function. Lesions in the limbic areas also cause significant immune changes, which may be related to specific neurotransmitter changes. Bilateral electrolytic lesions of the preoptic-anterior hypothalamic area result in thymic involution and a decrease in the number and blastogenic reactivity of splenocytes. In contrast, lesions in the hippocampus increase thymic and splenic mitogenic responsiveness and cellularity, whereas those in the amygdala do not change the cell numbers, but significantly enhance the response of splenocytes and thymocytes to mitogen stimulation. Hypophysectomy abrogates all changes in splenic number and function induced by hypothalamic and limbic lesions; it also abolishes the effects on thymocyte number and function of ablating the hippocampus and amygdaloid complex. Hypothalamic lesions in hypophysectomized animals result in an increase in the number of thymocytes but suppress mitogenic activity. These results indicate that neuroimmunomodulation is mediated predominantly by the limbic system, but may also involve the pituitary gland. In addition, lesions in the lateral hypothalamic area result in time-dependent blood NK cell cytotoxicity changes. Experimentally it has been found that the activity of NK cells against target cells changes from suppression of activity through elevation followed by further suppression on the second, fifth and 21st post-lesion day, respectively, as compared to the sham-operated animal.

A decrease in the weight of the spleen, and in the number of B cells, is also observed in these lesioned animals. On the other hand, the lesion of the medial hypothalamus does not cause any significant change in NK cytotoxic activity. The mechanism for this change in NK activity may be due to the action of the autonomic nervous system, caused by an enhanced sympathetic firing rate and increased concentration of circulating catecholamines. Lateral hypothalamic lesions also cause a number of endocrine abnormalities such as an increase in glucocorticoid secretion.

Changes in neurotransmission following brain lesions are the other major factor in neuroimmunomodulation. After the lesion of the medial septal nucleus, the cholinergic area, splenocyte and thymocyte proliferation is significantly suppressed from day 5 to day 25, and then recovers in parallel with the reduction of the lesion. Lesions of the locus coeruleus, the noradrenergic cell body region, or the central administration of the catecholaminergic neurotoxin, 6-hydroxydopamine (6-OHDA), cause an inhibition in the production of haematopoietic stem cells and a decrease in antibody response to a sheep red blood cell (SRBC) challenge. Thus, the brain modulates the immune system in two ways, either through direct innervation from the CNS to the immune system or by various neurotransmitters, neuropeptides and endocrine hormones that indirectly influence the immune process.

NERVOUS INNERVATION OF THE IMMUNE SYSTEM

Structural and histological analyses reveal that the spleen, thymus, lymph nodes and bone marrow are essentially innervated with both afferent and efferent nerve fibres. The autonomic nervous system is believed to serve as a major link between the brain and the immune system. Many studies have inicated that both sympathetic and parasympathetic innervation are involved. The evidence cited for a parasympathetic innervation includes acetylcholinesterase (AChE) staining of terminals in the thymus along the vagus nerve to brain stem nuclei. Preganglionic neurons that compose the autonomic nervous system are located in the brain stem and spinal cord. Their axons exit in the CNS and synapse in peripheral autonomic ganglia. These ganglion cells send postganglionic fibres to terminate in the immune organs. For the sympathetic nervous system (SNS), the preganglionic cells are located in the lateral horn and intermediate grey matter of the thoracolumbar spinal cord. The postganglionic nerve fibres of the SNS are mainly noradrenergic. Noradrenergic postganglionic innervation of rat spleen originates mainly in the superior mesenteric coeliac ganglion and noradrenergic fibres are present among cells in T-dependent areas, including T_H, T_C, macrophages and B cells. Noradrenaline (NA) interacts with these immune cells in two ways. (i) Electron microscopic studies have demonstrated direct contacts of nerve terminals with lymphocytes and macrophages in the white pulp of the spleen and (ii) NA can diffuse through the parenchyma after release from nerve terminals and combine with adrenoceptors on the target cells of the immune system.

In *lymph nodes*, noradrenergic innervation is found in the subcapsular zone, paracortical and cortical regions and medullary core, but is absent from follicles, the B-cell-containing areas. NA may affect B cells by receptor activation or by NA-induced cytokine release from other cells. It is known that the rat thymus gland (thymic capsule, cortex region and connective tissue septa) is innervated by noradrenergic varicose axon terminals (tyrosine hydroxylase- and dopamine-beta-hydroxylase-immunostained nerve fibres). This innervation is mainly associated with the vasculature and also separated from the vessels along the thymic tissue and branches into the thymic parenchyma. Synapses between thymocytes and neuronal elements have not been observed. These nerve terminals are able to take up, store and release NA upon axonal stimulation in a $[Ca^{2+}]$-dependent manner. The release is tetradotoxin-sensitive, while reserpine pretreatment prevents the release of NA following axonal stimulation, indicating vesicular origin of the transmitter.

In the bone, noradrenergic nerve fibres enter the marrow with the arteries, travel with vascular plexuses deep in the marrow where they may affect haematopoiesis and cell migration.

EFFECTS OF NEUROTRANSMITTERS ON IMMUNE FUNCTIONS

The hypothalamus receives neuronal afferents from numerous sources including inputs from limbic structures, such as the amygdala and hippocampus, and from brain stem regions involved in the regulation of the cardiovascular system and other autonomic functions. These afferents use a vast array of neurotransmitters and neuropeptides to influence the activity of the hypothalamic neurons. Hypothalamic neurons synthesize and secrete the hypothalamic releasing and release-inhibiting factors into the hypophyseal portal circulatory system. The afferents can modulate the activity of the hypothalamic neurons by forming synapses on the neuronal cell body, the nerve terminals in the median eminence or both. The neurotransmitters involved are the biogenic amines including NA, dopamine (DA) and adrenaline (A). In addition, serotonin (5-HT), acetylcholine (ACh), opioids and gamma-aminobutyric acid (GABA) are involved in controlling pituitary functions. These neurotransmitters exert effects on immune functions via neurotransmitter receptors on the immune cells.

Serotonin SRBC – Sleep ·RBC

5-HT may modulate immune functions via the central serotonergic pathways. The serotonergic system may provide an inhibitory effect on the immune responses. However, the direct effects of 5-HT upon the immune system have not been systematically investigated. Systemic administration of a 5-HT precursor, or an increased brain 5-HT concentration, before rats are injected with SRBC, results in a decrease in the amount of anti-SRBC antibody secreted by splenocytes. Conversely, pretreatment with inhibitor of 5-HT biosynthesis markedly enhances antibody production. Selective depletion of brain serotonin through intracerebroventricular (i.c.v.) injection of the neurotoxin 5,7-dihydroxytryptamine prior to SRBC immunization preserves the antibody response. In *in vitro* studies, 5-HT at a concentration of 10^{-4}–10^{-10} M impairs the cytotoxicity of human NK cells in whole blood and at 10^{-3}–10^{-4} M inhibits lymphocyte proliferation and antibody production from B cells. These effects are similar to those observed after administration of the 5-HT2 receptor antagonist, ketanserin. The role of serotonin as an immune modulator was also investigated by measuring the functional competence of T cells from control mice versus mice whose intracellular stores of serotonin had been depleted by pretreatment with *p*-chlorophenylalanine (PCPA). The level of expression of the alpha-chain interleukin-2 receptor (IL-2R) was reduced on splenic CD4+ cells but not on CD8+ cells in 5-HT deleted mice. Culture with the T-cell mitogen concanavalin A (Con A) failed to induce expression of IL-2R on either CD4+ or CD8+ cells of PCPA-treated mice, although IL-2R was induced on control cells. The proliferative response to Con A by these spleen cells from PCPA-treated mice was also reduced compared to that by control spleen cells. Both expression of IL-2R and proliferation in response to Con A by spleen cells from serotonin-depleted mice were increased or completely restored by supplementation of the cultures with serotonin. Studies to identify the mechanisms for the reduction in T-cell activation when serotonin levels were reduced implicated a defect in the capacity of macrophages from PCPA-treated mice to participate in T-cell activation. Splenic macrophages from control mice were able to restore the blastogenic capability of lymphocytes from PCPA-treated mice, although macrophages from PCPA-treated mice were unable to support normal lymphocyte blastogenesis unless the cultures were supplemented with serotonin. These results show the requirement of autologous serotonin for optimal T-cell activation and suggest the importance of serotonin in macrophage accessory function for T-cell activation.

The 5-HT1A receptor subtype is one member of the 5-HT1 receptor family and is constitutively expressed on lymphoblastic (Jurkat) cells and elevated on human T lymphocytes after mitogenic activation. There is evidence that human T lymphocytes and monocytes also release 5-HT after stimulation with mitogens or interferon (IFN)-γ. In both lymphocytes and the CNS, the 5-HT1A receptor is coupled to the regulation of adenylate cyclase. The 5-HT1A receptor agonists inhibit the activation of adenylate cyclase. Using human peripheral mononuclear or murine spleen cells, it has been shown that the inhibition of 5-HT synthesis inhibits IL-2-stimulated human T-cell proliferation and that addition of 5-hydroxytryptophan, a precursor of 5-HT, reverses inhibition of T-cell proliferation. The 5-HT1 receptor antagonist, metitepine, and the 5-HT1A antagonist, pindolol, also block T-cell proliferation. Inhibition by metitepine is reversed by 5-HT and by the selective 5-HT1A receptor agonist, 8-hydroxy-2-(di-*n*-propylamino) (8-OH-DPAT). In addition, selective 5-HT1A receptor antagonists cause elevation of cAMP in human T cells.Following the production of Th1 cytokines (such as IL-2 and

IFN-γ) in murine spleen cells is inhibited by an immune challenge, the immune murine spleen cells are inhibited by 5-HT1A receptor antagonists *in vitro* but not by 5-HT2 receptor antagonists. These results suggest that 5-HT acts as an immunomodulator through the 5-HT1A receptor. Complex relationships may also occur between other serotonin receptors and immune function.

Dopamine

Radioactively labelled DA uptake occurs into the bone marrow, spleen and lymph nodes of normal murine *in vivo*. DA D1- and D2-like receptors exist in the rat and pigeon thymus and in human peripheral blood lymphocytes. The selective D1-like antagonist [^{3}H]-SCH 23390 is used to label the D1-like receptors (D1 and D5 sites) and pharmacological analysis suggests that binding of [^{3}H]-SCH 23390 to sections of thymus and to human peripheral blood lymphocytes belongs mainly to the dopamine D5 receptor subtype. Light microscope autoradiography, performed on sections of rat and pigeon thymus, reveals that these receptors are located primarily in the cortical layer. D2-like receptors (D2, D3 and D4 sites) have been studied in sections of rat thymus and in peripheral blood lymphocytes by using the putative D3 receptor agonist [^{3}H]-7-OH-DPAT as a ligand. Both rat and pigeon thymus and human peripheral blood lymphocytes express a putative D3 receptor. Similar evidence has been reported from studies performed in human peripheral blood lymphocytes. The demonstration of different subtypes of DA receptors in a primary immune organ such as the thymus, and in circulating immune cells, supports the hypothesis of an involvement of DA in the control of immune function.

Mouse spleen cells and macrophages contained on average 7×10^{-17} and 2×10^{-17} M of DA per cell, respectively. NA has also been found in the mouse spleen cells. Several mouse B- and T-cell hybridomas were also shown to contain endogenously produced DA in concentrations ranging from 7×10^{-20} to 2×10^{-18} mol DA per cell. The DA production in lymphocytes can be blocked by the tyrosine hydroxylase inhibitor alpha-methyl-*p*-tyrosine, whereas incubation with the precursor 3,4-dihydroxy-L-phenylalanine (L-DOPA) increased the DA content. Incubation with L-DOPA, DA or NA dose-dependently suppressed mitogen-induced proliferation and differentiation of mouse lymphocytes. Even pretreatment of lymphocytes with L-DOPA and DA for a short period (several minutes) strongly suppresses lymphocyte proliferation and cytokine production. Incubation of lymphoid cells with L-DOPA, DA or NA dose-dependently induces apoptosis which, at least partly, explains the suppressive effects of catecholamines on lymphocyte function. These results demonstrate that catecholamines: (i) are actively produced by lymphocytes and (ii) have the capacity to act as auto- and/or paracrine regulators of lymphocyte activity through induction of apoptosis.

The central dopaminergic system appears to exert a net stimulatory influence over the immune system, a conclusion that is based on changes in the immune system of patients suffering from such neurological diseases as Parkinsonism. Depletion of striatal dopamine suppresses tumour necrosis factor (TNF) release from macrophages and enhances tumour growth. The pharmacological characterization of the recognition site suggests similarities mainly with the D2 and D4 rather than D3 subtype of dopamine receptor. Furthermore, dopamine treatment was able to reduce the intracellular cAMP levels of lymphocytes stimulated with forskolin, thus suggesting a potential functional significance of this dopamine receptor in mediating neural–immune interactions.

Noradrenaline and Adrenaline

In the sympathetic nervous system (SNS), NA and A mostly exert their suppressive effects on the immune system, while in the CNS, NA has an immunoenhancing influence. Depletion of NA in the CNS causes the impairment of the anti-SRBC response of rats; the intravenous injection of NA or A has been shown to change T-cell subpopulation and NK cell activity in humans, NA or A administration significantly increases NK cell numbers and activity in the circulation, but reduces CD3+ and CD4+ numbers and the CD4/CD8+ ratio. Concurrently, the IL-6 concentration in the blood is markedly increased, which is positively correlated with the increase in adrenaline concentration. This increase in IL-6 can be blocked by the beta-adrenergic receptor antagonist l-propranolol but not by d-propranolol. These results suggest that both sympathetic-adrenal hormones are equally potent modulators of natural immunity and provide further evidence that catecholamines might be responsible for the observed alterations in immune functions after phases of acute stress.

Under physiological conditions circulating adrenaline may be involved in the control of IL-6 production, and thereby may modulate inflammatory responses. *In vitro* studies show that NA, at concentrations of 10^{-8}–10^{-5} M, significantly reduces T-lymphocyte proliferation. This inhibition could be completely blocked by either the α-adrenergic antagonist phentolamine or β-adrenergic antagonist propranolol. Thus, NA probably modulates lymphocyte function though α- and/or β-adrenergic receptors.

Gamma-aminobutyric Acid (GABA)

Different GABA or benzodiazepine receptors may also exist on immune cells. The GABA/benzodiazepine (Bdz) receptor chloride channel complex has been proposed to play a modulatory role in immune function. Activation of the GABA receptors with the agonist muscimol, or activation of the Bdz receptors with diazepam, has stimulatory effects upon immunogenesis.

A decrease in GABA–Bdz–receptor–ionophore complex activity leads to a suppression of the immune response. This may be achieved by blocking the receptor complex with bicuculline, a competitive inhibitor of the GABA receptors, or by administration of a specific antagonist of the Bdz receptors flumazenil or Ro 15–3505. Blockade of chloride channels with picrotoxin has a similar effect.

Activation of the GABA-ergic system causes an increase in bone marrow content of T-helper cells. The immunomodulatory action of the GABA-ergic system is of central origin and can occur only when the hypothalamic–pituitary system is intact. Section of the pituitary stalk prevents accumulation of the T_H cells in the bone marrow. If DA or 5-HT is depleted in the brain, the immunomodulatory effect of GABA also fails.

Alprazolam, a triazolobenzodiazepine with high affinity for "central" benzodiazepine receptors, also has an effect on several parameters of immune function in mice. NK cell activity, mixed leucocyte reactivity and mitogen-induced lymphocyte proliferation were all significantly increased two hours after administration of low doses (0.02–1.0 mg/kg) of alprazolam. Twenty-four hours later similar, but less robust, immunoenhancing effects were observed. Higher doses of alprazolam (5–10 mg/kg) did not affect these measures of immune function. This immunoenhancing effect of alprazolam does not appear related to changes in the corticosterone concentration. In contrast, injection of the vehicle caused a profound suppression of these immune parameters two hours later, but was no longer apparent 24 hours later. The immunosuppression appeared to correlate with a stress-induced rise in serum corticosterone concentration. Subchronic treatment with diazepam also reduces the concentration of NA and 5-HT/5-hydroxyindole-acetic acid (HIAA) ratio, effects which may contribute to the suppression of immune functions. *In vitro*, the influence of GABA on specific immunity indices has been studied in animals. GABA was shown to facilitate the appearance of the Thy-I-antigen (one of the Ig-gene superfamily of surface glycoproteins) on the surface of mouse bone marrow cells and stimulate immune response of mice to thymus-dependent antigens. However, GABA had no effect on the immune responsiveness to thymus-independent Vi-antigens in these animals. This supports the hypothesis that the GABA/benzodiazepine receptor chloride channel complex primarily modulates immune function.

Acetylcholine

The murine thymus has been demonstrated to contain both cholinergic receptors and acetylcholinesterase activity. The possibility that ACh–lymphocyte interaction can occur is supported by the observation that lymphoid tissues are richly innervated by parasympathetic nerve fibres. In the brain, ACh seems to play an immunoinhibitory role. For example, the inhibition of ACh biosynthesis in the CNS causes the enhancement of the humoral immune response of rats to SRBC. By contrast, the inhibition of AChE activity in the CNS results in the suppression of immune response. ACh effects can be blocked by atropine, a muscarinic antagonist, but not by hexamethonium, a nicotinic antagonist. However, *in vitro* ACh at concentrations of 10^{-9} to 10^{-4} M significantly increases the mitogen-induced splenic cell proliferation. This action of ACh only occurs either before or just after T lymphocytes are activated through muscarinic cholinergic receptors.

Opioids

Opioid receptors have been identified on granulocytes, monocytes, lymphocytes and terminal complexes of complement. Endogenously released opioids increase lymphocyte proliferation, NK cell cytotoxicity and cytokine release. Opioid peptides appear to be dynamic signalling molecules that are produced within the immune system and are active regulators of an immune response. Furthermore, the receptors for these peptides occurring on immunocyte membranes share characteristics with neuronal opioid receptors, including molecular size, immunogenicity, and the use of specific intracellular signalling pathways. The mechanism of morphine-induced humoral immunosuppression is less certain, but the effects of opioids on the immune system are reversed by (–) naloxone. *In vitro* morphine has suppressing effects on the generation of antibody-forming cell to SRBC. When granulocytes are incubated with morphine, the migration, superoxide release and aggregation of neutrophils are largely inhibited. These changes are also prevented by naloxone pretreatment.

This experimental evidence suggests that NA, A, DA, and opioids are predominantly immunosuppressive, while ACh is immunostimulant. It has been suggested that NA and ACh play an opposite role in immune modulation, which is advantageous in maintaining an equilibrium in immune function.

IMMUNE RESPONSES CAUSE CHANGES IN NEUROTRANSMITTERS

Many years ago, the brain was considered to be a "closed" system that was completely separated from the periphery by the protection of the brain–blood barrier (BBB). Recent studies have revealed that activated leucocytes can cross into the CNS in much higher numbers during neuropathological disorders. Cytokines produced by lymphocytes, monocytes and other leucocytes can also enter the brain in several ways. IL-1 and TNF-α penetrate through the BBB by a saturable transport system, while IL-2 enters by a non-saturable system. In the preoptic nucleus of the hypothalamus and some other brain areas, receptors for IL-1, IL-6 and TNF-α have been detected.

These receptors combine with cytokines from the periphery and then transfer them into the brain.

Cytokine receptors have been widely located in many brain regions. Furthermore, astrocytes, microglia and neurons in the brain can also produce different cytokines, which mediate the development, differentiation, repair and ageing of the CNS. The relationship between peripheral cytokines and central cytokines is unclear but it is possible that some cytokines in the periphery may pass through the BBB and trigger central cytokine release.

Neurotransmitter Changes During Immunization

The response of the CNS to immunization is similar to its response to stress, which further demonstrates that the immune system acts as a sensory organ for the brain. The most consistent change in central biogenic amines caused by immunization and stress is an increase in NA, 5-HIAA and homovanillic acid (HVA) concentrations in several brain regions. A SRBC immune challenge increases NA, A, 5-HT, 5-HIAA and HVA concentrations and the NA : 3-methoxy-4-hydroxy-phenylglycol (MHPG) ratio, while a decrease in DA occurs in the hypothalamus and hippocampus. In the brain stem, immunization increases 5-HT, but reduces 5-HIAA concentrations. Influenza virus infection also increases the NA : MHPG ratio and the brain tryptophan concentration. The systemic administration of bacterial endotoxin produces an increase in the excellular concentration of 5-HT and 5-HIAA in the hippocampus. In contrast to central monoamine changes, a SRBC challenge reduces NA but elevates the DA concentration in the thymus and spleen. In addition to these neurotransmitter changes, during immunization the firing rate in the hypothalamus is largely increased.

Interactions of Cytokine and Neurotransmitters

Cytokines are a group of polypeptides produced from different leucocytes in response to a wide range of physiological and pathological stimuli. During an inflammatory or infectious response, the increased concentrations of cytokines may change neurotransmission and cause abnormalities in the CNS. These cytokines not only play different roles in immunomodulation, but may be also have different influences on neurotransmitter functions. Many cytokines have been found to act as neurotransmitters or neuromodulators.

IL-1 is the most studied cytokine with regard to the brain–immune communication. Peripheral administration of IL-1 causes most changes in neurotransmitter metabolism, effects which are similar those observed after a bacterial endotoxin injection or influenza virus infection, as exemplified by an increase in the ratio of NA : MHPG, 5-HIAA : 5-HT, 3,4-dihydroxyphenylacetic acid (DOPAC) : DA and in the concentrations of tryptophan, 5-HIAA, HVA and

MHPG in the hypothalamus. These changes can be blocked by IL-1 antagonists or the IL-1 receptor antagonist (RA). In the paraventricular nucleus (PVN) of the hypothalamus, IL-1 stimulates NA release and activates the hypothalamus to release corticotrophin-releasing factor (CRF), which stimulates ACTH release. IL-1-induced elevation in ACTH release can be completely prevented by pretreatment with a CRF antibody or CRF antagonist. In the hippocampus, similar changes in monoamines and their metabolites are observed. IL-1 also enhances GABA functions by increasing the conductance of Cl^- and inhibiting Ca^{2+} currents in the hippocampal neurons. Central administration of IL-1 also largely increases hypothalamic 5-HIAA concentration, decreases NA concentration in the spleen, suppresses macrophage activity and lymphocyte proliferation, and stimulates ACTH release.

IL-6 has similar effects to IL-1 on neurotransmission. Parenteral administration of IL-1 markedly increases IL-6 concentration in the blood. In the prefrontal cortex and hippocampus, systemic IL-6 administration also increases serotonergic and dopaminergic activity, while in the nucleus accumbens, both IL-1 and IL-6 reduce MHPG : NA ratio and increase 5-HIAA concentration. At high doses, peripheral IL-6 can also enhance the ACTH-induced release of corticosterone. However, there are some differences between the effects of IL-1 and IL-6 on CNS funtions. For example, IL-6 significantly reduces DA release from the nucleus accumbens, whereas IL-1 lacks this effect.

Most effects of IL-2 seem to be on the dopaminergic, noradrenergic and cholinergic systems, but not on the serotonergic system. Systemic injection of IL-2 significantly enhances NA and DA turnover in the hypothalamus and prefrontal cortex, and reduces DA release from the nucleus accumbens; *in vitro* incubation of IL-2 with striatal slices stimulates DA release. Moreover, in hippocampal and frontal cortical slices, IL-2 decreases ACh release. Similarly, interferon (IFN)-α activates the opioid receptors that then inhibit the presynaptic release of DA.

The mechanisms whereby these cytokines modulate neurotransmission include the activation of cAMP, protein kinase C, increased synthesis of nitric oxide, release of arachidonic acid and a change in Ca^{2+} or K^+ flux.

The central function of many other cytokines remains to be elucidated. Like some neuropeptides, the effects of the cytokines vary with the dose. For example, different doses of IL-2 result in a bell-shaped dose–response curve in DA release, i.e. low dose IL-2 increases DA release, while high dose reduces DA release. In general, it therefore appears that low doses of cytokines may beneficially affect the immune system, while high doses may be toxic.

IMMUNE–ENDOCRINE INTERRELATIONSHIPS

There is a well established interaction between the immune system and endocrine system. Different types of hormone receptors are distributed on immune cells, which modulate immune functions when hormones combine with them. Conversely, cytokine receptors have also been found on cells and tissues of the endocrine system and can thereby modify the activity of the endocrine system. Moreover, leucocytes under normal and inflammatory conditions, or following neurotransmitter activation, can produce different hormones while endocrine cells, under normal or stress conditions, also can produce different cytokines. Thus, hormones and cytokines are the common language for communication between the endocrine system and the immune system.

The Endocrine System Mediates the Immune System

As mentioned above, classical neuroendocrine hormones and their receptors are expressed in tissues and cells of the immune system. ACTH, arginine vasopressin (AVP), CRF, growth hormone (GH), luteinizing hormone (LH), luteinizing hormone-releasing hormone (LHRH), thyrotrophin-stimulating hormone (TSH) and prolactin (PRL) are all expressed in the thymus gland. Among these hormones, CRF is the key in neuroendocrine-immune modulation during inflammation and stress. In the CNS, CRF is produced by CRF neurons in the hypothalamus and pituitary, while in the periphery, CRF is produced by the spleen, various immune cells, such as T cells and macrophages, and acute or chronic inflammatory sites. The function of CRF in the periphery appears to act as an autocrine/paracrine proinflammatory mediator. After CRF binds to its receptor on the leucocytes, cAMP is activated, which stimulates monocytes/macrophages to secret IL-1, IL-6 and ACTH. ACTH released into the circulation acts on the adrenal gland and thereby increases the synthesis of glucocorticoids.

CRF-induced acute phase responses include enhanced leucocyte chemotaxis, enhanced production of superoxide by phagocytic cells, enhanced B-lymphocyte proliferation and increased expression of the IL-2 receptor. However, CRF also causes immunosuppression following systemic or central administration. Many of these effects are mediated centrally, but later indirectly by the action of CRF on the brain–hypothalamus–sympathetic nervous system and the hypothalamic–pituitary–adrenal (HPA) axis.

Many other hormones also modulate immune function and the most imporant ones will now be considered.

Corticosteroids

Autoimmune diseases and immune deficiency have a close relationship with the corticosteroids. Failure to produce an adequate quantity of corticosteroids, or failure to respond to corticosteroids, may promote the development of autoimmune disease. On the other hand, the immunosuppressive and anti-inflammatory effects of glucocorticoids are considered as a physiological negative feedback loop during an immune and inflammatory response. Hypersecretion of these hormones may suppress normal immune functions and exogenous corticosteroid administration results in thymocyte death and thymus atrophy. Corticosteroids also regulate the development of T_H type 1 (Th1) and type 2 (Th2) subset and suppress the production of the Th1 cytokines, IL-2 and IFN-γ and the Th2 cytokine IL-4. Hypersecretion of corticosteroids also inhibits some functions of lymphocytes and granulocytes, for example by reducing lymphocyte proliferation and neutrophil phagocytosis.

Sex Hormones

Thymus development during pregnancy is always under the influence of sex hormones. Gonadectomy increases the thymic mass, while oestrogens have the opposite effect. There is an increased incidence of autoimmune diseases in women, which provides further evidence that sex hormones play a role in immune modulation. Among sex hormones, LHRH plays a key role in immune modulation. Thus LHRH agonists can reverse thymic atrophy and age-related decline in lymphocyte proliferation, while LHRH antagonists reduce lymphocyte proliferation, the CD4+ percentage and thymus weight. In addition, oestrogen depletes immature thymocytes and enhances humoral antibody response, whereas testosterone suppresses both cellular development and antibody production.

Growth Hormone and Prolactin

Both GH and PRL stimulate thymocyte maturation and differentiation; hypophysectomy leads to thymic hypoplasia and severe immunodeficiency.

Thyrotropin-stimulating Hormone and Thyroid Hormone

Experiments on animals show that thyroidectomy causes a reduction in thymus weight, the number of lymphocytes, the production of thymus hormones and antibody responses. Following drug-induced hypothyroidism, the response of NK cells to IFN stimulation is completely blocked. These changes can be reversed by thyroid hormone treatment. Hyperthyroidism, on the other hand, increases thymus hormone production and induces autoimmune phenomena. Short-term treatment with thyroxine (T4) largely enhances NK cell activity, mitogen-induced lymphocyte proliferation and the antibody response to the SRBC. Thyroid-stimulating hormone (TSH) receptors occur on both thyroid tissue and immune cells and have similar effects to thyroxine administration. Therefore, the hypothalamic–pituitary–thyroid (HPT) axis appears to play an important role in the regulation of immune system.

The direct regulatory function of the endocrine system on the activity of immune cells is also evidenced from *in vitro* studies. Thus, preincubation of cortisol markedly reduces NK cell activity, while ACTH when added to NK cells *in vitro*, synergistically augments IFN-γ and IL-2 induced stimulation of NK cells and reverses the suppression caused by cortisol. This raises the possibility that *in vivo* release of ACTH may act to counterbalance some of the immunosuppressive effects of glucocorticoids, thereby avoiding any overshooting of steroid-dependent immunosuppression.

In vivo, the activity of pituitary hormones is adjusted by a feedback mechanism, so that when ACTH increases the glucocorticoid concentration, ACTH release is inhibited. Similarly, when CRF, ACTH or glucocorticoids exert their effects on immune cells, the synthesis and release of these hormones and cytokines from leucocytes is reduced. The cytokines act through cytokine receptors in the hypothalamus and the pituitary. Thus, the hypothalamus and pituitary not only regulate their hormone secretion according to the hormone concentration in the circulation, but also change hormone secretion by cytokine modulation. For example, inhibition of T-cell proliferation by cortisol is antagonized by IL-1, IL-6 and IFN-γ, and in human monocytes, IFN-γ reverses the suppression of IL-1 synthesis by glucocorticoids.

The Immune System Influences the Endocrine System

Peripheral lymphocytes and other leucocytes can produce different types of hormones (Table 2.4). This observation is probably pivotal to a biochemical understanding of how and why there is bidirectional communication between these two systems. Interestingly, the secretion of these hormones is regulated by hypothalamic regulators of pituitary hormones. For instance, GHRH up-regulates T-cell and B-cell-produced GH, effects which are blocked by somatostatin. Similarly, TRH is able to stimulate TSH synthesis from leucocytes, and such synthesis is blocked by triiodothyronine (T3) and thyroxine (T4). Thus, immune cells seem similar to pituitary cells that have ability to respond to hypothalamic-releasing factors and this response can be adjusted by a negative feedback loop. Not only that, there is a specific expression of the type of hormone in response to different kinds of immune stimulation. For example, Newcastle virus and CRF cause the production of propiomelanocortin-derived peptides with ACTH (1–39) and β-endorphin, while bacterial endotoxin elicits the production of ACTH (1–24, 1–26) and α- and γ-endorphin. These hormones may have completely different immune actions. For example, ACTH (1–39) and α-endorphin, but not ACTH (1–24) or β-endorphin, inhibit *in vitro* antibody production, whereas, β- (but not α-endorphin) enhances mitogen-induced lymphocyte proliferation. Therefore within the immune system, such differential processing could have unique immunomodulatory consequences. The mechanism for this

Table 2.4 Endocrine peptides produced by leucocytes

Hormones	Constitutive	Cellular or tissue source
ACTH	+	Lymphocytes and macrophages
Enkephalins	−	T-helper cells
TSH	−	T cells
GH	+	Lymphocytes
PRL	+	Lymphocytes
VIP	+	Leucocytes
CRF	+	Lymphocytes and thymus
AVP	+	Thymus

ACTH, adrenocorticotrophic hormone; TSH, thyroid-stimulating hormone; GH, growth hormone; PRL, prolactin; VIP, vasoactive intestinal peptide; CRF, corticotrophin-releasing factor; AVP, arginine vasopressin; + stimulate; − inhibit.

differentiation may be involved in the activation of different leucocyte types or different enzymes within immune cells.

Another group of modulators for endocrine secretion is the cytokines. Cytokines exert many actions on the HPA axis, HPT axis and hypothalamic–pituitary–gonadal (HPG) axis. Intravenous (i.v.), intraperitoneal (i.p.) or intracerebroventricular (i.c.v.) administration of IL-1 increases ACTH secretion. However, i.c.v. IL-1 is much more potent, which suggests that the site of IL-1 action on the HPA axis is in the CNS; IL-6 and TNF-α have similar stimulatory effects on ACTH release as IL-1. The ACTH-stimulating effect of these proinflammatory cytokines is abolished by pretreatment with a CRF antagonist or a CRF antibody. Following chronic injection of IL-1 for 10 days, the hypothalamic CRF concentration is largely increased. The mechanism by which IL-1 mediates CRF in the hypothalamus to stimulate ACTH release may be related to its effect on prostaglandin (PG)E2. Thus intraperitoneal administration of PGE2 (i.p. injection) also elevates ACTH secretion and causes fever; IL-1 administration markedly increases PGE2 concentration in the hypothalamus.

These cytokines not only stimulate the hypothalamus to secrete ACTH, but also stimulate the pituitary and adrenal gland to release ACTH and glucocorticoids; glucocorticoids exert a negative feedback on the HPA axis and inhibit leucocytes from producing these cytokines.

Circulating IL-1 has inhibitory effects on the HPT axis, acting both on the hypothalamic–pituitary system and on the thyroid. During inflammation, the increase in IL-1 can reduce plasma T3, T4 and TSH concentrations. Treatment with IL-1 for seven days causes a long-lasting inhibition of the thyroid independently of the pituitary TSH content. Furthermore, IL-1 stimulates the biosynthesis of somatostatin, which also inhibits TSH release in the hypothalamus. Of the other major cytokines, TNF and IFN have similar effects on the HPT axis as IL-1. Direct inhibitory actions of the cytokines on the pituitary and thyroid cells also occur. For example, IL-1 and TNF-α inhibit thyroid hormone release and thyroid cell growth by inhibiting cAMP formation.

The impairment of reproductive function is often associated with infection or inflammation. Cytokines, especially IL-1, have inhibitory actions on the HPG axis at the CNS and gonadal level. In animal studies, IL-1 administration (i.c.v.) significantly inhibits LH synthesis, which can be reversed by gonadotrophin-releasing hormone treatment; peripheral administration of IL-1 has no effect on LH synthesis and release. IL-1, TNF and IFN can also act directly on the gonads. *In vitro* studies show that they all inhibit oestradiol secretion, FSH-induced differentiation and LH-stimulated luteinization of granulosa cells. The action of IL-2 differs from these proinflammatory cytokines as much higher than physiological concentrations of IL-2 are needed to increase ACTH and glucocorticoid secretion. However, this effect cannot be blocked by pretreatment with a CRF antagonist or a CRF antibody, so there must be other mechanisms involved in IL-2 immunomodulation.

Other hormones, such as GH and PRL, are also changed during immune response or inflammation but the precise role of the cytokines in these actions is unclear.

THE INFLUENCE OF THE IMMUNE SYSTEM ON BEHAVIOUR

Sick individuals experience weakness, malaise, listlessness and inability to concentrate. They also show hypersomnia, anorexia, depressed activity and loss of interest in daily activities. These non-specific changes are called "sickness behaviour" and are considered to be the result of the debilitation process that occurs during infection. Recent evidence, however, indicates that these behavioural changes result from the direct mediation of the CNS by the immune system as a consequence of the infection. Cytokines have been used to treat various malignancies (i.e. leukaemia and renal cell carcinoma), infectious diseases (i.e. heptitis and HIV), neurodegenerative diseases (i.e. multiple sclerosis) and cancers. During treatment, it has been noted that many adverse neurological and behavioural changes appear. For example, subacute administration of IFN-α (1.5–5 MIU) results in a generalized slowing of behaviour, depressed mood and memory deficiencies. Electrophysiological studies reveal an increase in intermittent delta activity in the frontal cortex. In addition, chronic treatment with IFN-α impairs verbal memory and motor coordination and causes depressed mood, while IL-1β, used to treat some cancers, has been found to cause psychomotor slowing and speech difficulty. TNF-α is a highly neurotoxic agent and also causes significant neurobehavioural changes in patients; it induces transient amnesia or aphasia, and mild to moderate deficiencies in attentional ability, verbal memory and motor coordination. Conversely, IL-2, at very higher doses, causes agitation, paranoid and combative behaviour. However, the doses of these cytokines used in clinical treatments are much higher than physiological concentration (10^{6-9} fold) and therefore such adverse effects may only reflect their neurotoxicity in extreme conditions.

Using pharmacological doses, experimental studies in animals have shown many behavioural changes following cytokine administration. Exogenous IL-1 induces fever, increases slow wave sleep, anorexia and stress-like behaviour, as shown by decreased exploratory and social activity. After i.c.v. administration of IL-1β, rats also show anxious behaviour in the elevated plus maze, such as a decrease in time spent on the open arms (see Figure 3.2). Similar to IL-1, TNF-α administration induces anorexia, suppresses exploratory activity and social communication, and decreases the time spent on the open arm of the elevated plus maze. In addition, IFN-α reduces food intake and activity in novel environments. By contrast, IL-6 and IL-2 increase behavioural activities without inducing stressful and anxious behaviour.

However, there are many inconsistencies in the results from experimental studies of the effects of cytokines on behaviour due to the different doses of cytokines used, and the different species and routes of administration used. For example, a low dose of IL-2 (5–50 IU) causes sedation and sleep in rats, while IL-2 at 4×10^3 IU largely increases activity in the elevated plus maze and the "open field". Comparative studies show that lipopolysaccharide (LPS), endotoxin, i.p., or IL-1β i.c.v. administration all reduce locomotor activity in animals. This reduction in behaviour is paralleled by a significant increase in hippocampal 5-HIAA and 5-HT concentrations and an increase in the plasma corticosterone concentration. Serotonergic, endocrine and behavioural changes are antagonized by IL-1RA pretreatment. Conversely, IL-2 increases activity in the elevated plus maze and is negatively correlated with DA release from the striatum. Thus an important mechanism whereby cytokines mediate behaviour is by changing central neurotransmission and/or by modulating endocrine functions.

HOW BEHAVIOUR MAY AFFECT THE IMMUNE SYSTEM

Whether behaviour can change immune functions is unclear. However, there is evidence demonstrating immunomodulation through behavioural conditioning. This involves observing the effects of conditioned taste aversion on immunosuppression, and the effects of taste aversion conditioning on immunity and conditioning to allergic responses.

Conditioned taste aversion is a form of classical conditioning in which consumption of a mild but novel gustatory stimulus, the conditioning stimulus (CS), is paired with a substance that induces a physiological change, the unconditioning stimulation (UCS). After combination of CS and UCS for several occasions, on re-exposure to the CS alone, a taste avoidance behaviour is displayed and a recurrence of the physiological effects of the UCS occurs. As an example, to study the effect of conditioned taste aversion on immunosuppression, cyclophosphamide, an immunosuppressive drug, is injected into mice. During the period of drug administration, the animals are given saccharin-treated water. After 14 days combination, the mice are exposed to saccharin alone, and an unexpectedly high mortality is reported to occur among the conditioned mice. Conditioned animals also show an impaired immunity, such as low antibody production and immune cellular activities, especially to a SRBC challenge.

Rabbit anti-rat lymphocyte serum (ALS), when injected into rats, induces a transient immunosuppression due to lymphocyte cytotoxicity; saccharin is administered as the CS. After 14 days of CS and ALS injection, exposure to the saccharin alone causes a suppression in lymphocyte activity by 35% compared to control animals. In this case, saccharin does not act as an adverse CS and the UCS is not toxic. This type of experiment therefore establishes that immunosuppression is not dependent on the presence of an aversive CS and UCS.

Taste aversion conditioning, and enhanced immune function, have also been shown experimentally. Levamisole can elevate the ratio of T_H/T_S lymphocytes. After 14 days of levamisole with saccharin water, on re-exposing the animals to saccharin alone, a significant increase in the T_H/T_S ratio was observed. Similarly, repeated injections of ovalbumin (OVA) causes increases in the production of anti-OVA antibodies and lymphocyte proliferation. Following OVA combined with saccharin conditioning, on re-exposing the animals to saccharin alone an elevation in the response of anti-OVA antibodies and T-lymphocyte proliferation occurred. Furthermore, the severity in immune response is negatively correlated with the efficiency of learning.

Even colour can cause conditioned immune changes in humans. For example, when skin allergy to tuberculin administration is paired with an injection vial of a particular colour for several days, the administration of placebo in a vial of the same colour elicits a similar skin reaction to that associated with tuberculin challenge. In exposing guinea-pigs to an odour paired with an allergen challenge, it was also found that the concentration of histamine, a mast-cell-derived mediator of allergic reactions, was significantly increased. When conditioned animals were re-exposed to the odour alone, a similar increase in the histamine response occurred.

The mechanism responsible for these phenomena is unknown. However, many studies have demonstrated that conditioned immunomodulation is not a stress response as the elevation of plasma corticosterone does not contribute to conditioned immunosuppression. In addition, experimental evidence shows that immunosuppression can be achieved by means of a non-aversive UCS. Thus, following conditioning, a direct connection may arise between the CNS and immune system.

PSYCHONEUROIMMUNOLOGY AND THE INTEGRATION OF THE IMMUNE–ENDOCRINE NEUROTRANSMITTER–BEHAVIOURAL NETWORK

Figure 2.2 summarizes the possible relationship between the CNS, the endocrine system and the immune system.

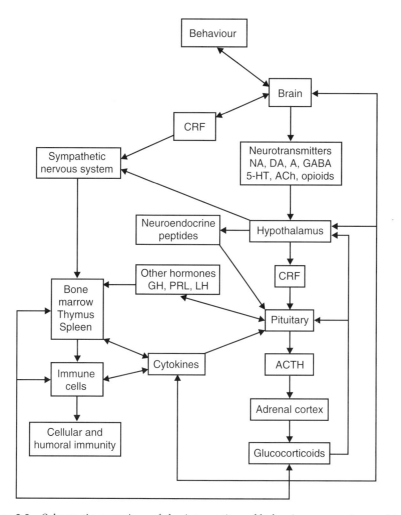

Figure 2.2 Schematic overview of the integration of behaviour, neurotransmitters, the immune system and the glucocorticoids. CRF, corticotrophin-releasing factor; PRL, prolactin; LH, luteinizing hormone; NA, noradrenaline; DA, dopamine; A, adrenaline; GABA, gamma-aminobutyic acid; 5-HT, 5-hydroxytryptamine; ACh, acetylcholine; ACTH, adrenocorticotrophic hormone.

1. A behavioural state or a stressor may stimulate the cortex and limbic system to release NA, DA, 5-HT, ACh and other neurotransmitters, as well as stimulating CRF neurons in the brain to secrete CRF, which activates the sympathetic innervation of the PVN of the hypothalamus. This innervation appears to play a critical role in the control of the rhythmic patterns of basal HPA and hypothalamic secretions of many neuroendocrine peptides. Depletion of PVN catecholamines inhibits the secretion of CRF and other peripheral hormones.

   CRF secreted from the hypothalamus stimulates the pituitary to release ACTH, which regulates the adrenal cortex to produce glucocorticoids. Glucocorticoids combine with their receptors on immune cells and mostly suppress immune function. In addition, immune organs and leucocytes can produce glucocorticoids which have feedback action on adrenal glands and pituitary.

   Cytokines released from leucocytes into the circulation may pass the BBB and combine with the cytokine receptors in the brain, hypothalamus and pituitary. In this way, the immune system modulates neurotransmission, behaviour and hormone secretion.

   IL-1 is the most potent peptide to stimulate the hypothalamus to release CRF.

2. The modulation of neurotransmitters, CRF and other hormones by the immune system is not only due to the action of glucocorticoids. The receptors of neurotransmitters, CRF and many hormones have been found on different types of leucocyte. Neurotransmitters and CRF released from the CNS, and hormones from pituitary into the blood can directly combine with these receptors to modulate immune cellular and humoral functions.

3. NA and CRF produced from the PVN may influence the activity of the SNS and increase NA and neuropeptide Y (NPY) release. Sympathetic nerves innervate lymphoid organs (such as the bone marrow, spleen and thymus) and endocrine organs (such as the adrenal gland). NA and NPY released from the SNS can also combine with their receptors present on lymphocytes, NK cells and adrenal cells. This may lead to the regulation of immune and endocrine functions.

In conclusion, it has been demonstrated that increased sympathetic tone during ageing, stress and depression is associated with an immune decline, whereas chemical sympathectomy has also been shown to suppress cell-mediated responses and enhance antibody responses. Thus, the aim of psychoneuroimmunology is to study the relationship between these three systems and to determine how changes in the interrelationship influence behaviour as a consequence of stress and psychiatric illness.

BIBLIOGRAPHY

Aroujo, D. M., Lapchak, P. A., Collier, B. and Quirion, R. (1989) Localization of interleukin-2 immunoreactivity and interleukin-2 receptors in the rat brain: interaction with the cholinergic system. *Brain Research* **498**: 257–266.

Benjamini, E., Sunshine, G. and Leskowitz, S. (1996) *Immunology: A Short Course* (3rd edn). John Wiley & Sons, New York.

Blalock, J. E. (1989) A molecular basis for bidirectional communication between the immune and neuroendocrine systems. *Physiological Reviews* **69**: 1–29.

Blalock, J. E. (1994) The syntax of immune-neuroendocrine communication. *Immunology Today* **15**: 501–511.

Cross, R. J., Brooks, W. H., Roszman, T. L. and Markesbery, W. R. (1982) Hypothalamic-immune interactions: effect of hypophysectomy on neuroimmunomodulation. *Journal of the Neurological Sciences* **53**: 557–566.

De Sarro, G. B., Masuda, Y., Ascioti, C., Audino, M. G. and Nistico, G. (1990) Behavioural and ECoG spectrum changes induced by intracerebral infusion of interferons and interleukin 2 in rats are antagonized by naloxone. *Neuropharmacology* **29**: 167–179.

Dunn, A. J. (1993) Role of cytokines in infection-induced stress. *Annals of the New York Academy of Sciences* **697**: 189–202.

Elgert, K. D. (Ed.) (1996) *Immunology: Understanding the Immune System*. John Wiley & Sons, New York.

Husband, A. J. (1993) Role of central nervous system and behaviour in the immune response. *Vaccine* **11**: 805–816.

Linthorst, A. C. E., Flachskamm, C., Muller-Preuss, P., Holsboer, F. and Reul, J. (1995) Effect of bacterial endotoxin and interleukin-1b on hippocampal serotonergic neurotransmission, behavioral activity, and free corticosterone levels: an in vivo microdialysis study. *Journal of Neuroscience* **15**: 2920–2934.

Madden, K., Sanders, V. M. and Felten, D. L. (1995) Catecholamine influences and sympathetic neural modulation of immune responsiveness. *Annul Review of Pharmacology and Toxicology* **35**: 417–448.

Meyers, C. A. and Valentine, A. D. (1995) Neurological and psychiatric averse effects of immunological therapy. *CNS Drugs* **3**: 56–68.

Namasivayam, A. and Devi, R. S. (1995) Dorsolateral hippocampus in immunomodulation. *Medical Science Research* **23**: 743–745.

Petitto, J. M., McCarthy, D. B., Rinker, C. M., Huang, Z. and Getty, T. (1997) Modulation of behavioral and neurochemical measures of forebrain dopamine function in mice by species-specific interleukin-2. *Journal of Neuroimmunology* **73**: 183–190.

Qiu, Y., Peng, Y. and Wang, J. (1996) Immunoregulatory role of neurotransmitters. *Advances in Neuroimmunology* **6**: 223–231.

Zalcman, S., Green-Johnson, J., Murray, L., Nance, D. M., Dyck, D., Anisman, H. and Greenberg, A. (1994) Cytokine-specific central monoamine alteration induced by interleukin (IL)-1, IL-2 and IL-6. *Brain Research* **643S**: 40–99.

3 An Outline of Research Methods Used in Psychoneuroimmunology

The methods used in psychoneuroimmunological research are essentially similar to those used in other research areas. As psychoneuroimmunological research involves the interaction between the central nervous system (CNS), endocrine and immune systems, the methods employed depend on the research emphasis. For easy summarization and understanding, the methods used are separated in five parts according to the study area or technique.

METHODS USED TO INVESTIGATE CNS FUNCTIONS

Most methods include a measurement of neurotransmitter synthesis, release and metabolism in different brain regions, electrophysiological activity in specific brain nuclei, and the primary gene *c-fos* (pro-oncogene) expression that may be related to an immune response in the brain. Cytokine production, cytokine-binding sites and cytokine mRNA expression in the brain should also be included.

MEASUREMENTS OF NEUROTRANSMITTERS AND THEIR METABOLISM

High performance liquid chromatography (HPLC) with electrochemical detection (ED) is normally employed for quantitation of biogenic amines, their metabolites and precursors in different brain regions, brain slices and specific brain nuclei. The HPLC system is highly suited to the screening of a large number of samples. To ensure long-term, uninterrupted performance, two robust chromatographic systems have been developed and optimized to separate neighbouring concentration peaks as widely as possible. This is achieved by using mobile phases of relatively low pH to retard acidic compounds, and optimal concentrations of the ion-pairing reagent to manipulate the retention times of amines on the RP-18 column; this also results in clear-cut separations from the solvent/tissue peak. The HPLC-ED system is able to quantify, in the noradrenergic system, the concentrations of noradrenaline (NA), adrenaline (A), the metabolite 3-methoxy-4-hydroxy-phenylglycol (MHPG) and the precursor, 3,4-dihydroxy-phenylalanine (DOPA). In the dopaminergic system, the HPLC-ED system can measure the concentrations of dopamine (DA), homovanillic acid (HVA), 3,4-dihydroxyphenylacetic acid (DOPAC), and precursor L-DOPA, and in the serotonergic system, 5-hydroxytryptamine (5-HT), the metabolite 5-hydroxyindole-acetic acid (5-HIAA) and precursor 5-hydroxy-l-tryptophan (5-HTP) and tryptophan. The samples for HPLC assay are usually obtained in several ways. Postmorten tissues are often used for measurement. Brain tissue is easily dissected into different regions, such as the cerebral cortex, striatum, hippocampus, amygdala, midbrain, brain stem, cerebellum and spinal cord, at 0–4°C. The limitation of this method is that the results only reflect neurotransmitter changes in whole tissue or specific brain regions. The micropunch technique is a more accurate way to obtain samples. Using this method, the brain is cut into several slices with a freezing microtome. Then, according to a brain map, different sizes of needles (dependent on the size of the nuclei) are used to punch out the specific nuclei position.

For studies on free moving animals, a push–pull or microdialysis probe is a useful method for sampling. The push–pull cannula, or microdialysis probe, is inserted into a specific nucleus in which the neurotransmitter changes are to be studied, for example following cytokine, lipopolysaccharide (LPS) or sheep red blood cell (SRBC) challenges. After the animals recover from surgery, the perfusion of artificial cerebrospinal fluid through the push tube or probe, enables the perfusate or dialysate samples to be assayed by HPLC-ED.

ELECTROPHYSIOLOGICAL PARAMETERS

In recent years, electrophysiological studies have concentrated on cytokine-induced changes in ion currents, fluxes of Ca^{2+}, K^+ or Na^+, membrane potentials and neuron firing. Some studies involve electroencephalography (EEG). Most electrophysiological methods can be applied to both neurons and leucocytes. Thus, the actions of neurotransmitters and hormones on electrophysiological characteristics of leucocytes and the action of cytokines on the electrophysiological property of neurons, can be determined.

In the CNS, hypothalamic and hippocampal neurons are generally employed. In the investigation of neuronal development, differentiation and ageing, the electrophysiological influence of cytokines on neurons, microglia and astrocytes has also received attention. Most research has been carried out on animals, for example, by recording single hypothalamic neurons to examine the effects of cytokines on the activity (spine and firing) of the median eminence (ME) using glass electrolyte-filled microelectrodes. By this method, it has been demonstrated that systemic interleukin-1 (IL-1) injection increases hypothalamic corticotrophin-releasing factor (CRF)-secreting neuronal activity five fold.

Intracellular recording and extracellular micropressure ejection techniques are suitable for recording the excitability of neuronal membranes. For instance, incubation of IL-1β with hippocampal neurons causes membrane hyperpolarization, while IL-2 results in membrane depolarization. The effect, of cytokines on the exitatory postsynaptic potential (EPSP) and inhibitory postsynaptic potential (IPSP) can also be achieved by extracellular recording with a monopolar glass stimulating electrode. The patch clamp technique is useful to determine K^+, Na^+ or Ca^{2+} currents in the whole-cell configuration following incubation with cytokines. The Ca^{2+} current is directly related to neuronal excitability. Using the whole-cell patch clamp technique, it has been found that IL-1β largely depresses the voltage-dependent Ca^{2+} current in hippocampal neurons. The stress effect of IL-1 may result from suppression of the Ca^{2+} current; this phenomenon is also often observed following a virus or bacterial infection. In thymocytes, using a patch clamp technique, NA has been shown to inhibit, in a concentration-dependent manner, outward voltage-dependent potassium current. This K^+ current suppression is related to NA-induced reduction of thymocyte proliferation and differentiation during stress.

In rats, EEG recordings have been employed to examine the synchronized and desynchronized period of cortical discharge which is induced by IL-1, IL-2 or interferon alpha (IFN-α). Stainless steel screws are placed into the skull. A screw placed into the frontal sinus or nose serves as the ground electrode, and a stainless steel cannula is implanted above the cortex. The screws are often attached to the terminals of an Amphenol plug and fixed to the skull with dental cement. EEG activity is recorded between cortical electrode pairs using a Grass polygraph. IL-1 administration has been shown to decrease significantly the synchronized EEG discharge and delay the onset of the first period of EEG synchronization, whereas, IFN-α and IL-2 largely increase synchronized EEG and sleep.

LOCATION OF CYTOKINE IMMUNOREACTIVITY, CYTOKINE RECEPTORS AND BINDING SITES IN THE BRAIN

So far, the location of most cytokine receptors and cytokine binding sites in the brain is still unknown, but the location of IL-1 and IL-2 receptors has been studied recently. The methods used include immunoautoradiography, radioimmunoassay and immunofluorescence micrography. To characterize the distribution of cytokine-like immunoreactivity, antibodies that have previously been shown specifically to recognize rat cytokine immunoreactivity (IR) and the Tac antigen-IR of the human cytokine receptors are employed. Immunoautoradiography is performed on brain slices that are coronal sectioned and preincubated in Tris–NaCl buffer. The brain slices are then incubated with antiserum directed against recombinant cytokines. This antiserum has been shown to detect rat cytokine-immunoreactive material in a radioimmunoassay of tissue from different brain regions. Cytokine immunolabelling of brain sections will be decreased if the cytokine anti-serum is preabsorbed with recombinant cytokine.

To localize the cytokine receptors, the brain section is incubated in sheep serum and then with a monoclonal antibody directed against the Tac antigen of the cytokine receptor. Immunolabelling of brain sections with the anti-Tac monoclonal antibody is undertaken if the antibody is preabsorbed with recombinant cytokine. For cytokine receptor autoradiography, the brain is removed and stored at $-80°C$; coronal sections are then cut onto gelatin-coated slides. The sections are then incubated in buffer containing radiolabelled cytokine (such as $[^{125}I]$) and the quantitation of cytokine immunoreactivity and receptor localization are undertaken using a computerized microdensitometer. Using these methods, it has been shown that IL-1 receptors are localized in neurons in the hippocampus, cortex, cerebellum and in the anterior pituitary; these areas are involved in the IL-1 stimulatory effect on ACTH secretion. IL-2 highest densities have been localized to the median eminence, hippocampus, and cerebellum; these locations may be related to affective modulation and memory functions.

CYTOKINE mRNA EXPRESSION, CYTOKINE GENE EXPRESSION AND c-fos EXPRESSION

Cytokine mRNA expression and gene expression have been associated with the inflammatory status of the brain. Genetic, physical and infection-induced changes in brain cytokine expression may have a causal relationship to psychiatric diseases. An *in situ* hybridization histochemical technique has been popularly employed to study cytokine mRNA expression in the brain. Using this technique, the brain tissues are sectioned to 30 µm by a microtome and mounted onto gelatin-coated slides. After drying in a vacuum, the slices are fixed and digested. ^{35}S-labelled cRNA probes are used to localize each transcript (cytokines and cytokine receptors) in the brain slices. Following hybridization, the mixture is spotted on each brain slice, the coverslips are sealed and incubated for 17–22 hours. After rinsing with Tris–NaCl citrate buffer, the sections are digested, rinsed and dehydrated. The sections are then exposed to X-ray film and developed for several days depending on the type of cytokine. The relative intensity of cytokine expression is then assessed on X-ray film images.

Recently, using this method, it has been shown that systemic administration of endotoxin LPS or proinflammatory cytokine IL-1β markedly stimulated IL-6 mRNA, IL-6 receptor (R) mRNA and IL-6 signal transducer gp130 mRNA expression in many brain regions which are functionally involved in neuroimmunomodulation.

The proto-oncogene *c-fos* is an "immediate-early gene" that is an important marker of cell function in response to stress. The *in situ* hybridization technique and immunocytochemical staining can be employed to determine the expression of *c-fos* mRNA. Brain slices are added to a cold cryoprotecting solution, rinsed in potassium phosphate-buffered saline (KPBS) and incubated with the anti-*c-fos* antibody or antiserum at 4°C for 60 hours. Thereafter, the brain slices are rinsed in KPBS and incubated with biotinylated goat anti-rabbit IgG at room temperature. After incubation with avidin–biotin–peroxidase complex, the slices are stained with a mixture of 3.3'-diaminobenzidine and hydrogen peroxide in PBS. Following staining with diaminobenzidine, the tissues are rinsed, mounted on gelatin/chrome alum-coated glass slides, dehydrated through graded ethanol solutions, cleared in Histoclear and cover slipped with Histomount. The presence of *c-fos* is evident as a blue-black reaction product in the cell nuclei.

Cytokines produced by neurons, astrocytes and microglia, and ACTH and glucocorticoids produced by neurons in the hypothalamus and the pituitary, can also be measured in the brain. The methods for detecting these substances will be introduced later.

METHODS FOR THE QUANTIFICATION OF HORMONES

Most hormone changes have been measured in the plasma or serum, but such changes can also be determined in the supernatant of tissue homogenates, such as the brain and immune organs. Leucocyte-produced hormones are normally assessed in cell culture medium or in whole blood after culture.

ACTH, CORTISOL AND CORTICOSTERONE ASSAY

The blood is mixed with EDTA or another anticoagulant, centrifuged and the plasma quickly frozen and stored at –70°C. Plasma ACTH, cortisol or corticosterone are subsequently determined in duplicate using commercially available assay kits.

Plasma corticosterone concentration may also be assayed by a fluorescence method. In this method, samples are mixed in chloroform. The chloroform phase is then transferred into a tube containing sulphuric acid : ethanol (32.5 : 17.5) and mixed. The samples were then kept in the dark for 45 min. An aliquot from the lower acid phase was removed and fluorescence measured in a spectrophotofluorimeter.

GROWTH HORMONE (GH) ASSAY

Rat GH may be assayed by radioimmunoassay. Purified rat GH is labelled with [125]I. The NIADDK reference preparation rGH-RP-2 is used as a standard, and the antiserum used is NIADDK-anti-rGH-S-5. Addition of label is delayed by 2 hours; this non-equilibrium protocol increases the sensitivity of the assay. Separation of the antibody-bound from free hormone is achieved by addition of protein A.

MEASUREMENT OF PROLACTIN (PRL) IN BLOOD

Rat PRL concentration is determined by a radioimmunoassay using anti-rat antiserum and rat PRL standard. The PRL assay sensitivity is 0.4–1.1 ng/ml. Radioimmunoassay kits are also available for human samples.

IMMUNOLOGICAL ASSAYS

Cellular immune aspects include mitogen-induced lymphocyte proliferation, granulocyte (neutrophil) phagocytosis and chemotaxis, superoxide anion production, natural killer (NK) cell cytotoxicity and monocyte/ macrophage activities.

MITOGEN-INDUCED LYMPHOCYTE PROLIFERATION

Mitogens are a group of lectins that are extracted from plants or bacteria. Using mitogens to stimulate lymphocytes imitates the antigen-induced lymphocyte response. Different mitogens have different stimulative properties. For example, phytohaemagglutinin (PHA) stimulates both T-cell and B-cell proliferation, and concanavalin A (Con A) stimulates T cells. Pokeweed mitogen stimulates B cells at low dose and both T and B cells at high dose. LPS stimulates macrophages. Therefore, different mitogens and doses may be used according to the cell types being examined.

   To separate lymphocytes, blood samples are layered onto a Nycoprep gradient (density = 1.077) and centrifuged at 600 g for 25 min at 20°C. Following centrifugation, one distinct band of white cells is obtained. This layer is removed and washed three times with cell culture medium. The lymphocyte suspension is placed in each well of a 96-well microtitre plate containing 0.2 ml of cell culture medium supplement with penicillin (2%) and heat-inactivated foetal calf serum (10%). To each well, one of the following reagents is added: cell culture medium for background activity and different concentrations of the mitogens. The cultures are then incubated at 37°C in a 5% carbon dioxide atmosphere. After addition of tritiated thymidine for several hours, the cells are harvested. The tritiated thymidine uptake is then measured in a scintillation counter. Mean scintillation counts per minutes (c.p.m.) are determined.

DETERMINATION OF NEUTROPHIL FUNCTIONS

Plasma substitute is mixed with blood and left at room temperature for 30 min for separation of red blood cells and leucocytes. For separation of neutrophils from the lymphocytes and monocytes, the supernatant from the first step is then layered on Histopaque (density 1.099) and centrifuged at 600 g for 25 min. Neutrophils are collected at the bottom of the centrifuge tube. The neutrophils are then harvested and washed three times with Hanks' balanced salt solution (HBSS). Phagocytosis is measured by flow cytometry.

A mixture of neutrophils in HBSS with Ca^{2+} and Mg^{2+} is mixed with 0.1 ml autologous plasma and 0.1 ml fluorescent latex particles (2 mm diameter) at a ratio of 50 beats/cell. After incubation at 37°C for 60 min, 2 ml cold HBSS (without Ca^{2+} and Mg^{2+}) are added and the cells are centrifuged at 400 g for 10 min. The neutrophil solution is diluted and measured by means of a FASCAN flow cytometer.

There are two substances that are used to stimulate neutrophil production of the superoxide anion. Zymosan, which has been activated by incubation with serum from same subject, initiates phagocytosis. Opsonized zymosan, similar to bacteria, can induce neutrophil phagocytosis. Phorbol myristate acetate (PMA) stimulates neutrophil oxidative metabolism. For detecting phagocytic activity, neutrophil-produced chemiluminescence is amplified by labelling luminol. Briefly, 200 µl of neutrophil suspension, 200 µl of the optimal concentration of luminol (0.1 mM) in 0.1 M NaOH and 200 µm of activated zymosan or optimal concentration of PMA are mixed together, and the chemiluminescence produced is recorded by a luminometer. Normally, the results from these two methods are parallel.

Neutrophil chemotaxis is also used as a marker of neutrophil function: 10^6/ml of neutrophils in HBSS (with Ca^{2+} and Mg^{2+}) are placed in the upper compartment, which is divided from the lower chamber by a nitrocellulose membrane filter with a 3 µm pore size. Casein, a chemotactic agent, is used in 1 mg/ml concentration and placed in the lower chamber. The chambers are incubated at 37°C for 60 min. Thereafter, the filter is fixed in ethanol and stained with Harris haematoxylin. The migration distance is determined and expressed as mm/h.

NK CELL CYTOTOXICITY

In experimental studies, isolated splenic cells are usually used for determination of NK cell cytotoxicity. In clinical studies, heparinized venous blood is used for separation of NK cells. A short-term ^{51}Cr-release assay is frequently used to determine NK cell cytotoxicity. Using U-bottomed microplates, effector cells are titrated, in triplicate, against 5.0×10^3 ^{51}Cr-labelled YAC-1 murine lymphoma target cells across the effector to target cell ratios of 100 : 1, 50 : 1 and 25 : 1. Incubation of target cells with 0.1 M HCl causes the total release of ^{51}Cr contained within the cells. Spontaneous release, the amount of radioactivity released in the medium alone, does not exceed 20% of the total amount released by 0.1 M HCl. The percentage of specific cytotoxicity is determined using the formula: (experimental c.p.m. – spontaneous c.p.m.)/(total c.p.m. – spontaneous c.p.m.) × 100.

ASSAY OF MONOCYTE/MACROPHAGE ACTIVITY

Monocyte/macrophage phagocytic activity may be determined under conditions mononuclear cells in which only monocytes/macrophages produce chemoluminescence after activation, or in purified monocytes by stimulated with mitogens or zymosan. As human blood cells contain 10% of monocytes, there are enough monocytes for determining activity. However, in animals, the spleen is rich with monocytes/macrophages, but there are insufficient monocytes in the blood for accurate assay. The separation of mononuclear cells is similar to the method for lymphocytes. The centrifuge speed will be slower depending on the species. PHA, Con A and PMA can be used to stimulate monocyte/macrophage phagocytic response. Monocytes/ macrophages may be separated from the rat or mouse spleen as follows. After decapitation, the spleen is quickly removed and immersed in the RPMI 1640 medium. By means of two sterilized glass slides, the spleen is cut and smashed into small pieces and finally into a cell mass. The splenic suspension is then layered onto Histopaque 1.077 and centrifuged at 600 g for 25 min at 4°C. The mononuclear fractions that occur at the interface are collected and washed three times with RPMI 1640 medium. The activity of monocytes/macrophages can then be determined by the method used for neutrophils.

For the purification of monocytes/macrophages in human blood, disodium-EDTA treated blood is mixed with dextran (6%) in a 10 : 1 ratio. The plasma layer containing the leucocytes is removed when the erythrocytes have sedimented after 15–30 min. The plasma is then layered onto the Nycodenz–NaCl gradient media (density 1.1466 g/ml) and centrifuged at 600 g for 15 min. After centrifugation the plasma is removed. The remaining plasma, together with slightly more than half the volume of the separation fluid, is collected. With this method of separating monocytes, the most important step is to adjust the density of the separation liquid by changing the concentrations of NaCl.

An alternative method for purification of monocytes/macrophages is to culture mononuclear cells at 37°C in a 5% CO_2 atmosphere for 1–2 h. Only monocytes/macrophages adhere to the bottom of the culture plate. Using warm RPMI-1640 with 10% foetal calf serum, non-adhering cells are removed. The adhered monocytes are released by adding 0.25% trysin to the culture plate and incubating for 10 min at 37°C. The monocyte/macrophage suspension is washed three times with RPMI-1640 medium or HBSS.

CYTOKINE ASSAY

Cytokines released from leucocytes may be detected in serum, plasma and whole blood. However, in normal or mild pathological conditions the concentration of some cytokines is virtually undetectable. Sometimes, stressors or infections do not affect cytokine synthesis by leucocytes unless specific antigens are present. To test the changes in cytokine release during stress, brain injury and psychiatric disorders, several methods have been developed. Purified mononuclear cells, monocytes or macrophages may be stimulated by mitogens and cultured for one to three days. Under these conditions the synthesis of cytokines is enhanced. Recently, a method for mitogen-induced cytokine release from whole blood has been developed. Whole blood incubated with mitogens at 37°C is a good model for studying the cytokine response to an antigen/immunogen invasion since leucocytes exist in an environment that is similar to the natural environment in the body. Not only does whole blood preserve cell-to-cell interaction but circulating stimulatory and inhibitory mediators are also present at their normal concentrations. The method consists of diluted heparinized blood 1 : 10 with cell culture medium containing 1% of penicillin, PHA (5 µg/ml), and LPS (20 µg/ml). For a blank, the blood from each sample is diluted with RPMI-1640 containing 1% penicillin. Samples (400 µl) are then pipetted into 24 well-plates prefilled with medium (1200 µl) and incubated for 24, 48 or 72 hours (depending on the peak time of cytokine release) in a humidified atmosphere at 37°C, 5% CO_2. After incubation, the plates are centrifuged at 1500 r.p.m. for 10 min. The supernatant is carefully removed under sterile conditions, divided into Eppendorf tubes, and frozen immediately at –70°C until the cytokines and their receptors may be assayed.

Most concentrations of human or murine cytokines and soluble cytokine receptors can be measured by the quantitative enzyme-linked immunosorbent assay (ELISA) technique. Monoclonal antibodies specific for each component are precoated onto 96-well microtitre plates. Standards and samples are pipetted into the wells and incubated at 37°C. Every cytokine receptor or soluble protein is bound by the immobilized antibody and incubated again at 37°C. After washing away any unbound substances, an enzyme-linked polyclonal antibody specific for each of these components is added to the wells and incubated at 37°C. Following a wash to remove any unbound antibody–enzyme reagent, a substrate solution is added to the wells for 10 min and colour development is in proportion to the amount of receptor or protein bound in the initial step. The colour development is stopped by addition of sulphuric acid and the intensity of the colour measured by the microtitre plate reader (absorbance at 450 nm).

Cytokine concentrations may also be determined by bioassay, a method that is being developed for rat and other animal studies. The principle of bioassay is to choose a special cell line which only survives in a culture medium containing one type of cytokine. The rate of cell proliferation will therefore depend on the concentration of the specific cytokine. Thus, by addition of sample to the cell culture medium, the cytokine concentration in this sample can be measured by counting the number of cells alive after incubation for several days.

ASSAYS FOR IMMUNOGLOBULINS, COMPLEMENTS AND ACUTE PHASE PROTEINS

These parameters are used to assess humoral immunity. Changes in immunoglobolin production, complements and acute phase proteins may result from changes in cytokine production and result in an inflammatory response. To determine these functions, fasting intravenous blood is drawn into a heparinized syringe. After centrifugation at 2000 g for 10 min, the plasma is aspirated and stored at $-20°C$. The immunogloblin IgG, IgA, IgM, complement C3 and C4, positive acute phase proteins (APPs), such as haptoglobin, alpha-1-acid glycoprotein and alpha-1-antitrypsin, are determined by means of a laser nephelometer analyser. Albumin, α_1, α_2 and γ globulins in the plasma are measured by gel electrophoresis. Five microlitres of each plasma sample is applied to each template slot and 2 min allowed for diffusion after the last sample has been applied. The gel is placed onto a gel bridge assembly containing the buffer and the sample is then subjected to electrophoresis for 35 min. The gel is stained and then washed with Pragon blue and acetic acid solution. The percentage of each protein is determined using the Apprais Densitometer System and the total protein can be measured in the plasma samples by using a Random Access Analyser. The quantity of each protein is calculated as a percentage of the total protein.

MEASUREMENT OF WHITE BLOOD CELL DIFFERENTIATION AND LEUCOCYTE SUBSETS

Changes in total leucocyte number and differentiation have been used as a general marker of infection or inflammation in general hospital routine. For example, increases in the total number of leucocytes, number and percentage of neutrophils are indications of an infection of inflammatory response. The total leucocyte count and leucocyte differentiation may be performed either by using a blood smear technique or by mean of a Technicon H2 system, an automated blood cell counter.

Leucocyte subsets are determined by means of flow cytometry. Monoclonal antibodies to certain leucocyte subset receptors are linked to fluorescent markers and mixed with a blood sample. These antibodies include anti-leu-2a (T-cytotoxic/suppressor cells); anti-leu-3a+3b (T-helper/inducer cells); anti-leu-4 (T cells); anti-leu-7 (T-cell and natural killer cell subsets) and anti-leu-lla (NK cells). A cell background control is used which is fluorescein-labelled mouse IgG subclass. The blood is incubated with mono-clonal antibodies at 0°C and then washed and fixed. The sample is then allowed to flow past a device that registers the number of cells characterized by each surface marker.

BEHAVIOURAL APPARATUS USED IN PSYCHONEUROIMMUNOLOGICAL RESEARCH

In Chapter 2, it was suggested that changes in immune function can affect behaviour. Immunological changes may result in anxious behaviour, hyper-activity, sedative behaviour, stress-like response or impairment of memory. Some of the standard behavioural methods used in psychoneuroimmunol-ogy are described below.

OPEN FIELD APPARATUS

This apparatus is used to test spontaneous motor activity of rodents in a stressful novel environment. The parameters observed in "open field" include locomotor activity, rearing, grooming and defecation. The apparatus consists of an open square or circular area. A grid is drawn on the floor of the open field for quantifying locomotor activity (Figure 3.1). Measurement of activities can be recorded automatically; light beams are shone across the floor, and photocells count the number of times these beams are broken by the moving animal. Animal behaviour in the open field is normally observed for 3–5 min.

ELEVATED PLUS MAZE

This apparatus is used for quantifying anxiety in rodents. The apparatus consists of an X-shaped maze elevated from the floor with two opposite enclosed and two open arms (Figure 3.2). The animal is placed in the centre of the maze, facing a closed arm. Entry into an arm is defined as the animal placing all four paws onto the arm. The cumulative times spent in, and the number of entries into the open or closed arms, are recorded for 5 min. An increase in the number of entries into, and time spent on, the closed arms is considered as an increase in anxious behaviour.

PASSIVE AVOIDANCE APPARATUS

Ths apparatus is used for testing the conditioned memory of an animal. There are two types of apparatus, the step through test and the step down test.

Step Through Test

The apparatus consists of a box divided by a wall into two compartments of equal size. The white chamber, illuminated by one 40 W incandescent light

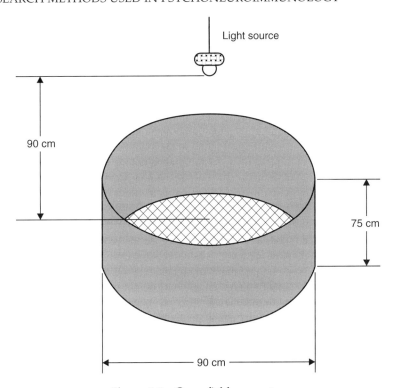

Figure 3.1 Open field apparatus.

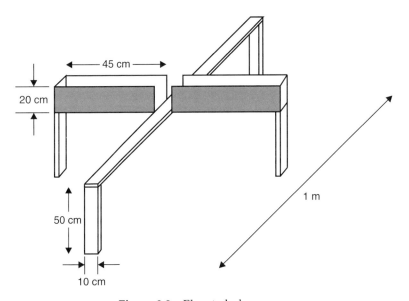

Figure 3.2 Elevated plus maze.

bulb, is connected to the rear black chamber, equipped with a grid floor, the two chambers being separated by a guillotine floor (Figure 3.3). The animals are subjected to a single adaptation trial (no shock) 24 h prior to the acquisition trials (with an unavoidable footshock when the animal enters the dark chamber). On the third day the retention test consists of placing the rat in the brightly lit compartment and the latency to enter the dark compartment is recorded during a 5 min period of observation.

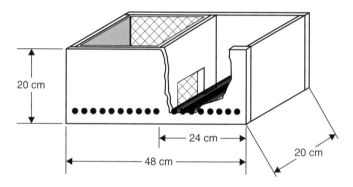

Figure 3.3 Step through passive avoidance.

Step Down Test

The chamber of this apparatus is equipped with a stainless steel grid floor through which an electric shock (50 V, AC, 60 Hz) is given. A platform is placed above the grid floor, on which an animal stays to avoid the electric shock. In the learning trial (day 1), animals are trained to stay on the platform for 10 min. They are punished by a footshock when they step down from the platform (error). The number of errors and the number of animals that do not step down during the latter 5 min of the learning trial were recorded.

MORRIS WATER MAZE

This apparatus is used for testing the spatial memory of an animal. The water maze is a large tank with warm water ($26 \pm 1°C$) (Figure 3.4). On day 1, the animal is placed in the water and allowed to swim freely for 1 min. On day 2, a platform is positioned below the water level in one of the quadrants of the maze and the latency to locate the platform is recorded; the animal is subjected to five trials. On day 3, the platform is left in the same position and the test of trials repeated. The time taken for the rodent to locate the hidden platform and the errors made before locating the platform are recorded. On day 4, the platform is repositioned in another quadrant of the maze and the latency to locate the platform is recorded over five trials. On day 5, the position of the platform and the test remains the same as on day 4.

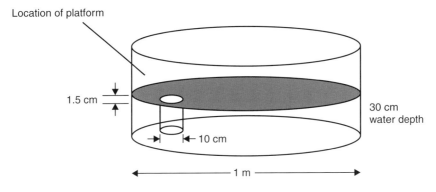

Figure 3.4   Morris water maze.

SELF-STIMULATION BEHAVIOUR

Animals are placed in a stereotaxic apparatus and implanted with a bipolar stimulating electrode located in the medial forebrain bundle at the level of the lateral hypothalamus. The intracranial self-stimulation (ICSS) apparatus consists of four identical black Plexiglas boxes. Two holes are located at the centre of the floor of each chamber. A ring of lights, covered with white translucent plastic, are embedded in the Plaxiglas floor and serve as a conditioning stimulus. Three infrared photobeam units are mounted in the perimeter of each hole and when the animal breaks the photobeam by placing its nose in the hole a small electric stimulation is delivered to the brain through a mercury-filled commutator connected to a constant current stimulator. A "nose-poke" response into the correct hole causes brain stimulation to be delivered, while responding to the incorrect hole is not reinforced. Once stable rates of responding are established the discrimination procedure is initiated. Light presentation is alternated between the holes at 30 s intervals over a 5 min session. Animals receive brain stimulation only when responding is directed towards the signalled hole. This procedure is maintained until the animal performs correctly on at least 90% of the total responses emitted. Following discrimination training, baseline descending and ascending rate-current intensity functions are determined. Once stable baseline functions are established, the animal may receive immune challenge and the effect of different types of challenge on the behavioural responses is assessed.

FEEDING BEHAVIOUR

Immune changes often affect feeding behaviour. Anorexia is one of the most common clinical manifestations of acute and chronic infection or inflammation. These pathophysiological processes stimulate proinflammatory cytokine synthesis and release, which causes anorexia by direct central actions. To determine eating and drinking behaviour, basal food and water intake during night time or total daily intake is measured before cytokine administration and then measured at different times after cytokine administration. Spillage of food and water should be minimized. The body weight is also measured. To determine the microstructure of eating and drinking, rats are housed in special test chambers equipped with electromechanical pellet dispensers controlled by pellet-sensing photobeams and photoelectric "lickometers". Changes in food and water intake before and after a cytokine injection can then be analysed during the experiment.

MODELS EMPLOYED IN PSYCHONEUROIMMUNOLOGY

Most models for the investigation of stress or psychiatric diseases can also be employed in psychoneuroimmunological research. In human subjects, the effects of stressful life events, physical stress, examination stress or public speech stress etc. may be used. In animals, electric footshock, swimming in cold water, noise stress, isolation, restrain or predator exposure have been used.

Depression models in rodents include developmental models, learned helplessness, reserpine-induced depression, the muricidal rat model and brain lesion models. Many stressors result in anxiety and may be used to develop anxiety models. Schizophrenia models may be developed by the use of stimulant amphetamines and psychotomimetics such as phencyclidine. Alzheimer's disease may be imitated by changing central cholinergic function or by neurotoxin lesions.

Changes in the immune system also cause many symptoms that resemble major psychiatric states in both humans and animals. These models are established by systemic or central administration of cytokines, LPS, bacteria, virus or SRBC. Moreover, the effects of ageing on the activity of the thymus and autoimmune diseases may have a causal relationship with immune disorders observed in psychiatric diseases. These aspects will be dealt with in more details in subsequent chapters.

BIBLIOGRAPHY

Anisman, H., Kokkinidis, L. and Merali, Z. (1996) Interleukin-2 decreases accumbal dopamine efflux and responding for rewarding lateral hypothalamic stimulation. *Brain Research* **731**: 1–11.

De Sarro, G. B., Masuda, Y., Ascioti, C., Audino, M. G. and Nistico, G. (1990) Behavioural and ECoG spectrum changes induced by intracerebral infusion of interferons and interleukin-2 in rats are antagonized by naloxone. *Neuropharmacology* **29**: 167–179.

Grealy, M. and O'Donnell, J. (1991) Secretion of growth hormone elicited by intravenous desipramine in the conscious, unrestrained rat. *British Journal of Pharmacology*. **102**: 369–372.

Koller, H., Siebler, M. and Hartung, H. P. (1997) Immunologically induced electrophysiological dysfunction: implications for inflammatory diseases of the CNS and PNS. *Progress in Neurobiology* **52**: 1–26.

Lapchak, P. A., Araujo, D. M., Quirion, R. and Beaudeit, A. (1991) Immunoautoradiographic localization of interleukin-2-like immunoreactivity and interleukin-2 receptors (Tac antigen-like immunoreactivity) in the rat brain. *Neuroscience* **44**: 173–184.

Lee, S., Barbanel, G. and Rivier, C. (1995) Systemic endotoxin increases steady-state gene expression of hypothalamic nitric oxide synthase: comparison with corticotropin-releasing factor and vasopressin gene transcripts. *Brain Research* **705**: 136–148.

Lin, J. and Krier, J. (1995) Human recombinant interleukin-1 beta inhibits nicotinic transmission in neurons of guinea pig plexus ganglia. *American Journal of Physiology* **269**: G981–987.

O'Neill, B. and Leonard, B. E. (1990) Abnormal zymosan-induced neutrophil chemiluminescence as a marker of depression. *Journal of Affective Disorders* **19**: 265–272.

Plata-Salaman, C. R. and Ffrench-Mullen, J. M. (1992) Interleukin-1 beta depressed calcium currents in CA1 hippocampal neurons at pathophysiological concentrations. *Brain Research Bulletin* **29**: 221–223.

Rivest, S., Torres, G. and Rivier, C. (1992) Differential effects of central and peripheral injection of interleukin-1b on brain c-fos expression and neuroendocrine functions. *Brain Research* **587**: 13–23.

Rothwell, N. and Dantzer, R. (eds). (1994) *Interleukin-1 in the Brain*. Pergamon Press, Oxford.

Seyfried, C. A., Adam, G. and Greve, T. (1986) An automated direct-injection HPLC-method for the electrochemical/fluorimetric quantitation of monoamines and related compounds opimized for the screening of large numbers of animals. *Biomedical Chromatography* **1**: 78–88.

Song, C. and Leonard, B. E. (1994) The effects of chronic lithium chloride administration on some behaviour and immune functions in olfactory bulbectomized rats. *Journal of Psychopharmacology* **8**: 44–47.

Song, C., Earley, B. and Leonard, B. E. (1996) The effects of central administration of neuropeptide Y on behavioural, neurochemical and immunological functions in the olfactory bulbectomized rat depression model of animal. *Brain, Behavior, and Immunity* **10**: 1–16.

Sonti, G., Ilyin, S. E. and Plata-Salaman, C. R. (1996) Anorexia induced by cytokine interactions at pathophysiological concentrations. *American Journal of Physiology* **270**: R1394–1402.

Vallieres, L. and Rivest, S. (1997) Regulation of the genes encoding interleukin-6, its receptor, and gp130 in the rat brain in response to the immune activator lipopolysaccharide and proinflammatory cytokine interleukin-1β. *Journal of Neurochemistry* **69**: 1668–1683.

Vizi, E. S., Orso, E., Osipenko, O. N., Hasko, G. and Elenkov, I. J. (1995) Neurochemical, electrophysiological and immunocytochemical evidence for a noradrenergic link between the sympathetic nervous system and thymocytes. *Neuroscience* **68**: 1263–1276.

4 Psychoneuroimmunology of Stress

Numerous clinical and experimental studies have shown that stress significantly alters immune functions in both humans and animals. However, while some investigators found that stress suppressed immune activity, others have reported that stress can enhance immune responses. These opposite effects on immune functions may be due to the many different factors involved in the interaction between stress and the immune system. These factors include the nature of the stressor, the severity of stress and its duration as well as the genetic, age and gender characteristics of the individual. Furthermore, different stressors may produce different degrees of autonomic nervous system activation and hormone release which may impact on the immune system in different ways. Stressors may be divided into those that are external or internal, psychological or physical, and psychogenic or neurogenic. The impact of these different types of stressors on the immune system will now be considered.

THE INFLUENCE OF EXTERNAL STRESSORS ON THE IMMUNE SYSTEM

In animal experiments, various stressors have been used to study the effects of external stressors on immune function. Environmental stressors, such as noise, bright light, odour and adverse housing conditions, are known to significantly reduce antibody production. Neurogenic stressors, such as electric footshocks, restraint stress and forced swimming in cold water, have been found to increase the number of total leucocytes and the number of neutrophils, and to suppress mitogen-induced lymphocyte proliferation, neutrophil phagocytosis and natural killer (NK) cell cytotoxicity; these stressors may also enhance B-cell and macrophage activities. Psychological stressors, such as social isolation, maternal separation and predator exposure, also markedly decrease some immune functions including mitogen-induced T-cell proliferation, NK cell cytotoxicity and macrophage activity.

In recent years, the effects of different types of stress on the concentrations of cytokines and cytokine receptors and leucocyte subsets have been investigated. For example, in animal studies, physical restraint, footshock and a conditioned aversive stimulus largely stimulate interleukin-1 (IL-1) and IL-6 production. Such changes are positively correlated with the concentration of the plasma corticosterone. Novel environment stress in the rat, for instance exposure to the "open field", also increases IL-6 release from macrophages.

In humans, experimental and epidemiological data have demonstrated that adverse life events, psychological distress and depression are associated with changes in the immune system, as shown by a reduction in cellular immunity. Most stressful life experiences, such as the death of a spouse or divorce, significantly reduce NK cell cytotoxicity and lymphocyte responses to mitogen stimulation. Likewise, the stress associated with other life events, such as caregiving for a family member with a severe disease, results in a reduction in the function of NK cells and lymphocytes.

The effect of physical stress has also been investigated in humans. These results have shown that strenuous exercise markedly reduces the number of T_H (CD4+), T_S (CD8+), NK and B cells and the production of IL-2 and IL-6, but increases the concentration of IL-1β and soluble IL-2R (sIL-2R). Following strenuous exercise, moderate exercise appears to attenuate these changes. Acute psychological stress, such as that caused by academic examinations, significantly increases the number of leucocytes, lymphocytes, neutrophils and monocytes, as well as the T-cell subpopulation of CD2+, CD3+ and CD8+s, but reduces CD4+ and the CD4+/CD8+ ratio. In human subjects, angioplasty stress also significantly increases the blood concentrations of IL-1, IL-2 and sIL-2R.

The effect of a stressor on the immune system also depends on the psychological condition and the personality of the individual. Thus, it has been found that academic examination-induced changes in total leucocyte number, leucocyte differentiation and subsets and changes in the plasma concentration of cytokines and receptors are positively correlated with scores on the Perceived Stress Scale (PSS) and/or State Trait Anxiety Inventory (STAI) in students.

Different cytokines may play different roles in the response to stress. Even though the relationship between most of the cytokines and cytokine receptors is still unclear, the IL-1 receptor antagonist (RA), a natural anti-stress agent, has been found to be increased during stress. Pretreatment with IL-1RA in rats prevents CRF release, physical restraint or immobilization-induced elevation of ACTH and corticosterone, and the consequent suppression of immune function. There is also an association between the cytokines produced by Th1 and Th2 lymphocytes. For example, the Th1 cytokines interferon gamma (IFN-γ) and IL-6 are increased by stress, while the Th2 cytokine IL-10 has a pronounced inhibitory effect on the production of these Th1 cytokines.

It has been shown that IL-1 causes many behavioural responses that simulate those caused by stress, directly stimulates corticotrophin-releasing factor (CRF) release from the hypothalamus and suppresses several immune cellular functions, while IL-2 has opposite effects to IL-1. In an animal model of depression, the olfactory bulbectomized rat, central administration of IL-2 reverses depression-like behaviour, neurotransmitter changes and immune suppression without increasing corticosterone concentration. Although the relationship between IL-1 and IL-2 during stress has been studied, a direct antagonistic effect between these two cytokines has not been found.

In humans, bereavement, divorce, loneliness and other stressful life events have been shown to provoke relatively long-lasting disturbances of various aspects of immune functioning, including reduced NK cell activity, lowered IFN-γ production, decreased mitogen-induced lymphocyte proliferation, altered expression of IL-2 receptors and impaired immune control regarding the reactivation of a latent herpes virus.

VARIABLE EFFECTS OF STRESS ON THE IMMUNE SYSTEM

THE INFLUENCE OF INTERNAL STRESSORS

As illustrated in Chapter 2, the immune system acts as a sensory organ for the brain. The response of the brain to a stressful stimulus, inflammation or infection is qualitatively similar. Conversely, abnormalities in the immune system can produce secondary stress responses in the central nervous system (CNS). For example, changes in neurotransmitters in the brain that are induced by a CRF injection are similar to those caused by the administration of IL-1β or endotoxin. In experimental studies, for example, changes in immune function following immunization cause changes in neuron firing rates recorded from hypothalamus and other brain regions. Monoamine neurotransmitters are also changed during an immune response, the change being closely correlated with these immune functions.

Internal stressors include tissue or organ damage and inflammatory or infectious diseases. In these cases, cytokines are released into the circulation, which then have an impact on immune functions. In addition, oxidative stress related to free radical damage in cells and tissues occurs in many diseases.

The influence of internal stress may also affect the interaction between stress and the immune system. For example, in patients with spinal cord injury or following a stroke, immune responses are strikingly decreased two weeks after the injury or stroke when compared with those of age-matched controls. NK cell function decreases and plasma ACTH values increase in patients two weeks after the injury or stroke. By contrast, urine free cortisol concentrations are elevated 24 h after the injury. Some aspects of cellular immunity are decreased for a considerable period. T-cell function is decreased by 60% three months after the injury and T-cell activation (IL-2R) is also diminished. With rehabilitation therapy, NK cell activity slowly returns to normal by seven months while IL-2R values improve in parallel with lymphocyte transformation. The depression of NK cell activity has also been reported to occur after stroke. In addition, the plasma concentrations of proinflammatory cytokines (IL-1, IL-6 and tumour necrosis factor alpha (TNF-α) are also increased. Rehabilitation therapy reverses these immune changes.

Patients subject to chronic stress, for example following diagnosis and surgical treatment for breast cancer, often experience psychological adjustment difficulties. This stress can affect the immune system, and thereby reduce the individuals ability to resist disease progression and metastatic spread. The relationship between stress and cellular immune responses has been studied in patients following breast cancer diagnosis and surgery. In one study, before beginning their adjuvant therapy, all patients completed a validated questionnaire for assessing stress. Several multiple regression models were used to test the contribution of psychological stress in predicting immune function. All regression equations controlled for variables that might exert short- or long-term effects on these responses and other potentially confounding variables were ruled out. The results of this study showed that the intensity of stress (1) significantly predicted lower NK cell lysis; (2) significantly predicted diminished response of NK cells to recombinant IFN-γ, and (3) significantly predicted the decreased proliferative response of lymphocytes to mitogens and to a monoclonal antibody directed against the T-cell receptor. The data show that the physiological effects of stress inhibit the cellular immune responses that are relevant to cancer prognosis, including NK cell toxicity and T-cell responses to mitogen stimulations.

Liver diseases are often associated with immune dysfunction, especially as they may affect cytokine production and acute phase protein synthesis. In patients with alcohol-induced liver injury and/or liver cirrhosis, cellular immunity is significantly depressed and characterized by the activation of the monocyte–macrophage system as shown by the increased production of TNF-α, IL-1 and IL-6. Increases in these cytokines could then result in changes in both cellular and humoral immunity, while the increased IL-6 further stimulates the liver to produce positive acute phase proteins. These changes are qualitatively similar to those observed in subjects exposed to stress, but in this case are the direct result of liver damage.

Other internal stressors, such as liver disease (hepatitis A, B and C), heart disease with consequent infection and lung diseases, are also associated with tissue damage, caused by oxidative stress. In patients with type C chronic hepatitis, IFN-γ production by mononuclear cells in response to the hepatitis C virus (HCV) core protein is increased. Production of IL-10 and IL-12 by mononuclear cells from patients with chronic HCV infection has been evaluated including asymptomatic HCV carriers with normal serum alanine aminotransferase (ALT) values, suggesting minimal liver cell damage. IL-10 is known to inhibit many functions of the immune system, suppressing Th1-type cell development for example, while IL-12 stimulates differentiation of Th1-type cells, facilitating cell-mediated immunity. Spontaneous IL-10 production is greater in patients with chronic hepatitis and liver cirrhosis than in controls, and is decreased during IFN treatment. Both HCV core protein and concanavalin A (Con A) enhanced IL-10 production by cells from HCV-infected patients. In chronic liver diseases, whereas the IL-12 concentration was not detectable in culture medium, addition of HCV protein resulted in increased IL-12 production. Addition of IL-10 to the cultures suppressed IFN-γ production in both the control and patient groups, but the effect of IL-12 on IFN-γ synthesis was significantly less in patients with type C chronic liver disease than in other patient groups or in controls. The findings suggest that secretion of IL-10 and IL-12 by cells from patients with different types of liver disease differs particularly in the response to IFN-γ synthesis.

T lymphocytes and immunoregulatory cytokines may be important in the host response to internal stressors. Thus, Th1 cytokines (IL-2 and IFN-γ) are required for host antiviral immune responses, including cytotoxic T-cell generation and NK cell activation, while Th2 cytokines (IL-4 and IL-10) can inhibit the development of these effector mechanisms. The concentrations of circulating IL-2, IL-4, IL-10, and IFN-γ are significantly elevated in HCV patients compared with normal controls. Treatment with IFN-α decreased the concentrations of IL-4 and IL-10, which paralleled a decrease in HCV RNA. These findings indicate that an activated T-cell response, as manifest by increased circulating immunoregulatory cytokines, is present in patients with HCV liver disease. Furthermore, treatment with IFN-α diminishes the Th2 cytokine response. Thus, modulation of T-cell function and cytokine production may be one mechanism whereby IFN-α therapy results in a reduced viral burden.

In experimental studies, it has also been shown that immune-mediated processes are involved in canine chronic hepatitis. Mononuclear cells from dogs with chronic inflammatory liver disease or with non-inflammatory liver diseases were evaluated for proliferative responses to pokeweed mitogen and canine liver membrane protein. It was found that mononuclear cell proliferation in response to liver membrane protein was significantly higher in dogs with chronic hepatitis than in control animals. Dogs with chronic hepatitis and dogs with non-inflammatory liver disease had greater proliferative responses to liver membrane protein than the control animals.

Tissue damage, inflammation and necrosis are also the hallmarks of myocardial infarction. Significant elevations of proinflammatory cytokines and serum acute phase proteins have been noted in coronary artery disease and angina pectoris.

Cardiac myosin-induced myocarditis has proved to be a valuable virus-free murine model for investigation of autoimmunological mechanisms in inflammatory heart disease. The disease was shown to be T-cell-mediated. The distribution of CD3+, CD4+, CD8+, CD19+, CD16+ and CD25+ lymphocyte populations in peripheral blood and the plasma concentrations of IL-1α, IL-2 and TNF-α have been investigated in 25 children with acute rheumatic fever. The percentages and absolute counts of CD4+, CD16+, CD25+ cells, the ratio of CD4/CD8 and plasma concentrations of IL-1α and IL-2 in these patients with acute rheumatic fever were shown to be significantly higher at admission than three months later. Furthermore, they were also significantly higher than in patients with chronic rheumatic heart disease or streptococcal pharyngitis, or in normal controls. It was found that production of IL-2 in acute and chronic rheumatic disease directly correlated with the percentages of CD4+ and CD25+ cells. In acute rheumatic fever, evidence of increased cellular immune response is indicated by the increased percentages CD4+ and CD25+ cells, the CD4/CD8 ratio, and increased plasma concentrations of IL-1α and IL-2. However, patients with chronic rheumatoid arthritis have very low concentrations of IL-2, IFN-γ and IL-2R, but higher levels of macrophage-produced cytokines, IL-1, IL-6 and TNF-α. Many studies have reported that rheumatoid arthritis is relatively rare among schizophrenics and is the only disease known which appears to protect against schizophrenia. One possible explanation for this may lie in the changes in cytokine production that occur in patients with rheumatoid arthritis.

CENTRAL EFFECTS OF STRESS-INDUCED CYTOKINES

Evidence of the adverse consequences of cytokine administration in different clinical conditions has accumulated in recent years. The side effects reported after the therapeutic use of cytokines have shown that activation of the immune response may sometimes have deleterious consequences. Several of these side effects appear as a direct consequence of the immune activation induced by cytokines, e.g. flu-like reactions, vascular leak syndrome and psychiatric abnormalities. Cytokine-induced exacerbation of underlying diseases or immune dysregulation were other complications of growing concern. IFN-α treatment has now been clearly linked with the exacerbation or occurrence of such autoimmune diseases as thyroiditis, systemic lupus erythematosus, haematological disorders and insulin-dependent diabetes mellitus; diseases involving altered cell-mediated immune functions such as inflammatory skin diseases, nephritis, pneumonitis and colitis also occur. By contrast, immunological side effects of IFN-β and IFN-γ have seldom been reported, but it must be emphasized that the extent of clinical experience with these cytokines is still very limited.

IL-2 has also been implicated in various conditions that may involve immunopathological processes such as thyroid disorders, rheumatoid arthritis, dermatological diseases and interstitial nephritis. Growth factors have been more specifically linked with the development, or with the exacerbation, of inflammatory skin diseases as a result of neutrophil, monocyte/macrophage or eosinophil activation (e.g. cutaneous vasculitis and generalized cutaneous eruption, Sweet's disease, bullous eruption and psoriasis). Exacerbation of autoimmune thyroiditis has been described following administration of granulocyte-macrophage colony-stimulating factor (GM-CSF). The immunogenicity of cytokines is also of relevance and the occurrence of antibodies binding IFN-α and IFN-β, IL-2 and GM-CSF has been reported. Finally, several isolated reports have recently suggested that IFN-α treatment may be associated with several immunosuppressive effects while IL-2 is clinically associated with an increased incidence of infectious complications. Changes in these cytokines, on the other hand, result in alterations in the CNS and endocrine system, which may alter the responsiveness of the immune system to external stressors.

STRESS, CANCER AND INFECTION

A causal relationship between stress, immune suppression and enhanced tumour development has often been suggested. In rodent studies, the effects of stress on Fisher 344 rats have been studied using a tumour model in which lung metastases of a syngeneic mammary tumour (MADB106) are controlled by NK cells. Animals exposed to acute stress showed a substantial decrease in NK cell cytotoxicity against this tumour *in vitro* and, when injected intravenously with this tumour, show a twofold increase in surface lung metastases. The critical period during which stress increases metastases appears to be the same as that during which this tumour is known to be normally suppressed by NK cells.

Physical restraint administered to C57BL/6 mice significantly alters the inflammatory response to influenza virus infection and depresses antiviral cellular immunity. Restraint-stressed animals show a pattern of reduced mononuclear cell infiltration and lung consolidation which coincides with elevated plasma corticosterone levels. Furthermore, cellular immunity to a virus infection is significantly depressed; IL-2 secretion is reduced by 96% and 59% in the mediastinal lymph nodes and spleens, respectively, as compared to a non-restrained group. However, the magnitude of the humoral immune response to influenza virus is unaffected by restraint stress. Thus antiviral IgG antibody concentrations in restrained/infected mice do not differ when compared to a non-restrained/infected control group 14 days post-infection.

Psychological stress is thought to undermine host resistance to infection through neuroendocrine-mediated changes in immune competence. Environmental stressors and psychological response to stress have been found to be positively correlated with the incidence of respiratory illness and changes in the number of CD4, CD8 and NK cells in preschool children. In summary, internal stressors (tissue damage and/or inflammatory response) markedly change immune functions, which may be perceived by the CNS as a stressful stimulus. These immune changes also alter the CNS response to external stressors. The mechanisms of the effect of internal stressors on CNS stress response could be due to (i) cytokine stimulation of the hypothalamic–pituitary–adrenocortical (HPA) axis via increased CRF secretion and/or (ii) the effect of cytokines on changes in neurotransmitter system in limbic and stress-related brain regions. These possibilities are shown diagrammatically in Figure 4.1.

VARIABLE EFFECTS OF STRESSOR SEVERITY, CONTROLLABILITY, TYPES OF STRESS AND PREVIOUS STRESS HISTORY ON THE IMMUNE SYSTEM

The severity, controllability, type and the timing of stressor administration relative to antigen administration may differentially influence the immune system. Immune responses to different types of stress are dependent on the severity of stressors. Severe stressors usually suppress immune function, and mild stressors sometimes stimulate immune activity or have little effect. For instance, mild and short-term handling in rats enhances lymphocyte responses to the stimulation of T-cell and B-cell mitogens, while immobilization stress (for 2–3 h) suppresses these responses. Similarly, 5 min of restraint in a novel environment, prior to sheep red blood cell (SRBC) inoculation, enhances the subsequent splenic plaque-forming cell response to SRBCs, while more intense stressors, such as footshock, suppress the IL-1 response to endotoxin challenge. In general, a very mild stressor, such as a single footshock in a passive avoidance training paradigm or exposure to a novel environment, also significantly enhances immune responses to SRBC inoculation. However, with further stressor application, this disappears and a very marked suppression of immune function becomes evident.

In animal experiments, it has been reported that uncontrollable stress impairs the immune system more effectively than controllable stress. For example, escapable footshock or a loud noise have no effects on NK cell cytotoxicity and lymphocyte proliferation, but inescapable shock or noise significantly reduces NK cell and lymphocyte function. However, some authors reported that although stressor controllability determined the response to a B-cell mitogen, it did not affect the response to a T-cell mitogen. Other investigations have demonstrated that antibody titres and plaque-forming cell responses were equally effective in eliciting immunosuppression after controllable or uncontrollable footshock.

Humans are subject to diverse stressors, and psychological, physical and immune stressors may produce different responses in the immune system. Similarly in experimental studies, it has been demonstrated that changes in

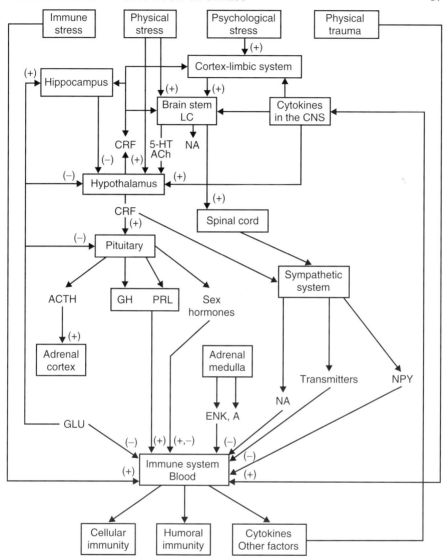

Figure 4.1 Schematic overview of the interaction of different stressors, the central nervous, endocrine and immune system. (+), stimulation; (–), inhibition; CRF, corticotrophin-releasing factor; A, adrenaline; NA, noradrenaline; 5-HT, serotonin, ACh, acetycholine; ACTH, adrenocorticotrophic hormone; GH, growth hormone; PRL, prolactin; NPY, neuropeptide Y; LC, locus coeruleus; ENK, enkephalin; GLU, glucocorticoids.

behaviour, endocrine and immune parameters caused by psychogenic stressors (exposure of a mouse to a rat or exposure of a rat to a cat) are different from those caused by neurogenic stressors (restraint or footshock). For example, exposing a mouse to a rat does not affect lymphocyte proliferation, but footshock stress increases or decreases lymphocyte response to mitogens depending on the rodent strain. In the same strain of rat, the restraint stressor-induced increase in ACTH secretion is more pronounced than that induced by the rat being exposed to a predatory ferret. These differences may be due to the fact that different types of stressors activate different target organs or brain regions. Thus, psychological stressors may directly stimulate the cortex and limbic system, physical stressors stimulate both the brain stem and the immune system (for example, pain and temperature cause immune responses) while immune stressors directly activate the immune system (Figure 4.1). However, there is presently insufficient evidence to indicate whether different stressors evoke the same neurotransmitter changes in the exerimental subject.

Stressor-induced alterations in immune activity may also be influenced by the organism's previous encounters with the stressor. For example, restraint stress applied on two days following antigen administration does not produce any immunosuppression, while the same stressor exposure on two consecutive days prior to inoculation provokes immunosuppression. In addition, if CD-1 mice are exposed to a stressor 72 h after SRBC inoculation, and the spleen and blood examined at the time of the peak immune response 24 h later, a marked suppression of the immune response is apparent. However, stressor applied at other intervals following inoculation is without effect. Interestingly, injection of 2-deoxyglucose, which acts like a stressor by producing an insulin-like state, reduces the splenic mitogen response to both Con A and phytohaemagglutinin (PHA). If animals are immobilized for 1 h prior to the 2-deoxyglucose administration, the extent of immunosuppression is comparable to that produced by the 2-deoxyglucose alone, but if restraint is applied 12 days earlier, then the drug-induced immunosuppression is more pronounced. Given that the initial stressor (immobilization) is appreciably different from the second stressor (2-deoxyglucose), it seems likely that the observed changes in the immune response reflect the sensitization, rather than conditioning, of mechanisms that are provoked by stressors to produce the immunosuppression. Furthermore, it appears that the stressor may have time-dependent effects on immune activity, wherein the immunosuppressive effects of an acute stressor sensitize the immune system with the passage of time. Such an effect would also appear to be specific to an immune process.

DIFFERENCE BETWEEN ACUTE AND CHRONIC STRESS

Acute stressors often cause significant changes in the CNS and endocrine system, which may be absent following a chronic exposure to stress. Similarly, in the immune system, chronic stress may result in different changes from those caused by acute stress. It is still unclear whether the immune response to a chronic stressor represents dynamic changes, such as the recruitment of processes which facilitate immune function, or just adaptation or habituation. As mentioned above, an acute stressor suppresses mitogen-stimulated lymphocyte proliferation, which is not observed after a repeated stressor application. In addition, an acute stressor, such as immobilization for 1 min, slightly reduces the number of total leucocytes and lymphocytes, but increases the number of neutrophils. After continuing the immobilization stress for seven days, the total number of leucocytes is reduced by 70% and the number of lymphocytes by 85% of the control values, while the neutrophil number returns to normal values. In some strains of mice, an acute stressor, such as footshock, provokes an immunoenhancement, which declines with repeated stress. Consequently, acute footshock-induced suppression in NK cell activity and lymphocyte response to mitogen stimulation are attenuated after repeated stress. For example, splenic NK cell cytotoxicity is largely decreased after animals are immersed in cold water, an effect that is reversed after eight days of treatment. Immobilization (for one to four days) also results in suppression of NK cell activity, but when the stress is continued over 10 days, the NK cell activity is comparable to that of the non-stressed animal.

Immunological parameters before, during and after spaceflight have been measured in both humans and animals. Spaceflight can result in a blunting of the immune mechanisms of crew members and also of animals. The changes in immune functions in short-term flights resemble those occurring after acute stress, while those occurring during long-term flights resemble chronic stress. In addition, this blunting of the immune function may arise as a consequence of a relative increase in potentially infectious microorganisms in the space cabin environment. This combination of events results in an increased probability of infections arising among the crew members.

Acute and chronic psychological stress also exert different effects on the immune system. The effects of antecedent chronic life stress on psychological and physiological responsivity have been investigated after an acute challenge with a psychological stressor. Male volunteers, with and without chronic life stress events, were administered a 12-minute laboratory stressor (mental arithmetic) or an appropriate video control. Acute psychological stress induces subjective distress, increases the circulating concentrations of adrenaline (A), noradrenaline (NA), β-endorphin, ACTH and cortisol, and causes a selective redistribution of NK cells into the peripheral blood as compared with the control condition. Although the two groups were almost identical at baseline in psychological, sympathetic, neuroendocrine and immune aspects, the chronic life stress group showed greater subjective distress, higher peak levels of A, lower peak levels of β-endorphin and of NK cell lysis, and a more pronounced redistribution of NK cells in response to the acute psychological challenge than the controls. Furthermore, the acute stressor induced a protracted decline in NK cytotoxicity in the chronic stress group but had no effect in the controls. Thus it appears that when individuals who are subject to chronic life stress are confronted with an acute psychological challenge, an exaggerated psychological response and peak sympathomedullary activity occurs that is associated with decrements in NK cell function and is protracted beyond termination of the stressor and the sympathomedullary recovery.

It has been hypothesized that handled and non-handled animals may exhibit differences in the plaque-forming cell (PFC) response to SRBC inoculation under conditions of acute and/or chronic stress. Neonatally handled animals exhibit lower HPA responses to a number of acute stressors in adulthood compared to non-handled animals. These differences emerge as a function of chronic, intermittent cold stress. Exposure to acute (for 4 h) cold stress decreases PFC responses in both handled and non-handled animals compared to non-stressed handled and non-handled animals. The decrease in PFC response produced by chronic, intermittent cold stress is similar in handled and non-handled animals and similar to that found in acutely stressed animals. When handled animals under chronic stress are re-exposed to cold stress, the PFC response is not different from acutely stressed or chronically stressed handled and non-handled animals. However, by contrast, the PFC response in non-handled animals under chronic stress re-exposed to cold stress is lower than in all other groups studied. Thus, neonatal handling prevents prior chronic stress-induced suppression of the PFC response to a subsequent stress. This data suggests that there may be subpopulations of individuals in whom prior chronic stress does not exacerbate the immune suppression produced by acute stress. However, those chronically stressed individuals in whom immune suppression does occur may be more vulnerable to infection and disease. Such findings illustrate the importance of early life experience on the ability of the immune system to adapt to the effects of stress in later life.

GENETIC VARIATION OF IMMUNE RESPONSES TO STRESSOR APPLICATIONS

Many studies have revealed strain differences in biogenic amine concentrations and in the neurochemical impact of stress. Genetic variation in the response to stress may also play a critical role in susceptibility to inflammatory diseases and the development of the immune response. In various strains of mice and rats, the difference in neuroendocrine and immune functioning has been well established. As an example, in three different strains of mice, experimental influenza viral infection has been used to study the effects of restraint stress on pathogenesis and the development of the immune response. In response to stressors, BALB/cByJ mice display much higher concentrations of plasma ACTH and corticosterone, more pronounced changes of

CRF in the hypothalamus and the central amygdala, greater monoamine variations in several brain regions than C57BL/6J and C57BL/6ByJ mice. Thus it has been suggested that BALB/cByJ mice might be useful in modelling stressor-induced depressive illness. When comparison are made of the effects of footshock on immune parameters between three strains of mice (C57BL/6ByJ, BALB/cByJ and CD-1), it has been found that footshock does not affect lymphocyte proliferation in C57BL/6ByJ mice. In contrast, the stressor significantly decreased lipopolysaccharide (LPS)-induced B-cell proliferation in BALB/cByJ mice, and increased lymphocyte proliferation in CD-1 mice. Moreover, among C57BL/6ByJ and BALB/cByJ strains, a single footshock largely suppressed NK cell cytotoxicity, but not in the CD-1 mice.

The effect of genetic composition on the immune response has also been seen in rats. Thus in strains of rats that have been selectively bred for differences in seizure development upon stimulation of amygdala (kindling), it has also been shown that stressors have different effects on immune functions. For example, in response to restraint stress, those rats that rapidly developed a seizure exhibited protracted struggling, greatly increased ACTH and corticosterone levels and greatly elevated splenic lymphocyte proliferation when compared to those rats that were resistant to seizure development. However, after exposing the rats to a predator (a ferret), macrophage activity was largely suppressed in the latter group, but not in the former group. It now appears that not only do stressors cause different responses in different strains of mice or rats, but the baseline of immune cellular activities in different strains may be also different. For example, rats that are resistant to seizure development have much higher macrophage activity than those that readily develop seizures. Similarly, CD-1 mice have higher macrophage and NK cell activities than BALB/cByJ and C57BL/6ByJ mice. In humans, immune responses to stressors may also be dependent on genetic composition, culture and diet. But so far, there have been few investigations showing racial difference in immune responsiveness.

Different immune responses to the stimulation of stressors in the different strains may be dependent on genetic differences in the immune system. Recent advances in immunology include the identification of two subsets of T_H cells. As mentioned previously, Th1 cells produce IL-2 and IFN-γ, which are important for the generation of cell-mediated immunity, whereas, Th2 cells produce IL-4, IL-5, IL-6 and IL-10 which promote humoral immune responses. C57BL/6 mice respond to a number of intracellular pathogens with a strong Th1 cell response, resulting in a protective cell-mediated immune response. However, the same antigens elicit from BALB/c mice a response that is largely Th2 cell-driven, with production of IL-4 and IL-10, resulting in a humoral immune response. BALB/c mice are relatively sensitive to infection, but can be made resistant by treatment with anti-IL-4 antibody. Conversely, resistant mice can be made susceptible by treatment with anti-IFN-γ antibody.

Another potential variable in the immune response to stress and the antigen challenge may be the endocrine status of the animal. For example, three inbred strains of mice (C57BL/6, DBA/2 and C3H/HeN), when infected with influenza A/PR8 and subjected to repetitive cycles of restraint stress for 12 h during the development of the immune response, show a reduction in cellular immune and inflammatory responses; yet only the DBA/2 strain demonstrates a stress-associated reduction in influenza viral-induced mortality. This would appear to be related to greater elevation of corticosterone in DBA/2 mice than in the other two strains. Presumably the increase in corticosterone modulates the activity of the immune system, as discussed in Chapter 2.

In rats, disease susceptibility is also strongly strain dependent. For example, Lewis rats are the most susceptible, while many other strains are resistant to diseases, probably because the corticosterone response to a stressor is greater in Lewis rats. In support of this, adrenalectomy in Lewis rats causes a reduction in their susceptibility to experimental allergic encephalomyelitis. The results of such studies suggest that humans, those individuals with genetically determined high glucocorticoid stress responses will be most at risk from infectious disease and other immune-related abnormalities.

THE INFLUENCE OF AGEING ON IMMUNE RESPONSES TO STRESSORS

Aged humans and animals show a chronic and sustained increase in the activity of the sympathetic nervous system, as shown by by the increase in the circulating concentrations of catecholamines. In addition, microneurographs have shown that the resting burst rate of sympathetic nerves innervating the muscle increases with advancing age. Ageing is also accompanied by a decline in immune responses to an antigen stimulation, immune dysregulation and a loss of self-tolerance.

In an animal model of ageing, NK cell activity, T-cell proliferation and T-cell-mediated responses including some antibody responses diminish with age. However, the activity of antibodies that are not related to T-cell-mediated antigen responses largely increases with age. Normal ageing is also accompanied by a decreased activity of phagocytic cells such as neutrophils and monocytes, which are of importance in the defence against infection. The production of cytokines by peripheral blood cells (for example, the increases in IL-1 and IL-6 and decrease in IL-2) has been widely reported to occur in elderly persons. Detailed studies have been conducted in rodents to examine the impact of ageing on immune responsiveness. In 3- and 24-week-old C57BL/6 mice, the regulation of IL-1 and IL-1R in the brain–endocrine–immune axis during maturation shows that basal levels of IL-1β in the hippocampus, spleen and testis of 24-week-old mice are significantly higher than those in 3-week-old mice, whereas IL-1α binding levels in the pituitary, spleen and testis of 3-week-old mice are significantly higher than those in 24-week-old mice. To further evaluate the changes in IL-1 receptors in ageing, IL-1α binding in 2-, 5-, 10-, 18- and 24-month-old mice has been measured. IL-1α binding in the testis was higher in 24-month-old mice than in the other groups, whereas binding of the cytokine in the hippocampus and spleen was unchanged. Following administration of a bacterial endotoxin, LPS, dramatic increases in IL-1β concentrations are observed 2 h after LPS injection in the pituitary, spleen, testis and plasma in both 3- and 24-week-old mice. By contrast, the concentration of IL-1β in the hippocampus increases in response to LPS injection only in 24-week-old mice. IL-1α binding in the hippocampus was significantly decreased in the 24- but not in 3-week-old mice after LPS challenge; IL-1α binding in the spleen and the testis is significantly decreased in both age groups following LPS administration.

From such experiments it would appear that ageing may change the integration between the CNS, endocrine and immune systems and affect immune responses to stressors. It has been determined in aged rats (24–28 months) that, compared to young rats, a series of different stressors applied over seven days accelerates the growth of a tumour induced by Fisher foetal rat cells that had been transformed with Fujinami sarcoma virus. Similarly, when animals that have been trained in a conditioned emotional response paradigm (i.e. footshock delivered in a specific environment) are subsequently exposed to the shock apparatus, this provokes a more pronounced NK cell activity and lymphocyte proliferation in 22-month-old Fisher rats than in 7-month-old rats. In addition, one week of isolation caused a greater suppression of splenic and peripheral blood NK cell activity in 12-month-old rats that in the 3-month-old rats.

Similar changes have been reported to occur in mice. Thus, exposure to uncontrolled footshock results in immunosuppression in both 3-month-old and 9-month-old mice, but the suppression can be provoked more readily in older animals. Moreover, shock-induced enhancement of the PFC response and antibody titres is much higher in older than in young animals. Following an overnight restraint stress, a greater decrease is observed in the number and proliferative activity of splenic T cells in older mice. The decrease in young mice is rather temporary and followed by a quick recovery. Whereas the number of NK cells in the spleen is no different between young and old mice before giving the stress, a significant decrease is observed in old mice after the stress. NK activity is much lower in older than in younger animals.

The pattern of metastasis of B16 melanoma cells also differs between young and old mice. Metastatic colonies in the lungs are larger in number and size in young mice than in old mice. After stress, the number increases but the size remains unchanged in old mice, whereas the size increases and the number remains unchanged in young mice. Thus the same restraint stress produces a more serious effect on the immune cells in older than in younger mice and gives rise to a differential effect on the pattern of tumour metastasis between them.

The mechanism whereby the ageing process modulates the immune responses to stress may include thymus ageing, CRF and endocrine changes, increased sympathetic outflow and changed central catecholamine metabolism. The thymus is the first organ to start ageing mammals. The thymus gland reaches its maximum at sexual maturity in humans then gradually shrinks, reaching only 5% to 10% of its original size by the age of 45. Thymus involution is associated with a decrease in circulating thymus hormones and an increase in the number of immature T lymphocytes in the thymus and in the peripheral blood. This results in changes in the proportion of T-cell subsets, decreased IL-2 and IFN-γ, reduced lymphocyte proliferation and NK cell activity; the also has an influence on B-cell maturation. The concentration of immunoglobulins in the blood is also changed with age, leading to increased IgG and IgA and a decrease in IgM. Therefore, in aged humans or animals stress-induced suppression of lymphocyte and NK cell functions, and enhanced PFC response to inoculation are likely to result from thymus ageing.

It is well established that CRF plays an important role in regulating sympathetic outflow and immune functions during stress. Indeed, a hypersecretion of hypothalamic CRF may occur in ageing. It has been shown that in aged rats CRF release from the hypothalamus increases after acetylcholine (ACh) stimulation while CRF receptors are decreased in the hypothalamus and the pituitary. The increase in CRF release can enhance sympathetic activity and stimulate ACTH secretion, changes which are similar to those observed during a stress response. In 3-month-old and 23-month-old Fisher rats, the basal concentration of A is similar, but central administration of CRF causes a more rapid, pronounced and persistent release of A and NA from sympathetic nerve in older than in younger rats. Furthermore, basal neuropeptide Y (NPY) concentrations in the blood and CRF-induced NPY secretion are significantly higher in aged rats, even though CRF administration elevates basal plasma corticosterone secretion in both aged and young animals.

Aged rats have reduced NK cell activity at baseline compared to values in young animals. Following CRF administration, NK cell cytotoxicity is further decreased in aged animals, but not in young animals. In elderly humans, there is also a negative correlation between the concentrations of circulating catecholamines, NPY and NK cell activity. As the corticosterone concentration is elevated by CRF in both aged and young rats, the decreased NK cell activity following CRF administration is probably a reflection of the increased sympathetic tone and catecholamine release. A reduction of NK cell cytotoxicity in ageing animals, and the further decrease following stress, may be causally related to the acceleration of tumour growth in aged rats after exposure to stress. Thus, the age-related increase in sympathetic activity and the decrease in immune functions might result from an age-associated increase in the release of CRF and/or augmentation of an ultra-short positive feedback loop of CRF on its own release. However, the inflammatory cytokines IL-1 and IL-6, which increase with age probably result from catecholamine hypersecretion. Also IL-1 and IL-6 stimulate ACTH and glucocorticoid secretion, which may also contribute to the increased morbidity and mortality seen in chronically stressed or aged subjects.

The immune system acts as a type of sensory organ that provides the brain with information of immunological activation; the brain then interprets immune activation as a stressor. Central catecholamine changes associated with immune activity is similar to that observed following stressor exposure. Many studies have shown that aged animals exhibit more pronounced stress-provoked alterations of central neurotransmitters compared to young animals. For example, when SRBCs were used to challenge the immune system of 15- and 3-month-old mice, both groups showed a reduction in hypothalamic and locus coeruleus (LC) NA and increased 3-methoxy-4-hydroxy-phenylglycol (MHPG) concentrations that coincided with the peak immune response. However, the increase in the NA metabolite MHPG was greater in the hypothalamus and occurred earlier in the LC of the aged mice. Changes have also been found in other neurotransmitters following stress. When using a conditioned emotional response paradigm to compare the neurotransmitter, endocrine and immunological responses to stress of 7- and 22-month-old Fisher 344 male rats, the basal dopamine (DA) metabolism in old non-stressed rats was shown to be significantly reduced in the medial frontal cortex, neostriatum, nucleus accumbens and hypothalamus, but not in the amygdala; following the conditioned emotional procedure however, an increase in DA turnover occurred in the medial frontal cortex, nucleus accumbens and amygdala in both the young and old rats. Similarly, while there were no differences in the concentrations of NA and 5-hydroxytryptamine (5-HT) in unstressed young and old rats, stress resulted in a decrease in medial frontal cortical 5-hydroxyindole-acetic acid (5-HIAA) and hypothalamic 5-HT concentrations in old but not in young animals. These observations suggest that there are age-related differences in the response of central sympathetic NA and 5-HT systems to stress. However, many other factors are also involved in the CNS integration of the immune response to stress. Firstly, ageing of the brain causes changes in neurotransmitter synthesis and metabolism. Secondly, ageing of the endocrine system induces down- or up-regulation of some hormone receptors in different brain regions. Thirdly, ageing of the immune system changes the communication between the brain and the immune system.

STRESS, SEX STEROIDS AND AUTOIMMUNE DISEASES: THE ROLE OF GENDER IN THE IMMUNE RESPONSE

The influence of stress on the onset of autoimmune diseases is a new field of psychoneuroimmuno-endocrinology. Experimental allergic encephalomyelitis (EAE) is an acute autoimmune disease of the CNS, which can be induced in susceptible species of animals by injection of CNS tissue. Physical restraint may exert a suppressive effect on EAE symptoms. Similarly, administration of adrenal hormones also shows the same protective effects. In Lewis rats subjected to sound stress for 19 days after immunization, the onset of EAE clinical symptoms is delayed, an effect which may be due to the action of ACTH and adrenal hormones on the immune system. In other experimental studies, it has been shown the central administration of a catecholamines or a serotonin depleting agent elevates the plasma concentration of ACTH and corticosterone and significantly suppresses EAE, while sympathectomy, which reduces the splenic concentration of A and the CD8 T-cell subset, significantly increases severity of EAE.

Recently many studies have shown that stress is able to accelerate the onset of disease in both human and animal models of autoimmune disease. For example, stressful life events seem to increase the onset of multiple sclerosis, and both psychological and physical stress has been implicated in the onset of autoimmune thyroid disease. However, results from studies of stress and the development of rheumatoid arthritis (RA) are contradictory; in general, personality factors and emotional stress seem to be implicated in the onset of the disease. Finally, in diabetes mellitus, traumatic or stressful events have been shown to precipitate the disease. For example, diabetic patients who have undergone surgery exhibit a dramatic deterioration, probably because the activation of the HPA axis by surgery increases the energy requirement and thereby increases the body's insulin demand. Psychological stress has also been associated with deterioration in these patients, probably due to an increase in sympathetic activity. In addition, it has been shown that there is an abnormally high frequency of depression in children with diabetes. Before the onset of the disease, most diabetic patients have experienced stressful events such as febrile disease, accident, pregnancy and various social problems. In such cases, it would appear that the stressful events increase the energy demands of the body and thereby indirectly reduce the amount of insulin available to meet these demands.

In non-obese diabetic mice and other rodents, the serum glucocorticoid concentration is higher in females than in males. After a single restraint stress, female diabetic mice exhibit a greater response in glucocorticoid secretion than male mice. After repeated stress, males also respond significantly less than females, suggesting an adaptation phenomenon. In general, it appears that diabetic mice exhibit a greater increase in concentration of corticosterone than non-diabetic animals; females show a greater response than males. Cytokines also have a greater impact on the adrenal glands in diabetics. IL-1 administration induces an increase in corticosterone in both male and female mice, this increase being much more pronounced in female non-obese diabetic mice. It thus appears that an inflammatory–

autoimmune response plays an important role in the impact of stress on the HPA axis.

Clinical evidence has shown that the majority of patients suffering from various types of autoimmune diseases are female. For instance, the ratio of female to male patients with Hashimoto's thyroiditis is 25–50 to 1. In systemic lupus erythematosus (SLE) and Sjögren's syndrome, the female to male ratio is 9 : 1. In addition, more women suffer from rheumatoid arthritis (RA), scleroderma, myasthenia gravis and multiple sclerosis than men. Indeed, females seem to have a more vigorous immune response, a more developed thymus, higher immunoglobulin concentrations, stronger primary and secondary immune responses, greater resistance to the induction of immunological tolerance and a greater ability to reject tumours and homografts than men. Experimental studies also show that SLE disease progression is more rapid in female mice than in male mice, and the mortality is also higher; ovariectomy reduces the evolution of the disease, suggesting that oestrogens may play an important role. By contrast, prepubertal orchidectomy enhances the expression of lupus in male animals and gives rise to a mortality pattern similar to that observed in females. The involvement of sex hormones in the progression of SLE has also been shown in men. Thus, female sex hormone replacement therapy (oestradiol or progesterone) accelerates, whereas androgens (dihydrotestosterone) delays, the evolution of SLE. Women with SLE have been shown to have decreased levels of androgens and an abnormal metabolism of androgens and oestrogens. In addition, patients with Klinefelter's syndrome associated with SLE or Sjögren's disease also show higher serum concentrations of luteinizing hormone (LH), lower testosterone levels and a decreased number of CD3 and CD8 cells but an increased CD4/CD8 ratio. An increase in the CD4/CD8 ratio has also been observed in patients with schizophrenia or normal subjects exposed to severe stress. In contrast to their role in SLE, oestrogens seem to ameliorate rheumatoid arthritis in women. Thus, during stressful responses, glucocorticoids and sex hormones may interact and exert a composite influence on the immune system.

The effect of the type of stressor (whether physical or psychological) on humoral immunity and neuroendocrine responses in male and female rats has also been studied. Animals were divided into four groups according to the following criteria; (1) voluntary running (high physical/low psychological stress); (2) immobilization (low physical/high psychological stress); (3) mixed stress (running and immobilization) and (4) cage control group. Five weeks after the start of the study, all animals were immunized with SRBC and sacrificed one week later. There was no specific effect of stress on any of the immune or endocrine parameters. However, strong gender differences emerged within the stress conditions. The stressed female rats displayed an enhanced antibody response to SRBC and a higher percentage of peripheral blood lymphocytes than their male counterparts. However, there were no significant differences between the male and female control animals with respect to these variables. Both stressed and control female rats consistently displayed elevated levels of plasma corticosterone and adrenal NA across all conditions. In addition, female rats had heavier adrenal and spleen weights.

There are three possible mechanisms that may be involved in the different responses to a stressor between males and females. First, it is known that neurotransmitter content and metabolism are sexually differentiated and under the influence of sex steroids in adulthood. For example, brain 5-HT content differs between sexes and in addition, differences in the impact of cortisol, ACTH and prolactin have been found in humans. These differences may affect immune functions and change the immune responses to stress. Second, the receptors for sex steroids are distributed on the reticuloepithelial cells of thymus, lymphocytes and macrophages. Some of the sex steroid induced changes may be non-receptor-mediated and act directly on the cell membrane. *In vitro*, androgens inhibit mitogen-induced lymphocyte proliferation in a dose-dependent manner. Third, stress and autoimmune diseases may directly induce the release of inflammatory cytokines which change the response of the CNS, the immune system and endocrine system to stressors (Figure 4.1).

MODULATION OF THE EFFECTS OF STRESS ON THE IMMUNE SYSTEM BY PSYCHOTROPIC DRUGS

It has been well established that acute and chronic stress is the major inducer of psychiatric disease and for this reason, the effects of psychotropic drugs on stress-induced changes in the CNS, endocrine and the immune system have been extensively studied.

In clinical studies, the effects of anxiolytic drugs on stress-induced changes in the immune system have been investigated. Twenty-five healthy males were subjected to an acute stressor, a first-time tandem parachute jump. Subjects were randomly assigned to a benzodiazepine (alprazolam) and a placebo. To evaluate the role of the spleen in stress, some splenectomized subjects also performed a parachute jump. It was found that the increases in blood adrenaline and cortisol caused by stress were attenuated by alprazolam treatment. Although the number and activity of NK cells significantly increased in the placebo group immediately after stress, alprazolam treatment did not alter the increase in NK cell numbers but did inhibit the increase in NK activity. In splenectomized subjects, the NK cell numbers, but not NK activity, increased as in the placebo treated subjects. The results of this study suggest that stress-induced change in NK cells partly depends on the spleen and that alprazolam differentially affects stress-induced changes in NK cell function. In addition, other studies have shown that chronic treatment with alprazolam significantly reduces stress-induced increase in virus titres and pulmonary vascular permeability.

In animal experiments, alprazolam has also been shown to have anti-stress effects. Mice exposed to surgical stress induced by laparotomy exhibit stress-induced suppression of the NK cell activity; chronic alprazolam treatment, in a dose-dependent manner, attenuated this suppression. These immunoenhancing effects of alprazolam were more intense when the drug was administered before surgery. In addition, mice exposed to a chronic auditory stressor and injected daily with alprazolam also showed a reduction in stress-induced suppression of *in vitro* and *in vivo* phagocytosis. Pretreatment with a benzodiazepine antagonist resulted in the suppression of the effects of alprazolam in the stressed mice.

The mechanism whereby the benzodiazepines modulate stress and immune changes may be related to their effects on the activation of the HPA axis and CRF secretion. This has been shown experimentally when the benzodiazepines diazepam or alprazolam were administered to a group of rats prior to central infusion of CRF; another group received only CRF. Rats that were administered CRF alone showed a significant reduction of splenic NK cytotoxicity as compared to rats in a control group, but pretreatment with diazepam or alprazolam blocked CRF-induced suppression of NK-cell activity. These results suggest that central-type benzodiazepines antagonize stress-induced immune suppression and may attenuate the reduction of cellular immune function in stress by reducing CRF secretion.

Both the serotonergic and dopaminergic systems have been found to play an important role in modulation of the immune response during stress. For instance, the effects of the partial 5-HT1A agonist buspirone on influenza A (PR-8/34) virus specific immune injury has been evaluated in CD-1 mice exposed to a chronic auditory stressor. Treatment with buspirone resulted in a decrease of the stress-induced increase of virus titres and pulmonary vascular permeability as well as in a reduction of the mortality of mice.

The effects of buspirone treatment on the delayed-type hypersensitivity (DTH) response of female mice exposed to an auditory stressor has also been evaluated two days before or two days after immunization with SRBCs. Results show that the DTH response to SRBCs was inhibited by the stress and this difference is greater when stress is given before SRBC sensitization. Treatment with buspirone significantly reduces the effects of stress on the DTH response in these experiments. By contrast, buspirone does not significantly affect affect the DTH response in unstressed mice. Other neuroendocrinological effects of buspirone in stressed mice may also affect the immune system. Thus, stress, through both known and unknown neuroendocrine pathways, can damage elements of the immunological system, which may leave animals vulnerable to the action of viruses. On the other hand, buspirone has been found to help in countering the adverse effects of stress.

The effects of the serotonin-reuptake releasing agent dexfenfluramine on stress-induced changes in ingestive behaviour, body weight and the humoral immune response have been were investigated in rats that had been submitted to repeated intense stress for 20 consecutive days. Some of the animals had also been treated with 5 mg/kg/day dexfenfluramine or saline (control) for 28 days. The humoral immune response of rats to SRBCs was assessed from the antibody titres on days 4, 8, 12, 16, 20 and 28 and the concentrations of antibodies and corticosterone measured on days 0 and 12. Rats treated with dexfenfluramine had a significantly reduced body weight five weeks after the end of treatment, whereas the decrease in body weight induced by stress at that time had disappeared. It was found that stress does not decrease the animals' immune response despite the increase in corticosterone secretion on day 0, a response that lasted for at least 12 days. Dexfenfluramine reduced corticosterone concentrations on day 12, but antibody production was significantly reduced in all the rats receiving dexfenfluramine. This study suggests that many of the effects of stress are mediated independently of the serotonergic system, wheras the synthesis of antibodies may be decreased as a result of an increase in serotonergic function. The role of the serotonergic system in modulating the effect of stress on the immune system is further indicated by the following experimental research. Male rats that had been immunized with SRBCs and stressed by repeated restraint were treated with a precursor, 5-hydroxytryptophan (5-HTP), or with an inhibitor of serotonin synthesis (parachlorophenylalanine (PCPA)). Repeated stress alone was shown to reduce the PFC response. Treatment with 5-HTP also reduced the PFC response and increases brain serotonin turnover, as indicated by increased concentration of 5-HIAA. Treatment with PCPA suppressed the PFC response, but was accompanied by decreased levels of brain serotonin and 5-HIAA content. The results of this study suggest that the serotonergic system may be only partially involved in modulating the impact of the endocrine system on cellular immunity. This evidence suggests that the serotonergic system is involved in neuroimmune modulation during stress.

To date there are relatively few investigations that have studied the effects of psychotropic drugs on stress-induced changes in cytokine production. *In vivo*, benzodiazepines have been shown to inhibit macrophage activity and reduce production of the proinflammatory cytokines IL-1, IL-6 and TNF. The anti-manic drug lithium carbonate has been shown to significantly increase the serum concentration of sIL-2R after chronic treatment, while the novel antidepressant rolipram suppresses TNF-α and IFN-γ production and prevents autoimmune encephalomelitis.

The neuroleptic chlorpromazine has been shown to inhibit TNF and increase IL-10 production *in vitro*. *In vitro* studies have also demonstrated that chlorpromazine incubated with mononuclear cells significantly enhances IgG synthesis without altering IL-1 release. By contrast, several non-steroidal anti-inflammatory drugs, such as indomethacin, piroxicam and D-penicillamine, significantly decrease IgG and slightly reduce IL-1 production. The site of action of these drugs may include both central and immune targets. Many psychotropic drugs have direct actions on immune cells and organs. For example, a tricyclic antidepressant-like binding site has been found on lymphocytes.

So far, the influence of antidepressants and other psychotropic drugs on the interaction between stress and the immune system has not been widely studied. Clearly, there is a need to investigate the interaction between stress, noradrenergic, serotonergic and other neurotransmitter systems and the mechanism whereby antidepressants modulate the immune system.

SUMMARY

The mechanisms involved in the interaction between stress and the immune system clearly include pathways whereby the CNS modulates immune function and those pathways in which the immune system modulates the CNS (Figure 4.1). This bidirectional communication has been described in Chapter 2. Briefly, a stressor stimulates the cortex and limbic system or other brain area to release neurotransmitters. These transmitters then activate the hypothalamus to release CRF, neurotransmitters and neuropeptides, which evoke endocrine secretions from the pituitary. These hormones include glucocorticoids, growth hormone (GH), prolactin (PRL), while the adrenals produce enkephalins, NA and A, and the sex hormones. These hormones then differentially affect immune function. At the same time, a stressor may stimulate the brain stem and activate the sympathetic nervous system. Changes in the levels of NA, NPY and other peptides released from the sympathetic terminals in the immune organs cause changes in immune functions. CRF released from the hypothalamus has a dual effect by acting on both the brain and the sympathetic system (Figure 4.1).

Many studies have demonstrated that CRF may play the most important role in stress response. CRF administration causes extensive impairment of immune functions resembling those observed in stress and depression. It has been reported that footshock, restraint and anaesthesia markedly suppress NK cell cytotoxicity and lymphocyte proliferation. This suppression is prevented by central pretreatment of a CRF antagonist or antibody. There are two ways, central and peripheral, that CRF modulates immune functions. It has been shown that intracerebroventricular administration of CRF for five days significantly suppresses lymphocyte proliferations and neutrophil phagocytosis, and increases the number of neutrophils and leucocyte aggregation. Central CRF administration also largely reduces NK cell number and activity. Central administration of CRF 20 min before immunization (T-cell-dependent antigen keyhole limpet haemocyanin) to rats reduces IgG protection.

The peripheral effect of CRF on immune functions may act through CRF receptors. These receptors have been found on monocyte-macrophages and

T-helper lymphocytes, but not on T-suppressor cells. When splenocytes are cultured *in vitro* with IL-2, proliferation is significantly increased. After addition of CRF (10^{-9} M), IL-2 stimulative effects on splenocytes are suppressed in a dose-dependent manner, which effect may be related to the increase in intracellular cAMP induced by CRF. When CRF and α-helical CRF are added together to the culture, IL-2 stimulatory function is restored. Another *in vitro* study showed that CRF at a dose of 10^{-14} M stimulated migration of human monocytes. In contrast to the central effect of CRF on MNK cell activity, the peptide (10^{-9} M) *in vitro* significantly enhances NK cell cytoxicity. The *in vitro* mechanism is due to the fact that CRF stimulates IL-1 release from NK cells, then triggers the release of β-endorphin, which further stimulates NK function.

There are four mechanisms by which CRF integrates ACTH, catecholamine and immune fuctions during stress (Figure 4.1). First, acute or chronic stress may stimulate the cortex and limbic system to release NA, DA, 5-HT, ACh and other neurotransmitters, as well as stimulating CRF neurons in the brain to secrete CRF, which activates catecholamine innervation of the paraventricular nucleus (PVN) of the hypothalamus. This innervation appears to play a critical role in the control of the rhythmic patterns of baseline HPA secretions and in HPA stress responses. Deletion of PVN catecholaminergic innervation was shown to inhibit the secretion of CRF and other peripheral hormones. CRF secreted from the hypothalamus stimulates the pituitary to release ACTH, which regulates the adrenal cortex to produce glucocorticoids. These hormones are released into the blood and combine with their receptors on immune cells, which mostly suppresses immune functions. CRF modulation of the immune system is not only by means of glucocorticoids. CRF receptors have been found on different leucocytes and the adrenal gland. CRF that is released from the CNS into the blood can combine directly with these receptors and modulate immune cellular and endocrine functions. In addition, NA and CRF produced from PVN may influence the activity of the sympathetic nervous system (SNS) and increase NA and neuropeptide Y release. It is well known that sympathetic nerves innervate lymphoid organs, such as the spleen and thymus and the adrenal gland. It has been found that 23 hour food deprivation for 1–5 days induced gastric ulcers and atrophy of the spleen and thymus, as well as a rise in plasma cortisol and catecholamine concentrations in mice. Noradrenaline and neuropeptide Y released from the SNS can also combine with their receptors present on lymphocytes and NK cells. Therefore, the innervations also exert regulative effects on immune and endocrine functions. It has been demonstrated that increased sympathetic tone during ageing, stress and depression is associated with an immune decline, whereas *in vivo* chemical sympathectomy suppresses cell-mediated responses and enhances antibody responses. Finally, stress-induced increases in CRF biosynthesis and secretion in the CNS stimulate NA, 5-HT, ACh and

A release into the blood, which also interact with their receptors on the immune cells.

Immune stress or internal stress (infection and inflammation), autoimmune disorders and physical trauma directly stimulate the immune system. These signals are transferred by different types of cytokines As mentioned in Chapter 2, different cytokines may differentially affect neurotransmitter metabolism and hormone secretion, which then alter the CNS and endocrine responses to a stressor. The relationship between these various process is shown diagrammatically in Figure 4.1.

BIBLIOGRAPHY

Anisman, H., Lu, Z. W., Song, C., Kent, P., McIntyre, D. C. and Merali, Z. (1997) Influence of psychogenic and neurogenic stressors on endocrine and immune activity: differential effects in fast and slow seizing rat strains. *Brain, Behavior, and Immunity* **11**: 63–74.

Ben-Eliyahu, S., Yirmiya, R., Liebeskind, J. C., Taylor, A. N. and Gale, R. P. (1991) Stress increases metastatic spread of a mammary tumour in rats: evidence for mediation by the immune system. *Brain, Behavior, and Immunity* **5**: 193–205.

Benschop, R. J., Jacobs, R., Sommer, B., Schurmeyer, T. H., Raab, J. R., Schmidt, R. E. and Schedlowski, M. (1996) Modulation of the immunologic response to acute stress in humans by beta-blockade or benzodiazepines. *FASEB Journal* **10**: 517–524.

Boitard, C., Caillat-Zucman, S. and Timsit, J. (1997) Insulin-dependent diabetes and human leucocyte antigens. *Diabetes and Metabolism* **23**: S22–28.

Boitard, C., Timsit, J., Larger, E. and Dubois, D. (1997) Immune mechanisms leading to type 1 insulin-dependent diabetes mellitus. *Hormone Research* **48**: S58–63.

Boyce, W. T., Chesney, M., Alkon, A., Tschann, J. M., Adams, S., Chesterman, B., Cohen, F., Kaiser, P., Folkman, S. and Wara, D. (1995) Psychobiologic reactivity to stress and childhood respiratory illnesses: results of two prospective studies. *Psychosomatic Medicine* **57**: 411–422.

Brady, A. J. (1995) Neutrophils in heart disease – stormtroopers of the immune system. *European Heart Journal* **16**: 151–152.

Buske-Kirschbaum, A., Jobst, S., Psych, D., Wustmans, A., Kirschbaum, C., Rauh, W. and Hellhammer, D. (1997) Attenuated free cortisol response to psychosocial stress in children with atopic dermatitis. *Psychosomatic Medicine* **59**: 419–426.

Cacciarelli, T. V., Martinez, O. M., Gish, R. G., Villanueva, J. C. and Krams, S. M. (1996) Immunoregulatory cytokines in chronic hepatitis C virus infection: pre- and posttreatment with interferon alfa. *Hepatology* **24**: 6–9.

Fixler, D. E. (1996) Respiratory syncytial virus infection in children with congenital heart disease: a review. *Pediatric Cardiology* **17**: 163–168.

Glaster, R. and Kiecolt-Glaster, J. (Eds) (1994) *Handbook of Human Stress and Immunity*. Academic Press, San Diego.

Herzum, M. and Maisch, B. (1992) Humoral and cellular immune reactions to the myocardium in myocarditis. *Herz* **17**: 91–96.

Homo-Delarche, F., Fitzpatrick, F., Christeff, N., Nunez, E. A., Bach, J. F. and Dardenne, M. (1991) Sex steroids, glucocorticoids, stress and autoimmunity. *Journal of Steroid Biochemistry and Molecular Biology* **40**: 619–637.

Leonard, B. E. and Miller, K. (Eds) (1995) *Stress, the Immune System and Psychiatry*. John Wiley & Sons, Chichester.

Limas, C. J. and Goldenberg, I. F. (1995) Soluble interleukin-2 receptor levels in patients with dilated cardiomyopathy. Correlation with disease severity and cardiac autoantibodies. *Circulation* **91**: 631–634.

Lopes-Virella, M. F. and Virella, G. (1996) Modified lipoproteins, cytokines and macrovascular disease in non-insulin-dependent diabetes mellitus. *Annals of Medicine* **28**: 347–354.

Narin, N., Kutukculer, N., Ozyurek, R., Bakiler, A. R., Parlar, A. and Arcasoy, M. (1995) Lymphocyte subsets and plasma IL-1 alpha, IL-2, and TNF-alpha concentrations in acute rheumatic fever and chronic rheumatic heart disease. *Clinical Immunology and Immunopathology* **77**: 172–176.

Sansonno, D., Iacobelli, A. R., Cornacchiulo, V., Lauletta, G., Distasi, M. A., Gatti, P. and Dammacco, F. (1996) Immunochemical and biomolecular studies of circulating immune complexes isolated from patients with acute and chronic hepatitis C virus infection. *European Journal of Clinical Investigation* **26**: 465–75.

Sheridan, J. F., Feng, N. G., Bonneau, R. H., Allen, C. M., Huneycutt, B. S. and Glaser, R. (1991) Restraint stress differentially affects anti-viral cellular and humoral immune responses in mice. *Journal of Neuroimmunology* **31**: 245–255.

Takao, T., Hashimoto, K. and De Souza, E. B. (1995) Modulation of interleukin-1 receptors in the brain–endocrine–immune axis by stress and infection. *Brain, Behavior, and Immunity* **9**: 276–291.

Tarazona, R., Gonzalez-Garcia, A., Zamzami, N. M., Marchetti, P., Frechin, N. et al. (1995) Chlorpromazine amplifies macrophage-dependent IL-10 production in vivo. *Journal of Immunology* **154**: 861–870.

Vial, T. and Descotes, J. (1995) Immune-mediated side-effects of cytokines in humans. *Toxicology* **105**: 31–57.

Wegmann, D. R. (1996) The immune response to islets in experimental diabetes and insulin-dependent diabetes mellitus. *Current Opinion in Immunology* **8**: 860–864.

Zavala, F., Taupin, V. and Descamps-Latscha, B. (1990) In vivo treatment with benzodiazepines inhibits murine phagocyte oxidative metabolism and production of interleukin-1, tumor necrosis factor and interleukin-6. *Journal of Pharmacology and Experimental Therapeutics* **255**: 442–450.

5 Stress, the Immune System and Depression

Stress and depression have similar effects on the central nervous, endocrine and immune systems. Thus, it has been suggested that stress acts as a predisposing and precipitating factor in the onset of affective illness. Over the last decade, there has been increasing evidence to suggest that immunological activation and hypersecretion of proinflammatory cytokines may have a causal relationship with aetiology of depression. Immune diseases can result in stress-like behaviour and increase the susceptibility of the brain and endocrine system to a stressor. Conversely, stress changes immune functions, which may play an important role in the onset of depression.

IMMUNE, NEUROTRANSMITTER AND ENDOCRINE ABNORMALITIES IN DEPRESSION

CHANGES IN IMMUNE FUNCTIONS IN DEPRESSION

Depression is associated with extensive impairment of both cellular and humoral immunity. Many investigations have provided evidence that stressful life events also significantly change immune functions.

Immune Suppression in Depression

At the early stage of research into depression, it has been found that depression is accompanied by a suppression in immune cellular functions. Patients with major depression show blunted lymphocyte proliferation responses to mitogen or antigen stimulation and decreased numbers of lymphocytes. This suppression seems more related to a T-cell-mediated response since phytohaemagglutinin (PHA) and concanavalin A (Con A) induced lymphocyte proliferation is decreased in depressed patients, but not significantly changed by pokeweed mitogen (PWM) and lipopolysaccharide (LPS) stimulation. Not all thes findings could be replicated, however. The inconsistent results may be due to differences in the severity of depressive symptoms and/or the occurrence of depression that is secondary to other conditions, such as anxiety, alcoholism or schizophrenia. Other factors, such as antidepressant and other drug treatments, hospitalization status and mitogen concentrations used, may also affect the lymphocyte response. For example, one study that included both bipolar and unipolar patients showed no differences between depressed patients and their controls in lymphocyte responses to one dose of mitogen, but when a higher dose was used, the bipolar patients exhibited a higher lymphocyte response than the controls or unipolar patients. Furthermore, reduced numbers of circulating lymphocytes appear to be more common among unipolar patients than bipolar patients or controls. Most clinical studies support a relationship between reduced immune function and the severity of depression. However, it has been shown that outpatients with depression have a decreased T-lymphocyte number, but do not have a significantly lower lymphocyte proliferative capacity than controls. Neutrophil phagocytosis has also been reported to be reduced in drug-free patients who were diagnosed with endogenous depression. In some animal models of depression (such as the olfactory bulbectomized rat and various learned helplessness models), neutrophil phagocytosis has been shown to be a sensitive marker of response to stress.

In depressive illness, the most consistent change found in cellular function is the decreased natural killer (NK) cell cytotoxicity, although the changes in the number of NK cells are not consistent in all investigations.

Immune-inflammatory Response in Depression

In contrast to the suppression of cellular immunity, many immune-inflammatory responses also occur in depressed patients. A higher incidence of antinuclear factors has been found in patients with endogenous depression, which indicates an autoimmune response. B cells produce antibodies, such as IgA, IgM and IgE, which are also increased in patients with major depression. Other aspects of cell-mediated immunity are also activated in depression. These include an increased number and phagocytosis of monocytes, an increased number of total leucocytes and neutrophils, increased number of activated T cells (CD25+ and HLA-DR+), CD4+ cells and increased ratio of CD4/CD8 cells.

The B-cell subset (CD19+) has also been found to be increased in depressed patients. The concentration of neopterin, a sensitive marker of activation of cell-mediated immunity, is significantly elevated in patients with depression compared to controls. Furthermore, the mitogen-induced production of pro-inflammatory cytokines from mononuclear cells interleukin-1 (IL-1), IL-6, tumor necrosis factor alpha (TNF-α), interferon gamma (IFN-γ) and cytokine receptors (IL-RA, sIL-6R and sIL-2R) is significantly increased in depressed patients. In addition, increased plasma positive acutue phase proteins (APPs) (haptoglobin, alpha-1-antitrypsin, alpha-1-acid glycoprotein and C-reactive protein) and a decrease in negative APPs (albumin and transferrin) have also been consistently observed in these patients. These changes suggest that immune activation occurs in depressive illness.

Increases in Monocyte/Macrophage and T-lymphocyte Activation in Depression

In depression, increased IL-2R, CD4+, CD25+ and HLA-DR+ T cells indicate an activation of T cells. The increase of IL-1, IL-6, TNF-α and IL-6R indicates an activation of monocyte/macrophage functions, which is consistent with the increased monocyte phagocytosis and monocyte number observed in depression. Moreover, both activated T cells and monocytes can produce IFN-γ, while the increase in IL-1RA has been positively related to the increse in the number of total leucocytes, neutrophils, and some T-cell and B-cell subsets.

The serum concentration of IL-1RA is also elevated during a stress response. In rats, pretreatment of IL-1RA can inhibit the increase in corticosterone and prevent immune suppression caused by stress. Thus, the increase in IL-1RA in depression suggest a stress-like response, which may trigger other immune and endocrine changes. In addition, an increase in the cytokine IL-6 derived from activated monocytes in depressed patients is positively correlated with an increased number of leucocytes, neutrophils, monocytes and B-cell subsets; the increase in plasma APP production appears to be due to the stimulation of monocymic cytokines to the liver.

Thus, the immune suppression observed in depressive illness may result from the enhanced action of proinflammatory cytokines on the secretion of glucocorticoids and prostaglandin E2 and from multiple feedback effects or immunosuppressive factors (Figure 5.1).

From such evidence it has been proposed that depression is accompanied by an immune inflammatory response which may be caused by excessive production of cytokines from activated monocytes/macrophages and T lymphocytes.

NEUROTRANSMITTER CHANGES IN DEPRESSION

There are several neurotransmitter hypotheses of depression. Schildkraut in 1965 proposed that there was a defect in catecholamine (noradrenaline (NA) and dopamine (DA)), a hypothesis that was later extended by van Praag and Coppen to include a serotonin (5 hydroxytryptamine; 5-HT) deficit. Later, changes in other neurotransmitters and their receptors were included to account for the complex changes that occur in this condition.

Changes in Catecholamines and Their Metabolite in Depression

The NA deficit hypothesis was derived largely from indirect pharmacological evidence of the behavioural and mood effects of drugs acting on these

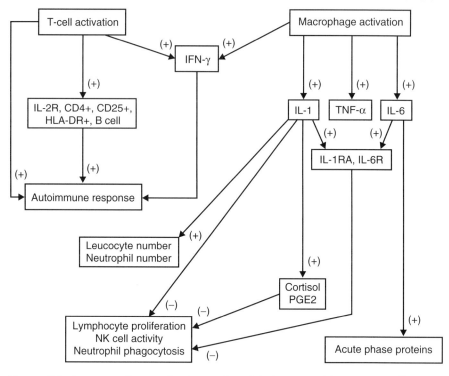

Figure 5.1 Immune changes in depression. (+), increase; (−), suppress; IL, inter-leukin, R, receptor; A, antagonist; NK, natural killer; TNF, tumour necrosis factor; IFN, interferon; PGE2, prostaglandin E2.

systems in laboratory animals and humans. For example, reserpine and tetrabenazine could cause depletion of NA in the brain and result in de-pressed symptoms in some individuals. As both NA and DA are metabol-ized by monoamine oxidase (MAO), an event that is enhanced by reserpine, both NA and DA are implicated in depression. Moreover, in clinical studies, some depressed patients show a decrease in both NA and DA, and the DA metabolite homovanillic acid (HVA) concentration in the cerebrospinal fluid (CSF). By contrast, psychotic depression results in an increase in DA and HVA in the CSF. Stress and the glucocorticoid dexamethasone also increase HVA in the nucleus accumbens of rats, which can account for some of the neurotransmitter changes seen in depression. It has also been shown that in Parkinson's disease, neuroleptic treatment and withdrawal from chronic amphetamines are associated with depression.

Monoamines and their metabolites have been studied in various biolog-ical fluids, as an indirect measure of the central monoamine activity. In relation to the noradrenergic system, NA and 3-methoxy-4-hydroxy-phenylglycol (MPHG) have been most studied. However, results have not always been consistent in depressed patients. For more than two decades, urinary MHPG has been found to be decreased in patients with unipolar depression, but increased in bipolar depressed patients. Longitudinal studies of bipolar patients during both phases of the illness have reported a lower urinary MHPG excretion during a depressive phase and a higher concentration during mania. In addition, in some studies it has been reported that patients who respond to amitriptyline treatment excrete significantly more MHPG than non-responders. Therefore, these results may indicate a change in the metabolism and/or release of NA. However, the results from studies or CSF and plasma concentration of MHPG are not always consistent. Several studies have shown that CSF concentration of MHPG is reduced in depression, but increased in postmenopausal women with depression. There may be important differences between different types of depression. In general plasma MHPG concentrations tend to be higher in depressed patients than in normal controls. An increase in the plasma NA concentration seems a more consistent finding, which may reflect the activity of the peripheral sympathetic system rather than the central nervous system (CNS). The evidence suggests that there is abnormal peripheral sympathetic activity in depression. In recent stress research, increases in plasma and CSF MHPG and NA concentrations have been found to be associated with stress stimulation. Thus it may be concluded that changes in central and peripheral sympathetic activity may reflect not only fundamental changes in noradrenergic function but also an abnormal response to external stressors.

Changes in Serotonin, its Precursor and Metabolites in Depression

5-Hydroxyindole-acetic acid (5-HIAA) is the major metabolite of serotonin and has been studied in CSF as a marker of central serotonergic activity in depression. Some investigators have shown that the 5-HIAA concentration is reduced in depressed subjects; in particular a low CSF concentration of 5-HIAA is often associated with suicidal behaviour. Thus is has been suggested that a reduced CSF 5-HIAA concentration could be a marker of suicidal behaviour in depressed patients.

Several studies have examined the binding of ^{3}H-imipramine to platelets from depressed patients. Normally, imipramine binds to the uptake site for 5-HT in platelets and neuronal membranes. In depressed patients, however, a significant decrease in the number of ^{3}H-imipramine binding sites has been observed when compared with controls. This suggests that 5-HT transport may be defective in depression. In support of this, other researchers have shown a significant decrease in the ability of platelets to transport 5-HT in depressed patients.

Serotonin is synthesized in the brain from unbound tryptophan that is actively transported from the blood. Thus, variations in brain tryptophan concentrations may reflect net synthesis of brain serotonin. In patients with depression, or with depression-associated alcohol abuse, the ratio between trytophan and other amino acids is decreased. This may account for the modest antidepressant effect of the 5-HT precursor, 5-hydroxytryptophan (5-HTP).

Partly as a consequence of the finding that NA and 5-HT are malfunctioning in depression, a number of tricyclic antidepressants and selective serotonin reuptake inhibitors (SSRIs) have been developed. These drugs improve many of the symptoms of depression. However, not all antidepressants appear to act directly on specific monoamines and their metabolites. These antidepressants may also act on other neurotransmitter systems and result in side effects. Both clinical and experimental studies have shown the shortcomings of these neurotransmitter hypotheses of depression. For example, the NA and 5-HT hypotheses are unable to explain (i) the delayed therapeutic action of tricyclic and SSRI antidepressants; (ii) the failure of L-DOPA and tryptophan as affective antidepressants; and (iii) why some antidepressant treatments decrease biogenic amines and their metabolism.

Changes in the Cholinergic and GABAergic Systems in Depression

Elevation in the activity of the cholinergic system has been observed in some patients with depression. Cholinomimetic agents, such as physostigmine, can induce depressive symptoms in patients and anhedonic behaviour in rodents, effects that are corrected by most antidepressants. Gamma-aminobutynic acid (GABA) has also been implicated in the pathogenesis of depression. It has been shown that antidepressants, lithium, carbamazepine and electroconvulsive therapy (ECT) reduce GABA turnover, and decreased CSF GABA concentrations have been found in depressed patients. In addition, GABA agonists (progabide and fengabine) are reported to show weak antidepressant effects.

Changes in Neurotransmitter Receptors in Depression

Chronic administration of most antidepressants results in changes at postsynaptic receptor sites; for example, the down-regulation of β-adreno-ceptors. Moreover, some behavioural and NA turnover studies indicate that presynaptic α_2-receptors become subsensitive following administration of some antidepressants. As there is evidence that the density of β-adreno-ceptors is increased in lymphocytes and cortical membranes from depressed patients, and those having committed suicide, the pathophysiology of depression is thought to be related to the supersensitivity of β-adrenergic receptors. Experimental studies have shown that chronic treatment with some antidepressants reduces the activity of NA-stimulated adenylated cyclase and the number of β-adrenergic receptors, thereby supporting the hypothesis that a malfunctioning β-adrenoceptor system is causally related to the depressed state.

The β-adrenergic receptor hypothesis of depression offers an advance over the monoamine deficit theory in that it is able to explain the time delay between start of antidepressant treatment and the therapeutic response. However, it must be emphasized that (i) the data are mostly from animal studies; (ii) the human data are based on peripheral changes; (iii) the down-regulation may be the side effects of drug treatment; and (iv) decreased cAMP response to NA is not specific for antidepressants.

In parallel to these studies of changes in noradrenergic receptors in depression, studies on 5-HT receptors have also shown that chronic treatment with various antidepressants results in decreased 5-HT2A receptors in the frontal cortex of rat brain. However, ECT has been found to increase 5-HT2A receptors in rat brain, while 5-HT2 receptors are also increased in the brains of suicide victims and on platelets from depressed patients. Other types of 5-HT receptors have also been reported to change in depression but the results of such findings are equivocal.

There is both clinical and experimental evidence that the dopaminergic system is also involved in depressive disorders. Clinical studies demonstrate that chronic antidepressant treatments and ECT reduce the sensitivity of presynaptic dopamine receptors and increase postsynaptic DA receptor functions in the mesolimbic/mesocortical pathways. The enhanced dopaminergic functioning caused by effective antidepressant treatments may acount for the pro-hedonic action of these drugs.

From the above evidence it can be seen that the monoamine deficit hypothesis requires major revision to account for the interaction between different neurotransmitters in depression, and the interrelationship between the immune–neuroendocrine–neurotransmitter axis and the aetiological basis of the disorder.

ENDOCRINE CHANGES IN DEPRESSION

Early endocrine studies in which urinary corticosteroids were assayed showed that adrenal corticoid activity was increased in depression. The hypersecretion of cortisol from the adrenals in response to ACTH stimulation, and the increased weight of the adrenal glands, is also well established. In addition, the suppression of cortisol secretion by dexamethasone is blunted in more than 50% of depressed patients and forms the basis of the dexamethasone suppression test (DST) as a marker of depression. Such evidence indicates that depression is accompanied by an abnormality in the hypothalamic–pituitary–adrenocortical (HPA) axis. Despite the initial enthusiasm for using the DST as a diagnostic marker of depression, an impaired HPA axis may also occur in Alzheimer's disease, bulimia nervosa, anorexia and alcoholism. Recently, many investigations have shown that the DST abnormality is a consequence of hypersecretion of corticotrophin-releasing factor (CRF) in the CNS. In depressed patients, the ACTH response to a CRF challenge is significantly blunted and the CSF concentration of CRF is increased. CRF is the primary physiological mediator of ACTH and β-endorphin secretion from the anterior pituitary. Within the hypothalamus, CRF-containing neurons project from the paraventricular nucleus (PVN) to the median eminence (ME). Activation of the CRF neural circuit occurs in response to immune, psychogenic and neurogenic stress, resulting in ACTH and related peptides. The elevated CSF concentrations of CRF are believed to reflect increased synaptic concentrations of the peptide, probably due to central CRF hypersecretion. Increased CRF during depression is reduced upon recovery following ETC and antidepressant (for example, desipramine and fluoxetine) treatment. Thus, the CRF challenge test may become a popular and more specific method to determine HPA axis functions in depression.

The markedly depressed mood and cognitive dysfunction of patients with primary hypothyroidism led to scrutiny of the hypothalamic–pituitary–thyroid (HTP) axis in depression. In approximately 25% of depressed patients, the thyroid-stimulating hormone (TSH) response to the thyrotrophin-releasing hormone (TRH) test is blunted. Furthermore, the CSF concentration of TRH is elevated in depressed patients in comparison with controls. In order to determine whether an increase in TRH secretion might underlie the blunted TSH response to TRH reported in depressed patients by causing TRH receptor down-regulation in the pituitary, rats were chronically treated with TRH. As expected, a blunted TSH response to TRH and decreased plasma concentrations of TSH, triiodothyronine (T3) and thyroxine (T4) were observed. This study has also been replicated in human subjects. Thus, it may suggest that elevated CSF concentrations of TRH are due to the hypersecretion of TRH.

An abnormality in growth hormone (GH) regulation has also been reported in depressed patients. For instance, in normal subjects, the α_2-agonist clonidine causes an increased GH response, whereas in depressed patients it shows a blunted response. This may result from α_2-adrenoceptor abnormality in depression. Similar to the lower response of GH to clonidine challenge, prolactin (PRL) has shown a diminished response to hypoglycaemia and opioid agonists. This may be related to the alteration of DA, 5-HT and/or opioid regulation in depression.

Clinically, approximately half of the women who complain of premenstrual syndrome have distressing physical, psychological and behavioural changes of sufficient severity to result in deterioration of interpersonal relationships and/or interference with normal activities. Hormonal changes during the menstrual cycle may lead to fluctuations in affective symptoms, which could exacerbate an underlying affective disorder, or trigger the expression of depression in a cyclical pattern. Ovarian steroid hormones are known to interact with the CNS and directly affect neuro-transmitters in their synthesis, release, reuptake, enzymatic inactivation, and also the sensitivity and presynaptic and postsynaptic neurotransmitter receptors. For example, it is known that an abnormal serotonergic function, as shown by the response of 5-HT1A receptors to the partial agonist buspirone, occurs in women with premenstrual dysphoric disorder (PDD). Such evidence suggests that sex hormones also play an important role in depression and in the regulation of aminergic function, especially in women.

STRESS AS A TRIGGER FACTOR IN DEPRESSION

Depression is often provoked or exacerbated by stressful life events (bereavement), environmental stress (chronic difficulties and risk factors) and early adversity (marital discord or child abuse). There is general agreement that the likelihood of suffering from a depressive episode is increased five- or sixfold in the six months following stressful life events. There is also evidence to suggest that exposure to chronic low grade stress may be a predisposing factor in depression. Many experimental and clinical studies have demonstrated that chronic or unavoidable/uncontrollable stress causes changes in behavioural and neurotransmitter function, endocrine and immune aspects that are similar to those occurring in depressed patients. However, it is still unclear whether the changes occurring in depression are indpendent of chronic stress or whether depression is a consequence of chronic stress.

NEUROTRANSMITTER CHANGES IN STRESS RESPONSE

The effects of stress on NA function have received great attention. In experimental studies, acute stress normally increases NA metabolism and synthesis in both the CNS and periphery, while severe or maladaptive chronic stress depletes NA content in the brain, but increases it in the periphery. The NA changes reported to occur in endogenous depression are similar to those observed after severe or maladaptive chronic stress.

Many stressors induce a reduction in central DA concentration. However, acute stress increases DA metabolites, HVA and 3,4-dihydroxyphenylacetic acid (DOPAC), changes which have not been reported in depressed patients. Some experimental stressors, such as acute footshock, also increase DA synthesis. The results of stress-induced changes in DA and it metabolites are dependent on severity of stress and the brain region studied. As such studies have not been undertaken in depressed patients, is it difficult to comment on their relevance to depression. There are similarities in both dopaminergic function and the behavioural changes seen following stress and in depression. Thus exposure of animals to an unavoidable or uncontrollable aversive experience leads to inhibition of DA release in the mesoaccumbens dopaminergic system and impaired responding to rewarding or aversive stimuli. These behavioural changes could model stress-induced expression and exacerbation of depressive symptoms such as anhedonia and feelings of helplessness in humans as well as syndromal depression provoked by traumatic experiences.

Several studies have reported that stress may influence the turnover and/ or concentrations of 5-HT. Most forms of acute and controllable stress have been found to increase brain 5-HT, 5-HIAA and tryptophan concentrations. However, severe and chronic stress exposure may reduce 5-HT and 5-HIAA concentrations in the hypothalamus and hippocampus.

Despite the very limited data on changes in aminergic function following exposure of patients to specific stressors, it is possible that different stressors may induce different neurochemical changes in different brain regions, changes which may be related to different subtypes of depression.

STRESS, DEPRESSION AND HPA ACTIVITY

Stress-induced changes in corticosteroid synthesis and secretion are qualitatively similar to changes occurring in depression. For example, in the wild olive backed baboon, the dominant male baboons have preferential access to mates and places of safety in the event of an attack by predators, while subordinate baboons lack both and receive the displaced aggression from frustrated baboons higher up the hierarchy. This situation is similar to chronic stress in the clinical context. Interestingly, hypercortisolaemia, dexamethasone resistance and blunted ACTH response to CRF have been found in the subordinate olive backed baboon. Similarly, rats exposed to noise or light *in utero* develop a fearful temperament in later life, as shown by reduced activity in a novel situation, an enhanced corticosterone response to mild environmental stress and enhanced punishment induced suppression of an appetitive response. Endotoxic shock *in utero* also results in desensitization of corticosteroid receptors and prolongs the corticosterone response to stress.

Early adversity in animals is known to result in some impairments in behaviour and HPA activity in later life. For example, maternal separation in rats during early postnatal life has been shown to cause an increased corticosterone response to stress and suppressed immune functions. Similarly, children who have experienced prior sexual or physical abuse show reduced ACTH responses to CRF with 24 h excretion of urinary free cortisol. These changes are also similar to those observed in depressed patients.

Stress-induced changes in HPA acivity and corticosteroid secretion are similar to those occurring in depression. Thus, stress causes hypersecretion of ACTH and corticosteroids due to stress-induced stimulation of CRF release from the paraventricular nucleus (PVN) of the hypothalamus. During a stress response, the expression of CRF mRNA has been found to be increased and in depressed patients, while the CSF concentration of CRF is increased. In the brains of depressed suicides, CRF expressing cells in the PVN are increased fourfold compared to non-depressed controls. Several investigators have reported that chronic stress causes a down-regulation in corticosteroid receptors which mediate negative feedback regulation of the HPA axis. Such a negative feedback control of the HPA response to stress is exerted by corticosteroids at different levels. For example, as plasma corticosteroid concentrations rise, corticosteroid receptors in the hippocampus are activated in order to mediate fast feedback inhibition of the HPA axis. The corticosteroids are known to act at two classes of receptors—the mineralocorticoid receptors (or type 1 receptors), which have high affinity for corticosteroids and so are fully occupied most of the time, and those glucocorticoid receptors which have a low affinity for corticosteroids (type 2 receptors) and which are mainly activated in response to stress. Chronic stress exposure reduces the densities of both types of receptor, especially in the hippocampus.

It is well established that depression is accompanied by an impaired negative feedback control of the HPA axis. In addition to the dexamethasone suppression test, the inhibition of ACTH in response to hydrocortisone is also used to test feedback inhibition at the level of the hippocampus; this response is also impaired in depression. In addition to changes in glucocorticoid secretion, chronic stress in both humans and animals results in hypertrophy of the adrenal glands. An enlargement of pituitary gland volume has also been found in depressed patients. These changes associated with chronic stress or depression can mostly be reversed by chronic antidepressant treatments in both depressed patients and animal models of depression.

STRESS, DEPRESSION AND THE IMMUNE SYSTEM

In experimental studies, cellular immune suppression observed following exposure to stress is similar to that observed in depressed patients. For example, decreased lymphocyte response to mitogens, NK cell cytotoxicity and neutrophil phagocytosis have been reported in experimental animals after exposure to footshock, restraint, cold water or novel environmental-induced stress. Mild and acute stress may stimulate some immune functions, while chronic and severe stress usually suppress cellular immune functions. Stress and depression also increase the number of leucocytes and neutrophils, and decrease the number of lymphocytes. For example, forced swimming stress in rats significantly increases the number of leucocytes and neutrophils. In addition, in human subjects, spaceflight suppresses lymphocyte proliferation and increases the number of leucocytes and neutrophils, while, those who have suffered bereavement, divorce and other chronic stressful life events show lower cellular immune functions.

As well as the changes in cellular functions, depression is accompanied by changes in plasma acute phase protein (APP) concentrations. Recently, it has also been found that acute stress significantly increases plasma positive APP concentrations, changes which may result from the increase in the secretion of proimflammatory cytokines. Increases in plasma IL-1, IL-1RA, IL-6, IL-6R and TNF-α have been reported in subjects after exposure to physical or psychological stress. These immune changes are more pronounced in response to uncontrollable and severe stressors. Thus, similar inflammatory immune responses that result from excess production of cytokines may also occur during a stress response. Moreover, stress not only impairs immune functions in the periphery, it also changes the expression of some proinflammatory cytokine mRNA. Stress-induced alterations in the expression of IL-1, IL-6 and TNF-α mRNA have been reported in different brain regions.

EFFECTS OF ANTIDEPRESSANTS ON IMMUNE FUNCTION IN DEPRESSION

There is some evidence that antidepressant treatments attenuate impaired immune functions in depression. For example, it has been shown that major depression and dysthymia (chronic, low grade depression) are associated with an increase in the number of NK cells in blood, but following effective treatment with SSRIs (fluoxetine and fluvoxamine), the symptoms of depression are alleviated and the NK cell number declines to control values. In patients with major depression, it was found that the NK cell numbers reached control values within four weeks, whereas six months of treatment were required for such an effect to be achieved in dysthymic patients.

In vitro studies of the effect of desipramine on human NK cell activity have shown that concentrations of 625 ng/ml or greater inhibit NK activity. Preincubation of lymphocytes with desipramine before assay did not increase the inhibitory effect; neither did removal of the drug from preincubated cells immediately before assay completely eliminate the inhibitory effect. These results demonstrate that desipramine may reversibly inhibit NK activity at serum concentrations that could occur in depressed patients.

Other clinical studies have shown that antidepressants (fluoxetine and amitriptyline) suppress lymphoid functions and promote tumour growth in some depressed patients. In these patients, cutaneous pseudolymphomas are also associated with antidepressant therapy, reflecting perturbation of lymphoid function.

In depressed patients with HIV, chronic imipramine treatment has been shown not to affect lymphocyte subsets. It has also been demonstrated that subchronic treatment with tricyclic antidepressants could attenuate the increased total leucocyte number and neutrophil number, but not reduce the increase in the CD2+, CD4+ and CD4/CD8 ratios. However, some investigators have reported that chronic treatment with tricyclic antidepressants causes an increase in the number of leucocytes and neutrophils.

In the olfactory bulbectomized rat model of depression, the increased number of leucocytes and neutrophils that occurs following the brain lesion was not attenuated by chronic desipramine or lithium treatment. By contrast, in the control rats, the percentage of neutrophils was increased by desipramine treatment. Clearly there are significant difference between animal models of depression and patients, which could be responsible for the difference in the effects of the antidepressants on leucocyte or bone marrow functions.

In the bulbectomized rats, desipramine treatment attenuates the hyperactivity of the rats in a stressful novel environment of the "open field", increases NA and NA turnover in several brain regions and reverses the impaired neutrophil phagocytosis that follows the lesion. However, this drug also has some toxic effects on the immune system. For example, it reduces the weight of the thymus and spleen, increases leucocyte aggregation and suppresses lymphocyte proliferation in the control animals. By contrast, chronic treatment with SSRI antidepressants (such as sertraline and fluvoxamine) can reverse behavioural, neurotransmitter and immune changes caused by bulbectomy without causing a reduction in the weight of the immune organs.

The results from the study of antidepressant effects on cytokine synthesis are inconsistent and so far there are few studies in depressed patients. Experimentally, acute desipramine treatment in the rat significantly increases TNF-α production in the hippocampus and TNF-α mRNA in the locus coeruleus; no changes are apparent after chronic administration. Furthermore, while central TNF-α administration reduces the release of [^{3}H]-NA from hippocampal slices in a dose-dependent manner, it enhances NA release after desipramine treatment for 14 days. This effect can be reversed by the α_2-adrenergic antagonist idazoxan. Therefore, the TNF-induced regulation of NA release appears to be associated with an alteration of α_2-adrenergic receptor responsiveness, which may help to explain the mechanism for the delay in action of antidepressants.

It is known that the serum concentration of sIL-2R (soluble IL-2R) is increased in depressed patients and those receiving chronic lithium carbonate also show a significant increase in serum sIL-2R, suggesting that lithium exposure enhances some immune functions and suppresses some autoimmune diseases such as psoriasis.

Other antidepressants, such as imipramine, fluvoxamine and maprotiline, have been reported to increase IL-1 expression in the hypothalamus, hippocampus, frontal cortex and brain stem of rats. This evidence would seem to contradict the view that antidepressants may alleviate depressive symptoms by inhibiting cytokine secretion in the brain or immune cells. However, *in vitro* studies have demonstrated that many antidepressants inhibit LPS-induced IL-1, TNF-α and IL-6 release from monocytes. The relationship between *in vivo* and *in vitro* effects of antidepressant treatments in terms of clinical significance, and which cytokine and CNS pathway is involved in the action of antidepressants that attenuate both symptoms of depression and the immune status, remains an enigma.

THE ROLE OF CYTOKINES IN THE AETIOLOGY OF DEPRESSION

It is now established that there are many immune changes occurring in depression, especially in the proinflammatory cytokines. However, are these changes the consequence or the cause of depression? In 1991, the macrophage theory of depression was proposed by Smith. This hypothesis suggested that an excessive secretion of monocyte/macrophage cytokines, such as IL-1, IL-6, TNF-α and IFN, may cause symptoms of depression. In recent years, support for this hypothesis has been gaining ground and it will now be considered in more detail.

CYTOKINES AND DEPRESSIVE SYMPTOMS

Depression has a close relationship with physical illness. It has been noted that patients with cancer, heart disease, stroke, rheumatoid arthritis, food allergy, systemic lupus erythematosus and also postpartum women are at a higher risk of developing depression compared to the normal population. All these conditions have a common factor in that macrophages are activated and the production and secretion of macrophage cytokines are increased. Indeed, an increased number and phagocytosis of monocytes and monocymic cytokines have been found in patients with major depression.

Cytokines have been used for treatment of some cancers. In these patients and also in volunteers, macrophage-produced cytokines (such as TNF-α or IFN-α) cause most of the symptoms required for a DMS III-R diagnosis of major depression. Thus, such patients experience moderate to severe fatigue, psychomotor slowing, anhedonia, anorexia and hypersomnia. Most become irritable and develop depressed mood.

In animals, both IL-1β and TNF-α, following central or systemic administration, increase anxious behaviour in the elevated plus maze, suppress exploration in the novel environment and increase corticosterone secretion. These cytokines also change the sleep pattern, induce anorexia, reduce body weight and cause anhedonic behaviour.

THE RELATIONSHIP BETWEEN CYTOKINES AND THE CNS IN DEPRESSION

As mentioned in Chapter 2, cytokines produced from peripheral leucocytes can pass the blood–brain barrier (BBB) into the brain by means of both a saturable and non-saturable transport system and by a receptor transportation system. During brain injury, infection or an inflammatory response, the BBB increases in its permeability. Furthermore, cytokines have been found to act on the CNS via the organum vasculosum of the laminae terminalis where the BBB is absent.

Cytokine receptors are widely distributed on astrocytes, glial cells and neurons in different brain regions. It is also known that astrocytes, glial cells and neurons can produce most monocyte/macrophage cytokines in the brain. It has been reported that the peripheral administration of bacterial LPS increases the expression of mRNA for IL-1β, IL-6 and TNF-α within the CNS and causes a depressive-like episode in rats. These results suggest that peripheral immune changes may alter CNS function via the effects of peripheral cytokines on central cytokine production. As has been mentioned, both systemically and centrally administered cytokines can change neurotransmitter synthesis, release and metabolism. For example, IL-1 and TNF-α increase NA release and NA turnover, and also HVA and 5-HIAA concentrations in several brain regions, while IL-6 increases turnover of DA and 5-HT. Some of these changes are similar to those observed in depression and stress. However, most of these results are from acute studies with high doses of cytokines, which may only reflect the effect of an acute immune stressor on the CNS. Clearly, future research should study the effects of chronic administration of different cytokines on neurotransmitter, endocrine and immune functions.

Studies of the relationship between inflammatory activation and serotonergic functions provide more direct evidence for an association between cytokines and depression. The plasma concentration of L-tryptophan is markedly decreased in depressed patients and brain 5-HT synthesis depends, in part, on the availability of L-tryptophan in the blood. As an immune response may cause decreased availability of free tryptophan to the brain, it has been proposed that lowered L-tryptophan in major depression could be a consequence of an increase in peripheral cytokines and immune activation. In support of this view, it has been demonstrated that in depressed patients, the decrease in plasma concentrations of L-tryptophan is negatively correlated to plasma concentrations of IL-6 and positive APPs.

CYTOKINES AND HPA ACTIVITY IN DEPRESSION

It is well known that IL-1 and TNF-α can stimulate the hypothalamus to synthesize CRF, which then stimulates the pituitary gland to secrete ACTH. ACTH in turn acts on the adrenal gland to synthesize and release corticosteroids. IL-6 and IFN can also stimulate the pituitary and adrenal gland to secrete corticosteroids. Increased production and release of cytokines resulting from physical illness, tissue damage and autoimmune diseases, like chronic stress, continually stimulates the HPA axis and thereby may change the negative feedback control of ACTH release and eventually down-regulate corticosteroid receptors in the CNS (see Figure 4.1). Thus the increased CRF, the blunted ACTH response and hypercortisolaemia that occur in depression may also result from excessive production of macrophage cytokines.

CYTOKINES, PGE2 AND CELLULAR IMMUNE SUPPRESSION IN DEPRESSION

Prostaglandin E2 (PGE2), a potent mediator of inflammation, is released in large quantities by activated macrophages. PGE2 has been reported to be increased in depression and following chronic stress. In the CNS, IL-1 has been shown to stimulate PGE2 secretion in many brain regions, and an increase in the blood concentration of PGE2 exerts immunosuppressive effects on the activities of lymphocytes, NK cells and neutrophils. It has been reported that in depression, the decreased lymphocyte response to a plant mitogen (concanavalin A) is inversely correlated with the plasma concentration of PGE2. Moreover, following the incubation of different concentrations of PGE2 with human monocytes or neutrophils it was found that low dose of PGE2 stimulated, but high dose inhibited, monocyte activity, while both low and high doses of PGE2 suppressed neutrophil phagocytosis.

In the CNS, PGE2 is involved in the onset of fever and inflammatory responses. PGE2 has been found to reduce NA release from central noradrenergic neurons to stimulate the HPA axis and thereby increase corticosteroid secretion. Tricyclic antidepressants and monoamine oxidase inhibitors (MAOIs) can reduce PGE2 synthesis in rat brain, an effect which may help to account for the immunomodulatory action of antidepressants following their chronic administration.

In addition to an increase in inflammatory cytokines in depression, some T-cell produced cytokines are also increased, such as IFN, TNF and IL-2R. However, it is not certain whether the macrophage cytokines induce T-cell-mediated immunity or whether T-cell-mediated immunity changes first. Nevertheless, it does appear that the immune changes seen in depression are similar to those seen in an autoimmune disease.

IS DEPRESSION AN AUTOIMMUNE DISORDER?

Many chronic autoimmune diseases are accompanied by depressive symptoms. For example, patients with systemic lupus erythematosus, autoimmune thyroiditis, postpartum thyroiditis, insulin-dependent diabetes, rheumatoid arthritis of Sjögren's syndrome show obvious emotional distress, anxiety, psychological problems and cognitive deficits. In mice with autoimmune disease, it has been found that neurobehavioural changes are similar to those observed in animal models of depression. In addition, several studies have shown that antidepressant treatments attenuate depressive symptoms and antoimmune responses. Of particular interest is the observation that the antidepressant rolipram is effective for treatment of multiple sclerosis (MS), a T-cell-mediated antoimmune disease. In this study, human CD4+ major basic protein (MBP)-specific T cells from patients with MS and encephalitogenic CD4+ MBP-specific rat T cells were incubated with different concentrations of rolipram. It was found that rolipram administration significantly and dose dependently suppressed TNF-α and IFN-γ release from the T-cell line of the patients, rats and their respective controls. At a very high dose, rolipram also suppressed lymphocyte proliferation. In experimental autoimmune encephalomyelitis (EAE) Lewis rats, chronic rolipram completely prevented the appearance of neurological symptoms and lowered the blood TNF-α concentration.

Unlike infection caused by a single antigen, most autoimmune disease is multifactorial and requires a combination of genetic and environmental factors. Figure 9.1 summarizes the possible contributing factors in autoimmune diseases, many of which also exist in depressive illness.

The production of autoantibodies is normally increased in an autoimmune disease. It is known that the synthesis of antibodies is controlled by both T cells and B cells, T cells controlling the generation of autoantibodies which are responsible for the development of immune tolerance. T-cell tolerance can be attenuated by exposure to neoantigens, chemicals or viruses. In depression, increased autoantibodies, antiphosphatidylserine and antipartial thromboplastin titres have also been detected. As with autoimmune diseases, other antibodies, such as IgA, IgE and IgM, are also significantly increased in depression. This may also result from B-cell activation via polyclonal stimulation (for example, by means of cytokines, LPS, some viruses and parasites).

The immune system is a dynamic system kept in balance by regulatory CD4 and CD8 T cells or Th1 and Th2 cells. These cells dampen the response to foreign and autologous antigens. Thus, if CD8 T cells are lost, but CD4 increased, the result can be the development of harmful autoantibodies or autoreactive T cells. Increased T_H cells during an autoimmune response may cause excess production of IFN-γ, resulting in tissue damage. Interestingly, depressed patients also have increased plasma concentrations of CD4, a decreased CD4/CD8 ratio and increased IFN-γ.

In an autoimmune disorder, abnormal cytokine synthesis can be a stimulant factor for the activation of T_H cells. Activated T_H cells then activate macrophages through the thymus-dependent (T_D) cells, which cause further inflammatory immune responses. This process may also occur in depression as both hypersecretion of cytokines and hyperactivated macrophage function have been found. There are qualitative differences between autoimmune disease and depression, however. Thus, in some autoimmune diseases, elevated plasma concentrations of IL-2 and sIL-2R have been reported, whereas, in depression, only increased sIL-2R has been found.

In the last decade, most psychoneuroimmunological studies have focused on depression-associated inflammatory responses. The macrophage theory of depression proposed that all these changes result from excessive synthesis of macrophage cytokines. Later, the macrophage–lymphocyte hypothesis of depression was proposed, which emphasizes that lymphocytes may be involved in the illness. The evidence presented here suggests that some changes in immune function is depression are similar to those observed in autoimmune illness. Other changes such as the suppression of cellular immune functions (lymphocytes and NK cells) in depression differ from changes seen in autoimmune diseases.

In conclusion, there is ample evidence to show that stress and depression affect the functioning of the thymus gland and the immune system. However, the relationship between Th1 and Th2 cell activity and cytokine production, T cells, macrophage activity and the thymus status in depression and stress have not been fully elucidated.

BIBLIOGRAPHY

Checkley, S. (1996) The neuroendocrinology of depression and chronic stress. *British Medical Bulletin* **52**: 59–67.

Crowson, A. N. and Magro, C. M. (1995) Antidepressant therapy. A possible cause of atypical cutaneous lymphoid hyperplasia. *Archives of Dermatology* **131**: 925–929.

Denburg, S. D., Carbotte, R. M. and Denburg, J. A. (1997) Psychological aspects of systemic lupus erythematosus: cognitive function, mood, and self-report. *Journal of Rheumatology* **24**: 998–1003.

Hickie, I. and Lloyd, A. (1995) Are cytokines associated with neuropsychiatric syndromes in humans? *International Journal of Immunopharmacology* **17**: 677–683.

Ignatowski, T. A. and Spengler, R. N. (1994) Tumor necrosis factor-a: presynaptic sensitivity is modified after antidepressant drug administration. *Brain Research* **665**: 293–299.

Kronfol, Z., House, J. D., Silva, Jr, J., Greden, J. and Carrol, B. J. (1986) Depression, urinary free cortisol excretion and lymphocyte function. *British Journal of Psychiatry* **148**: 70–73.

Lechin, F., van Der Dijs, B. and Benaim, M. (1996) Stress versus depression. *Progress in Neuro-Psychopharmacology and Biological Psychiatry* **20**: 899–950.

Maes, M. (1995) Evidence for an immune response in major depression: a review and hypothesis. *Progress in Neuro-Psychopharmacology and Biological Psychiatry* **19**: 11–38.

Maes, M., Smith, R. and Scharpe, S. (1995) The monocyte-T-lymphocyte hypothesis of major depression. *Psychoneuroendocrinology* **20**: 111–116.

Maes, M., Stevens, W., DeClerck, L., Peeters, D., Bridts, C. et al. (1992) Neutrophil chemotaxis, phagocytosis, and superoxide release in depressive illness. *Biological Psychiatry* **31**: 1220–1224.

Maes, M., Vandoolaeghe, E., Ranjan, R., Bosmans, E., Bergmans, R. and Desnyder, R. (1995) Increased serum interleukin-1-receptor-antagonist concentrations in major depression. *Journal of Affective Disorders* **36**: 29–36.

Maes, M., Wauters, A., Verkerk, R., Demedts, P., Neels, H. et al. (1996) Lower serum L-tryptophan availability in depression as a marker of a more generalized disorder in rotein metabolism. *Neuropsychopharmacology* **15**: 243–251.

Maes, M., Vandoolaeghe, E., van Hunsel, F. and Bril, T. (1997) Immune disturbances in treatment-resistant depression: Modulation by antidepressive treatments. *Human Psychopharmacology* **12**: 153–162.

McAdams, C. and Leonard, B. E. (1992) Effect of prostaglandin E2 and thromboxane A2 on monocyte and neutrophil phagocytosis in vitro. *Medical Science Research* **20**: 673–674.

McAdams, C. and Leonard, B. E. (1993) Neutrophil and monocyte phagocytosis in depressed patients. *Progress in Neuro-Psychopharmacology and Biological Psychiatry* **17**: 971–984.

Miller, A. H., Asnis, G. M., van Praag, H. M. and Norin, A. J. (1986) Influence of desmethylimipramine on natural killer cell acitivity. *Psychiatry Research* **19**: 9–15.

Musselman, D. L. and Nemeroff, C. B. (1996) Depression and endocrine disorders: focus on the thyroid and adrenal system. *British Journal of Psychiatry* **30**: S123–S128.

O'Neill, B. and Leonard, B. E. (1990) Abnormal zymosan-induced neutrophil chemiluminescence as a marker of depression. *Journal of Affective Disorders* **19**: 265–272.

Rabkin, J. G., Rabkin, R., Harrison, W. and Wagner, G. (1994) Effect of imipramine on mood and enumerative measures of immune status in depressed patients with HIV illness. *American Journal of Psychiatry* **151**: 516–523.

Ravindran, A. V., Griffiths, J., Merali, Z. and Anisman, H. (1995) Lymphocyte subsets associated with major depression and dysthymia: modification by antidepressant treatment. *Psychosomatic Medicine* **57**: 555–563.

Sakic, B., Szechtman, H. and Denburg, J. A. (1997) Neurobehavioural alterations in autoimmune mice. *Neuroscience and Biobehavioural Reviews* **21**: 327–340.

Schildkraut, J. J. (1965) The catecholamine hypothesis of affective disorders: a review of supporting evidence. *American Journal of Psychiatry* **122**: 509–522.

Smith, R. S. (1991) The macrophage theory of depression. *Medical Hypotheses* **35**: 298–306.

Sommer, N., Loschmann, P. A., Northoff, G. H., Weller, M., Steinbercher, A. et al. (1995) The antidepressant rolipram suppresses cytokine production and prevents autoimmune encephalomyelitis. *Nature Medicine* **1**: 244–248.

Song, C. and Leonard, B. E. (1995) The effect of olfactory bulbectomy in the rat, alone or in combination with antidepressants and endogenous factors, on immune function. *Human Psychopharmacology* **10**: 7–18.

Weisse, C. S. (1992) Depression and immunocompetence: a review of the literature. *Psychological Bulletin* **111**: 475–489.

6 Immune Abnormalities in Schizophrenia

Despite the many decades of research into the possible biological basis of schizophrenia, no single abnormality has been identified that is exclusively associated with the disease. Nevertheless, there is considerable agreement that there is a familial basis for the condition which appears to have a genetic rather than a purely environmental association. For example, the increased risk of suffering from schizophrenia is approximately proportional to the genetic similarity between the patients and their immediate relatives. Thus among first-degree relatives of schizophrenic patients, the disorder is approximately ten times more prevalent than in the general population, while the risk in first-degree relatives is approximately four times that of second-degree relatives. Similarly, in monozygotic twins the concordance rate is approximately 50% compared to 15% in dizygotic twins. This indicates that the extent of the genetic similarity correlates with the degree of concordance.

In recent years, it has become apparent that there are remarkable parallels between susceptibility to schizophrenia and autoimmune diseases such as insulin-dependent diabetes and Graves' disease. It would appear that the predisposition to such autoimmune diseases is determined by combinations of co-dominant genes and this may also apply to patients with schizophrenia. For example, schizophrenia, in common with many autoimmune diseases, is not expressed at birth but only appears later in life. Similarly, remission and relapses characterize both schizophrenia and autoimmune diseases. While the possible involvement of the immune system in autoimmune diseases and schizophrenia is undoubtedly complex, it is known that histocompatibility antigens (HLA) are frequently associated with autoimmune diseases and there is some evidence that schizophrenia is associated with particular HLA antigens. This will be discussed in more detail later in this chapter. Despite the circumstantial evidence which suggests that the frequency of some autoimmune diseases is higher in patients with schizophrenia than in the general population, it is still unclear whether they are causally linked to a genetically determined immunological defect. Furthermore, such an autoimmune hypothesis is difficult to reconcile with the popular view that schizophrenia is caused by hyperactivity of the dopaminergic system in the frontal cortex. Nevertheless, it has been speculated that dopamine receptor-stimulating autoantibodies occur in schizophrenic patients that are analogous to the thyroid-stimulating autoantibodies that cause hyperthyroidism in Graves' disease.

To date, however, there is only limited evidence for the existence of such antibodies. Nevertheless, there is an increasing body of evidence that implicates a disorder in the immune system as a contributory factor in the biological changes that underlie schizophrenia.

EVIDENCE FOR A DYSFUNCTION IN THE IMMUNE SYSTEM IN SCHIZOPHRENIA

There are numerous reports in the clinical literature of various aspects of cellular and humoral immunity in schizophrenic patients but there is also a frequent lack of consistency in the findings which has often led researchers to the conclusion that the abnormalities are the result of spurious findings, artefacts of treatment or epiphenomena of the illness. An alternative explanation is that the lack of consistency in the findings may stem from the heterogeneity of the condition so that particular immunological changes may only be relevant to one sub-group of patients. Furthermore, lack of consistency in the immune changes may occur because the state of progression of disease (for example, acute phase, late phase, in remission or relapse, presence or absence of medication) has not been precisely defined. Lastly, inadequate sample sizes and inconsistencies in the methods used to determine the immunological parameters can frequently lead to discrepant results. Such problems, of course, are common to most immunological research that has been undertaken in patients with major psychiatric illness but are more noticeable in schizophrenia research because of the greater paucity of data in comparison to areas such as depression and stress.

AUTOIMMUNE DISEASES AND SCHIZOPHRENIA

Over 60 years ago, Lehmann-Facius suggested that a humoral "antiself" factor might be involved in the pathogenesis of schizophrenia but it is only in the last 15 years that several investigators have independently emphasized the clinical and epidemiological similarities between autoimmune diseases and schizophrenia. However, direct evidence of an autoimmune basis to schizophrenia must rely on studying the relative proportion of T and B cells and their subpopulations, the presence or absence of cytokines as well as the immune response genes (such as human leucocyte antigens: HLAs). In addition, direct evidence of the involvement of the immune system in schizophrenia can be obtained by demonstrating the presence of antibodies that are directed against relevant brain antigens associated with schizophrenia. The evidence that implicates some of these immune factors in schizophrenia will now be considered.

CHANGES IN CELLULAR IMMUNITY IN SCHIZOPHRENIA

Lymphocyte subpulations in schizophrenia patients have been studied by more than 20 groups of investigators and the results of such studies have been variable. However, it would appear that many investigators have found an increase in the number of T-helper cells but this may be due to the presence of neuroleptics, as such a change does not appear in drug-free schizophrenia patients. With regard to B lymphocytes, three groups of investigators have reported an increase in the percentage and absolute number of these cells in patients. However, whether this is due to medication is not apparent.

As has already been mentioned, a major problem that arises in interpreting such changes in schizophrenic patients relates to the small sample sizes, lack of appropriate controls, the clinical status of the patients as well as such factors as race, gender and effects of medication. Until such factors are properly controlled, it is difficult to draw any firm conclusion regarding the relationship between possible abnormalities in lymphocyte function and the disease process.

Despite the lack of consistency in the results of studies in which the lymphocyte subpopulations were determined in schizophrenic patients, there is convincing evidence that some cytokines are abnormal in this condition. In many autoimmune diseases, there is evidence that the synthesis of IL-2 is decreased, especially during the active phase of an autoimmune disease. Furthermore, in studies of animals with autoimmune diseases, it is reported that the reduction in the concentration of this cytokine occurs shortly before the onset of the active phase.

There is consistent evidence from six different groups of investigators that mitogen-stimulated lymphocyte interleukin-2 (IL-2) synthesis is reduced in schizophrenic patients. This effect would not appear to be a consequence of neuroleptic medication and occurs early in the development of the disease before the patients are treated. However, while it would appear that the ability of lymphocytes to synthesize IL-2 following stimulation with mitogens is impaired in schizophrenic patients, the basal blood concentration of this cytokine appears to be unchanged. It should be emphasized that mitogen-stimulated IL-2 synthesis reflects the ability of lymphocytes to synthesize and release IL-2 *in vitro*, whereas the serum IL-2 concentration is an *in vivo* determinant. The physiological significance of the basal IL-2 concentration is difficult to assess because this cytokine acts as both an autocrine (i.e. affecting the secretory cell) and paracrine (i.e. affecting those cells in close proximity to where it is released) factor. In schizophrenia, the concentration of IL-2 is reduced in the blood. The reduction in the mitogen-stimulated release of IL-2 may be the result of an exhaustion of the capacity of the Th1 subset of CD4 cells to synthesize the cytokine or IL-2 synthesis may be suppressed by activated Th2 cells; as has already been mentioned, there is evidence of an increase in Th2 derived cytokines in non-medicated schizophrenic patients.

In addition to the reduction in the stimulated synthesis and release of IL-2 from monocytes and whole blood cultures that occurs in schizophrenic patients, there is also convincing evidence from several studies that the serum concentration of the IL-2 receptor (IL-2R) is increased in the unmedicated state; IL-2 is increased in the cerebrospinal fluid (CSF). There is also evidence that the IL-2 concentration is increased in the intestine of schizophrenic patients which may be related to an increase in allergies seen in such patients. Neuroleptic treatment appears to reduce the serum concentration of IL-2R. IL-2R is released from activated T cells and is widely accepted as a marker of T-cell activation. It is therefore somewhat surprising to find that the basal concentration of IL-2 is decreased in schizophrenic patients, rather than increased, which would be anticipated by the observation that the T cells are activated in schizophrenic patients. Furthermore, the significance of these findings may be confounded by a failure to control for the effects of smoking by patients; smoking has been shown to elevate IL-2R concentrations in healthy young adults. In addition, further studies are needed in neuroleptic naive patients and in those who have been off medication for sufficient time to be free of the effects of neuroleptics and their metabolites on immune parameters. The need for a long withdrawal period following neuroleptic medication is particularly important as the active metabolites of the phenothiazine neuroleptics are known to be excreted for at least 60 days after the last dose. Clearly, there is a need to extend these studies to monitor both IL-2 and IL-2R concentrations under carefully controlled conditions.

In addition to the finding that IL-2 and IL-2R concentrations are significantly altered in schizophrenic patients, the question arises whether these changes in cellular immunity are associated with any of the symptoms of the condition. There is evidence from one preliminary study of a significant inverse correlation between IL-2 synthesis and positive thought disorder and bizarre behaviour; conversely, the reduced IL-2 concentration may be positively correlated with the negative symptoms. If such a finding is replicated, it could indicate that IL-2 synthesis varies in different subtypes of schizophrenia and those with schizophreniform disorder.

A further consideration in this regard is whether the differences in IL-2 synthesis reflect the degree of non-specific arousal between subtypes of schizophrenia. A detailed discussion of the effects of psychological stress on the proinflammatory cytokines has been given in Chapter 4. It is therefore possible that differences in IL-2 synthesis and release may be related to the responsiveness of the patients to environmental and psychological stress.

Of the other cytokines that have been determined in schizophrenic patients, IL-6 has been shown to increase by at least three independent groups of investigators. There is also some evidence that the IL-6 receptor (IL-6R) is also increased, while the concentrations of both IL-6 and IL-6R are decreased in patients who have been treated with neuroleptics. However, whether the changes in IL-6 and IL-6R are causally related to the pathology of schizophrenia is uncertain. An increase in the blood concentration of IL-6 occurs in many autoimmune diseases as exemplified by systemic lupus erythematosus, rheumatoid arthritis and type I (insulin-dependent) diabetes mellitus, which indicates that IL-6 may be a factor in the development of autoimmune states. Thus the changes in the concentration of this cytokine in schizophrenic patients may indicate that there is also an autoimmune basis to this disease.

With regard to natural killer (NK) cell activity in schizophrenics, there are several contradictory reports regarding the changes that occur during the acute phase of the disease. Thus three studies have reported a reduced NK cell activity while two study groups reported no change. It would again appear that some of these differences could be due to the presence of neuroleptics as there is evidence that the reduction in NK cell activity at the start of neuroleptic treatment (with phenothiazines) was associated with a gradual increase in NK cell activity over the four to eight week period of therapy. In addition, in this study it was shown that there was an elevation of CD56, a cell surface marker of NK cells, which suggests that not only NK activity but also differentiation and distribution of NK cells might be altered in schizophrenia.

Results of changes in the CD4/CD8 ratio in schizophrenia are inconsistent, which may be at least partly due to the presence of neuroleptics. Thus the CD4/CD8 ratio in acute schizophrenics was reported to be elevated in those that were drug free but not in those that were on neuroleptic treatment.

In summary, it would appear that changes in cellular immunity occur particularly after acute exacerbation of the condition. These changes are qualitatively similar to those reported to occur in some autoimmune states. In this regard, it is of interest that the treatment of schizophrenic patients with azathioprine, a drug commonly used for the treatment of autoimmune and inflammatory disease, was found to improve the symptoms of schizophrenia, at least in a small pilot study. In addition, the elevation in CSF IL-2 might contribute to the hyperdopaminergic state which has long formed the hypothetical basis for the aetiology of schizophrenia.

ANTIBRAIN ANTIBODIES IN SCHIZOPHRENIA

One of the first-reports to suggest that antibrain antibodies occurred in the sera of schizophrenic patients and were causally related to schizophrenia was by Lehmann-Facius in 1939. It took a further 30 years before evidence was found to support this hypothesis, when it was shown that antibodies present in the sera of schizophrenic patients were able to selectively bind to limbic regions of the brain. Unfortunately, these findings could not be replicated by other investigators. Nevertheless, more recent studies have provided evidence that a serum globulin factor from schizophrenic patients could bind specifically to the septal region of the human brain. Such findings have led to the hypothesis that autoantibodies are produced in schizophrenia that stimulate dopmine receptors, thereby precipitating the acute (positive) symptoms of the illness.

Perhaps the most convincing evidence that schizophrenia is an autoimmune associated disease comes from the research that demonstrates the presence of antibrain antibodies. This implies that specific antibodies are raised in these patients and cause damage to specific brain regions, thereby rendering the patient vulnerable to the behavioural changes that characterize the disease. However, it must be emphasized that the studies of brain antibodies have probably created more controversy and scepticism regarding the autoimmune causes of schizophrenia than any other immune findings. The reason for this appears to lie in the clinical differences (e.g. patients in remission versus those in relapse, those on neuroleptic medication compared with those without medication), the nature and size of the patient samples investigated, and the differences in methods of analysis used. However, there do appear to be consistent findings with regard to the presence of specific antibodies against antigens derived from the hippocampus and several other brain areas that have been implicated in the pathology of schizophrenia. In addition to the hippocampus, these regions include the frontal and parietal cortex, the cingulate gyrus and parahippocampal gyrus. Antibodies against the septum have also been detected in the relatives of patients with schizophrenia.

The results of the studies showing the presence of anti-hippocampal antibodies are particularly exciting because of the evidence implicating an abnormality of the temporal lobe in schizophrenia. A disorder of this brain region is implicated by both neuropathological and imaging studies that demonstrate changes in the medial temporal lobes in this condition. This region of the brain includes the hippocampus, the parahippocampal gyrus and the entorhinal cortex. In addition to the presence of antibrain antibodies affecting those regions of the brain that appear to be dysfunctional in schizophrenia, the hippocampus is the only site in the brain known to contain a high density of IL-2 receptors. It would therefore seem reasonable to conclude that specific brain antibodies against temporal lobe antigens play a causal role in the psychopathology of schizophrenia, and that further studies of cell-mediated immunity directed at antigens in this region of the brain are worthy of further attention.

Few of the studies implicating the presence of antibrain antibodies in the sera of schizophrenic patient have been replicated. In a detailed study of the antibody reactivity to rat brain components in the sera for some 24 acutely ill schizophrenic patients using enzyme-linked immunosorbent assay (ELISA) and Western immunoblotting techniques, the prevalence of autoantibodies did not differ from that of the control group. Indeed, the large individual variation in antibody reactivity to brain structures occurred independently of the state of health of the patients or their controls; this may account for the conflicting results that have been reported in the literature when antibody reactivity in sera from schizophrenic patients has been compared with those of healthy controls. Nevertheless, there is some evidence that IgG reactivity to rat brain membrane antigens in some schizophrenics differs from controls because some 25% of patients have circulating antibodies directed against brain structures which have affinity for haloperidol and sulpiride. In addition, by means of the Western immunoblotting technique, it was found that specific polypeptide bands occurred in more than 50% of schizophrenic patients but in only 3 out of 50 sera sample from control subjects. Several of these polypeptide bands were found to be close to the 94 kDa position, the reported molecular weight of the D2 dopamine receptor. These results do not exclude the possibility that schizophrenic patients have autoantibodies that are reactive to the dopamine receptor but it is vital that such studies are repeated using sera samples from unmedicated patients in order to validate the hypothesis that autoantibodies are responsible for the dopaminergic hyperactivity.

In addition to the specific antibrain antibodies, several other antibodies have been found to be raised in schizophrenic patients. However, it would appear that in many of these studies the presence of these antibodies are a consequence of treatment with neuroleptics. Nevertheless there is evidence to show that in drug-free schizophrenic patients, the prevalence of anti-nuclear antibodies is higher than in appropriate controls. Such studies require replication.

HLA ANTIGENS IN SCHIZOPHRENIA

Genes of the HLA complex occur on the short arm of chromosome 6 and play a crucial role in the immune response. The response of T cells to an antigen is limited by HLA molecules of two major classes. Thus class I HLA antigens (termed HLA-A and HLA-B) restrict the activity of cytotoxic and suppressor (CD8+) T lymphocytes while HLA class II antigens (termed HLA-DR, HLA-DQ and HLA-DP) restrict helper (CD4+) T lymphocytes.

Several immune-mediated disorders have been associated with HLA antigens and there are several studies showing that HLA-A and HLA-B antigens are raised in schizophrenia. However, it would appear that there is only a weak positive association between schizophrenia and subtype HLA-A antigens so that the overall significance of the association between schizophrenia and HLA antigens is likely to be small and possibly of questionable significance.

While most studies have concentrated on the association between HLA class I antigens and schizophrenia, there is evidence that the HLA class II antigens are more relevant to the presence of an autoimmune process. Two of the four studies of the presence of HLA class II antigens have reported that a positive association exists between the presence of these antigens and schizophrenia. It has also been shown that there is a negative association between some of the alleles of the HLA-DQ region and schizophrenia in African-Americans. This observation may be of importance as there is considerable evidence for a negative association between schizophrenia and insulin-dependent diabetes and in addition a strong association between HLA-DQ genes and the risk of developing diabetes. From positron emission tomography studies, it is evident that the utilization of glucose in the prefrontal cortex is impaired. Thus it may be hypothesized that some HLA class II antigens may not only impair normal insulin function, thereby causing insulin-dependent diabetes, but as a consequence reduce the availability of insulin to the brain and thereby precipitate impaired glucose utilization in the frontal cortex.

EFFECT OF NEUROLEPTICS ON IMMUNE FUNCTION IN SCHIZOPHRENIA

In all areas of psychoimmunology, the direct influence of psychotropic drugs on immune parameters is an important consideration in attempting to unravel the complex immune changes that may be causally related to the disease process. Nowhere is this more apparent than in the treatment of schizophrenic patients with neurolepics, particularly as it is very uncommon to find drug naive patients in whom the basal immune state can be evaluated before the commencement of treatment. Nevertheless, the results of studies of the influence of neuroleptics (mainly the typical neuroleptics such as phenothiazines and haloperidol) are conflicting. *In vitro* studies have described an increase in lymphocyte proliferation to different mitogens in chlorpromazine-treated patients together with the occurrence of abnormal lymphocytes, while other investigators have reported a reduced lymphocyte proliferation following mitogen stimulation with phytohaemagglutinin (PHA) in phenothiazine-treated patients. There is also clinical evidence that chloropromazine and other phenothiazines increase the serum autoantibody (particularly antinuclear antibody) concentration. At least two studies have independently suggested that chlorpromazine, but not apparently other phenothiazines, specifically activates antibody synthesis.

There is a paucity of data regarding the effects of atypical neuroleptics on the immune system. However, there is a suggestion that the atypical neuroleptic clozapine may owe its therapeutic efficacy at least partly to this modulatory action on the immune system. For example, chronic treatment of schizophrenic patients with clozapine was shown to increase the IL-2R concentration in a dose-dependent manner, and decrease the blood concentrations of tumour necrosis factor alpha (TNF-α) and IL-6R to control values; these changes appear to be correlated with the rise in the concentration of the cytokine antagonist, the Clara cell protein, and the IL receptor antagonist. The immunosuppressive actions of clozapine and haloperidol were further supported by the finding that both drugs suppressed mitogen-induced lymphocyte proliferation *in vitro*. However, concentrations of the neuroleptics used to produce these effects exceeded the therapeutic range. When used in the therapeutic range, clozapine and haloperidol were shown to significantly increase the production of IL-1 receptor antagonist from human whole blood, a qualitatively similar effect to that observed following the treatment of schizophrenic patients with clozapine. This is an important finding because the IL-1 receptor antagonist is an endogenous factor which inhibits IL-1 activity and inflammatory response *in vivo*. In addition, it has an "anti-stress"-like action by inhibiting the IL-1 induced activation of the HPA axis. It would therefore appear that clozapine, and halperidol in high doses may reduce the over-activation of T lymphocytes and monocytes/macrophages which are responsible for the increased inflammatory response that occurs in the acute phase of a schizophrenic episode.

With regard to the other proinflammatory cytokines, a biphasic effect of clozapine has been observed *in vitro*, with supratherapeutic doses suppressing the PHA plus lipopolysaccharide (LPS) induced release of interferon gamma (IFN-α) from lymphocytes, while doses in the clinical range increased the release of this cytokine. By contrast, both therapeutic and supratherapeutic concentrations of haloperidol had no effect on the concentration of IFN-α. Doses of clozapine in excess of the therapeutic range have been shown to reduce the IL-6 and IL-IR antagonist concentration in whole blood *in vitro* and IL-10 release from whole blood following mitogen stimulation. Whether these effects are clinically relevant is presently unclear. It is well established that clozapine can cause agranulocytosis in a small percentage of patients but whether this is related to its immunosuppressive action is unknown.

One of the many factors which appear to complicate the interpretation of the results obtained from studies of the immune system in schizophrenics relates to the effects of neuroleptics. However, it has recently been observed that neither typical nor atypical neuroleptics had an effect on mitogen-stimulated lymphocyte responsiveness of schizophrenics, although there is some evidence that long-term treatment with neuroleptics is associated with an increase in the percentage of CD3+ and CD4+ lymphocytes. These findings await replication. Other studies of the effect of medication on the immune system have shown that the percentage of T cells is increased in the peripheral blood of schizophrenic patients, an effect that appears to be largely restricted to lower therapeutic doses of neuroleptics.

There is evidence to show that there are significant differences in the plasma concentrations of IL-1 alpha and IL-6 between drug-free patients and those taking neuroleptics. However, other studies have shown that the IL-6 receptor and the transferrin receptor (a transmembrane glycoprotein, the expression of which is regulated by the growth rate of proliferating cells and by the cell requirement for iron) are raised in the plasma of the schizophrenic patient but return to control values following effective neuroleptic treatment. Clearly, this area of research requires further exploration.

In general, it would appear that the effect of neuroleptics on immune function *in vivo* is slight and may have been overestimated by extrapolations from *in vitro* studies in which higher than therapeutic doses were used. Nevertheless, this is an area that requires further research.

CHANGES IN IMMUNOGLOBULINS IN THE CEREBROSPINAL FLUID

Changes in the protein concentration in the CSF in schizophrenic patients were first noted in 1928 and in more recent studies it has been found that the protein content of the CSF is raised above 50 mg% in 20% or less of schizophrenic patients. This increase in the protein content has been ascribed to an increased permeability of the blood–brain barrier that may occur in schizophrenia combined with a rise in the 1gG concentration that reflects the increased inflammatory process occurring in the brain. However, it should be emphasized that the raised IgG concentration only appears to occur in a minority of schizophrenic patients. In these patients, a positive correlation was found between the degree of affective blunting, alogia/paralogia and the rise in CSF IgG concentration. In addition, there is a suggestion that the rise in the CSF IgG concentration is associated with an increase in the negative symptoms of the disease. Such changes do not appear to have been due to neuroleptic medication.

Thus high CSF IgG concentrations, whether they are due to increased permeability of the blood-brain barrier or to increased synthesis of the antibody within the brain as a consequence of an inflammatory response, may reflect an unfavourable development in the disorder since negative symptoms tend to be chronic and to show a poor response to treatment. However, it must be emphasized that such changes only appear in a minority of schizophrenic patients and cannot be generalized to the majority of patients with this diorder.

CYTOKINE CHANGES IN THE CSF OF SCHIZOPHRENIC PATIENTS

While there is evidence of changes in some cytokines in the blood of schizophrenic patients which might contribute to the causation of some of the acute symptoms of the condition, studies of changes in the cytokine composition of the CSF are more likely to provide and understanding of the immune changes that occur in the brain of the schizophrenic patient. However, there is a relative paucity of data regarding such changes. Despite this limitation, it has been shown that there is a preponderance of type 2 cytokines in the CSF of children with schizophrenia. Type 2 cytokines, such as IL-4, IL-5 and IL-10, are derived from Th2 cells and, as has been mentioned in Chapter 2, are involved in growth and differentiation of B cells and function to protect against extracellular pathogens. By contrast, type 1 cytokines, as exemplified by IL-2, IFN-γ and TNF-β, are derived from Th1 cells and are involved in cell-mediated immunity, cytolysis and protection against intracellular pathogens. The other cytokines such as IL-1, IL-6 and TNF-α do not fit easily into the type 1/type 2 schema.

In schizophrenia in children, the early age of onset and the relative refractoriness of the condition to neuroleptic treatment suggest that such patients may represent a more severe form of the disease and therefore any changes in the immune system of such patients may be more easily separated from a normal population. The results of such a study show that IL-4 concentrations were detectable in the schizophrenic patients but not in those with obsessive compulsive disorder or attention deficit hyperactivity disorder (ADHD); the concentration of IL-5 was similar in patients with OCD, ADHD and schizophrenia. The apparent increase in the concentration of IL-4 was associated with a reciprocal decrease in IL-2 and a slight increase in IFN-α. This finding is of particular interest as IFN-α is an important component of the antivirus immune response and there is a suggestion that viral infections during pregnancy may be associated with an increased incidence of schizophrenia in the offspring. This will be further discussed later in this chapter.

Of the other studies of cytokines in the CSF, an increase in IL-2 concentration has been found in a group of non-medicated adult schizophrenic patients, a finding that contrasts with the reduction in the concentration of this cytokine in the blood of schizophrenic patients. As there is evidence from experimental studies that intracerebroventricularly administered IL-2 increases the brain dopamine concentration, it may be speculated that the increase in the concentration of this cytokine in the CSF may contribute to the hyperdopaminergic state which is implicated in the pathology of schizophrenia. Experimental evidence suggests that IL-2 enhances dopamine release evoked by the excitatory amino acids glutamate (via N-methyl-D-aspartate receptors) and kainate receptors. Dysfunction of the relationship between glutamate and dopamine may underlie the cause of schizophrenia. Furthermore, the increase in CSF concentration of IL-2 has been proposed as a significant predictor of schizophrenic relapse following the withdrawal of neuroleptics such as haloperidol. If replicated, this could be a clinically important finding, as neither the changes in the 5-hydroxyindole acetic acid (5-HIAA) or homovanillic acid (HVA) concentrations nor the anxiety state have been found to be of any predictive value for relapse. The fact that unlike the CSF the serum IL-2 concentration does not have predictive implications for relapse implies that the effects of the brain on serum IL-2 concentrations may either be masked by the known increase in the serum IL-2 receptors or that the activation of this cytokine is restricted to the central nervous system.

CHANGES IN ACUTE PHASE PROTEINS IN SCHIZOPHRENIA

As has already been discussed in Chapter 5, there is evidence that the acute phase response in patients with major depression is related to the increase in some proinflammatory cytokines. Both IL-1 and IL-6 are pleiotropic cytokines which are known modulators of the acute phase response in humans and animals. In depression, these cytokines are known to increase the synthesis of positive acute phase proteins (such as haptoglobin, alpha-l-acid glycoprotein, alpha-l-antitrypsin, haemoplexin, C-reactive protein and anti-chymotrypsin), while reducing the concentration of negative acute phase proteins (as exemplified by albumin and transferrin). Despite the well-established findings of an altered acute phase response in depression, there is a paucity of data regarding such changes in patients with schizophrenia. This is surprising, as there is evidence of monocyte and macrophage activation in patients with schizophrenia, and some preliminary evidence that alpha-l-acid glycoprotein, alpha-l-antitrypsin and haptoglobin concentration are raised. This preliminary finding has been recently confirmed when it was shown that patients with acute psychiatric illness (schizophrenia or mania) have elevated plasma acute phase proteins. These results further confirm the studies that demonstrate that schizophrenia is accompanied by immune activation. In addition, it would appear that the changes in the acute phase proteins are more pronounced in patients with schizophrenia than in those with major depression (for example, the plasma haptoglobin and alpha-1-acid glycoprotein concentrations are higher in schizophrenic than in depressed patients). Thus it may be concluded that the increased acute phase response is not specific to any one major psychiatric disorder but may reflect the response of the patient to the psychological stress that precedes or accompanies such major disorders. Furthermore, it would appear that the plasma concentration of the acute phase proteins are significantly higher in non-medicated schizophrenic and manic patients than in patients on neuroleptics or lithium; these medications have been shown to reduce the acute phase protein response. Whether the effects of psychotropic drugs on the acute phase proteins are due to their direct action on the synthesis of the proteins in the liver or related to changes in the clinical response of the patients to treatment is unknown.

DO VIRUSES PLAY A ROLE IN THE AUTOIMMUNE CHANGES IN SCHIZOPHRENIA?

There are numerous case reports of patients exhibiting the symptoms of schizophrenia following viral infections with herpes simplex encephalitis, varicella zoster encephalitis and subacute sclerosing panencephalitis. In addition, epidemiological data have indicated that schizophrenia is more frequent in patients born to mothers who have been infected with the influenza virus, the frequency of schizophrenia being apparently greater in children born during the winter months. Raised titres to viruses, such as herpes, simplex, measles, cytomegalovirus, varicella and bornavirus, have also been detected in higher concentrations in schizophrenic patients compared to controls. In some studies, these virus titres were found to be increased in the CSF, suggesting that the antibodies have been formed in the brain and CSF of the patients. However, it must be emphasized that not all investigators have found such changes. One possible explanation for the differences may be that the viruses are only detectable during specific phases of the virus infection so the fact that they are undetected does not necessarily exclude their involvement in the pathogenesis of the disease. A similar situation arises, for example, in the case of multiple sclerosis. Multiple sclerosis and schizophrenia show other similarities in that both conditions wax and and wane and frequently show an early onset.

It is not unreasonable to assume that viruses are only detectable during certain stages of a disease process and, if so, the fact that viruses or a viral genome could not be isolated from the brains or body tissues of schizophrenic patients does not necessarily mean that viruses are not involved in the pathology of the condition. In multiple sclerosis, which bears some similarity to schizophrenia in terms of the immune changes, raised virus antibody titres are thought to represent a local synthesis of antibodies against a number of different neurotropic viruses (such as rubella, varicella, etc). Such an antiviral response would indicate an immune dysregulation with an unspecific activation of antibody-producing B cells. Thus multiple sclerosis and schizophrenia may bear similarities not only in terms of the possible genetic predisposition and the waxing and waning of the symptoms during the course of the disease, but also in the occurrence of a schizoform psychosis in both groups of patients. It would therefore seem that the evidence for an activation of the immune system in schizophrenia is compatible with both a viral and an autoimmune hypothesis of schizophrenia. Virus infections may play a role in the aetiology of schizophrenia, at least in a minority of cases. This hypothesis would seem reasonable as viruses induce infected cells to change their identity, probably by expressing new cell membrane antigens, thereby leading to the infected cell being attacked by immune cells.

CONCLUSION

Even though the autoimmune hypothesis of schizophrenia was first postulated over 60 years ago, the evidence currently available neither verifies nor disproves its validity. Most of the studies have reported immune abnormalities in subgroups of patients. While most researchers have speculated that an immune mechanism may play a role in causing a brain dysfunction, other aetiological factors (such as genetic composition, developmental or viral factors) that may be essential for an autoimmune disease to develop have not been adequately addressed. Furthermore, most of the studies reported cannot convincingly establish whether the immune abnormalities are the cause or the effect of the disease since they are largely based on cross-sectional comparisons of patients. Clearly detailed longitudinal studies are essential to provide data on the possible changes in immune function before the occurrence of a relapse in the condition.

If it is eventually proven that schizophrenia is an autoimmune disease, the use of immunomodulators may be of therapeutic value. There is some evidence that the use of levamisole, a T-suppressor cell enhancing drug, has anti-schizophrenic activity at least in a subgroup of young schizophrenic patients. However, most of the immunosuppressive drugs that are currently available are fairly toxic, which limits the practical application of this approach. Treatment strategies aimed at using antigens to immunize patients with proven immune abnormalities may be one approach. In addition, treatments aimed at major histocompatibility complexes, T cell receptor molecules or reducing brain autoantigens may be therapeutically valuable.

Besides the obvious need to standardize protocols with regard to patient numbers and patient selection, more studies need be undertaken on patients who have never received neuroleptic medication as many of the results reporting changes in immune status have been undertaken on mixed populations of medicated and non-medicated individuals. This is an area of research that requires considerable attention. However, despite the variability of the evidence currently available, it does suggest that autoimmune processes may play a causal role in the occurrence of schizophrenia in a minority of patients.

The interconnections between the immune changes that may be involved in the pathology of schizophrenia are shown in Figure 6.1.

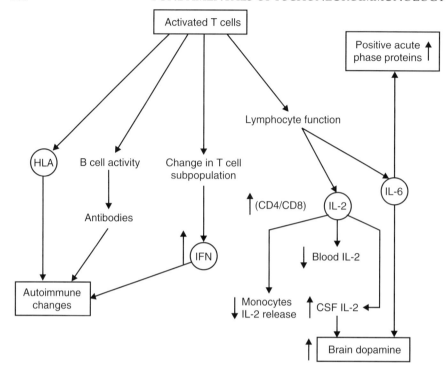

Figure 6.1 Interconnections between the immune changes and dopamine in schizophrenia. IFN, interferon; IL, interleukin.

BIBLIOGRAPHY

Galinowski, K. N., Barbouche, R., Truffinet, P. et al. (1992) Natural autoantibodies in schizophrenia. *Acta Psychiatrica Scandinavica* **85**: 240–242.

Garsuli, R., Rabin, B. S. and Brar, J. S. (1992) Antinuclear and gastric parietal autoantibodies in schizophrenic patients. *Biological Psychiatry* **32**: 735–738.

Gonguli, R., Brar, J. S. and Rabin, B. (1994) Immune abnormalities in schizophrenia: evidence for the autoimmune hypothesis. *Harvard Review of Pschiatry* **2**: 70–83.

Holden, R. J., Pakula, I. S. and Mooney, P. A. (1997) A neuroimmunological model of schizophrenia and major depression: a review. *Human Psychopharmacology* **12**: 177–201.

Lehmann-Facius, H. (1937) Ueber die Liquordiagnose der Schizophrenien. *Klinische Wochenschrift* **16**: 1646–1648.

Logan, D. G. and Deodhar, S. D. (1970) Schizophrenia, an immunological disorder? *JAMA* **212**: 1703–1704.

Maes, M., Bosmans, E., Calabrese, J. et al. (1995) Interleukin 2 and interleukin 6 in schizophrenia and mania: effects of neuroleptics and mood stabilizers. *Journal of Psychiatric Research* **29**: 141–152.

Maes, M., De Lange, J., Ranjan, R. et al. (1997) Acute phase proteins in schizophrenia, mania and major depression: modulation by psychotropic drugs. *Psychiatry Research* **66**: 1–11.

Mittleman, B. B., Castellanos, F. X., Jacobsen, L. K. et al. (1997) Cerebrospinal fluid cytokines in pediatric neuropsychiatric disease. *Journal of Immunology* **159**: 2994–2999.

Muller, N. and Ackeneheil, M. (1995) The immune system and schizophrenia. In: Leonard, B. and Miller, C. (Eds) *Stress, the Immune System and Psychiatry*, pp. 137–164. John Wiley and Sons, Chichester.

Muller, N. and Ackenheil, M. (1998) Pschychoimmunology and the cytokine action in the CNS: implications for psychiatric disorders. *Progress in Neuro-Psychopharmacology and Biological Psychiatry* **22**: 1–32.

Nepons, G. T. and Erlich, H. (1991) MCH class II molecules and autoimmunity. *Annual Review of Immunology* **9**: 493–525.

Roberts, G. W. (1990), Schizophrenia: the cellular biology of a functional psychosis. *Trends in Neuroscience* **13**: 207–211.

Schott, K., Batra, A., Klein R. et al. (1992) Antibodies against serotinin and gangliosides in schizophrenia and major depression. *European Psychiatry* **7**: 209–212.

Sundin, U. and Thelander, S. (1989) Antibody reactivity to brain membrane proteins in serum from schizophrenic patients. *Brain, Behavior, and Immunity* **3**: 343–358.

7 Psychoneuroimmunology of Anxiety Disorders

INTRODUCTION

The concept of anxiety as a psychiatric disorder arose many years ago when it became necessary to distinguish pathological anxiety (also called anxiety neurosis) from anxiety that was a novel human response to a stressful situation. With the advent of the Diagnostic and Statistical Manual of Mental Disorders (DSM) in the USA and the International Classification of Diseases (ICD) by the World Health Organization, anciety disorders became classified into several subtypes, as shown in Table 7.1. A major advantage of this classification is that it has led to better criteria for epidemiological assessment.

Table 7.1: Subtypes of anxiety disorder (anxiety neurosis)

Generalized anxiety disorder	(GAD)
Panic disorder	(PD)
Obsessive compulsive disorder	(OCD)
Post-traumatic stress disorder	(PTSD)
Social phobia	(SP)
Phobic disorders	(PB)
Mixed anxiety depression	(MAD)

In addition to the above classification, the DSM IV classification also includes the category of *acute stress disorder*, which is an immediate response to a major traumatic event and, unlike post-traumatic stress disorder, seldom lasts longer than one month after the traumatic event.

Irrespective of the type of anxiety disorder, stress (either psychological, environmental or physical) plays a part either as an initiating factor or as a consequence of the condition. This impacts upon both the endocrine and immune systems and although there is now substantial information indicating that stress can alter immune function (see Chapter 4), few studies have examined the parameters of the stressful experience and the precise mechanism whereby a stressor alters immune function.

One approach to elucidating the mechanism involved in stress reactions and anxiety disorders is to study the effects of anxiolytic drugs that are used to treat the symptoms of the disorder. The benzodiazepines are undoubtedly the most useful anxiolytics and specifically counteract the behavioural, neurochemical and hormonal changes that are induced by stress or anxiety. In the brain, it is well established that the anxiolytic effects of the benzodiazepines are mediated by the activation of benzodiazepine receptor sites which are located on the gamma-aminobutyric acid (GABA) type A receptor complex. Benzodiazepines facilitate central inhibitory neurotransmission by increasing the frequency of opening of the chloride ion channels by GABA. Drugs such as diazepam thus reduce the degree of anxiety or stress by inhibiting the release of corticotrophin-releasing factor (CRF), the major stress peptide that both activates the pituitary–adrenal axis and suppresses the immune response (Figure 7.1).

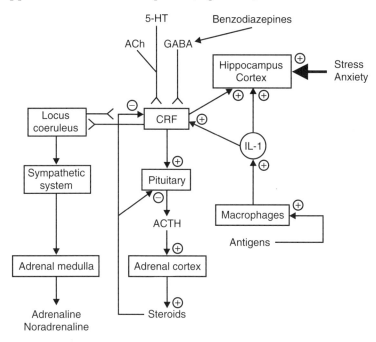

Figure 7.1 Diagram of changes in the endocrine and immune systems in stress and anxiety. ACh, acetylcholine; 5-HT, 5-hydroxytryptamine; GABA, gamma-aminobutyric acid; CRF, corticotrophin-releasing factor; IL-1, interleukin-1; +, stimulatory; –, inhibitory.

In addition to the indirect action of the benzodiazepines on the immune and endocrine systems which are modulated through the release of CRF, benzodiazepines can directly affect the peripheral organs, and the immune system in particular, by activating peripheral benzodiazepine receptors. These receptors are quite distinct from the central GABA-A receptors that are associated with the mitochondria and plasma membranes. In addition, they are located on glial cells in the brain and on lymphocytes in the immune system. Unlike the central benzodiazepine receptors which are responsible for the allosteric modulation of GABA synapses, the peripheral benzodiazepine receptors are involved in the control of cell proliferation, steroidogenesis and regulating the immune response. The affinity of benzodiazepines for the peripheral and central benzodiazepine receptors is of the same order of magnitude, which indicates that the immune system is directly influenced by therapeutic concentrations of these drugs.

THE ROLE OF PERIPHERAL BENZODIAZEPINE RECEPTORS IN ANXIETY DISORDERS AND IMMUNOMODULATION

Benzodiazepines have been shown to be potent stimulators of monocyte chemotaxis *in vitro*, an effect that occurs through the activation of the peripheral benzodiazepine receptors; the peripheral benzodiazepine antagonist PK-11195 can block this effect. Benzodiazepines have also been shown to stimulate the humoral immune response of mice to sheep red blood cells, to enhance the synthesis of interleukin-1 (IL-1) and tumour necrosis factor alpha (TNF-α); *in vitro*, benzodiazpines have been shown to inhibit the secretion of IL-1 and IL-2, which emphasizes the caution that must be taken in extrapolating from *in vitro* to *in vivo* studies. It is of interest that the benzodiazepine inverse agonist DMCM (methyl-6, 7-dimethoxy-4-ethyl-beta carboline), which causes anxiety in both animals and humans, has been shown to reduce the humoral immune response to a keyhole limpet haemocyanin challenge in rats.

In patients with generalized anxiety disorder (GAD), a significant decrease in the density of the peripheral benzodiazepine receptors occurred on the circulating lymphocytes which was largely normalized by effective treatment with chronically administered diazepam; acutely administered diazepam was without effect. These changes in the receptor density would appear to be specific for the anxiety disorder. The control and differentiation of normal and malignant cells *in vitro* is also known to be influenced by peripheral benzodiazepine receptors. The precise mechanism whereby the immunomodulatory and antiproliferative action of these receptors occurs is controversial and could occur either by the regulation of voltage dependent calcium channels or by the regulation of oncogene expression.

In addition to the direct action of benzodiazepines on peripheral benzodiazepine receptors located on immune cells, it is also possible that the immune system is indirectly affected by the increased synthesis of adrenal corticosteroids. There is also evidence that steroidogenesis is increased in the brain following the administration of benzodiazepines that stimulate peripheral benzodiazepine receptors. Such neurosteroids have an affinity from the GABA-A receptor complex and could therefore contribute to the anxiolytic and stress-reducing effects of these drugs.

The results of these clinical and experimental studies suggest that the peripheral benzodiazepine receptors play a prominent role in the cellular and humoral immune response. Anxiolytics that act on central and/or peripheral benzodiazepine receptors can modulate the immune system either indirectly by reducing the central secretion of CRF, the major stress hormone, by acting on central GABA-A receptors, or directly by stimulating the peripheral benzodiazepine receptors on immune cells. There is experimental evidence to suggest that an endogenous ligand for central benzodiazepine receptors exists, the diazepam binding inhibitor, which has anxiogenic properties. The identity of endogeous substances that act as anxiolytics, and which are therefore agonists at central and peripheral benzodiazepine receptor sites, is uncertain.

IMMUNE CHANGES ASSOCIATED WITH PANIC DISORDER

Panic disorder, frequently associated with agoraphobia, is a syndrome in which severe anxiety is the core of the disease, with panic attack initiating severe stressful episodes. Panic attacks are also often associated with severe depressive episodes. The coexistence of anxiety, depression and severe episodes of stress suggests that the immune function in patients with panic disorder would be severely impaired. Somewhat surprisingly, there is evidence that the lymphocyte count and lymphocyte subsets (T, B, CD4, CD8, natural killer (NK) cells) are relatively normal, although variable results have been obtained regarding the lymphocyte proliferative response to mitogens with reports of an increase, decrease or no change relative to control values. With respect to the changes in number of T and B cells in patients with panic disorder, it should be noted that some studies have reported an increased number of NK cells, B cells and lymphocyte expressing HLA-DR.

A major problem in interpreting these results arises from the fact that several of the patients studied suffered from depression in addition to panic attacks; such heterogeneity of the clinical status could have profoundly influenced the results. Thus in a group of 17 patients with panic disorder without concomitant depression, Brambilla and coworkers showed that mitogen stimulation of T lymphocytes was normal despite the fact that the patients suffered from severe anxiety and had frequent panic attacks. In these patients, there was also evidence of an elevated plasma ACTH concentration and a blunted cortisol response to dexamethasone. Thus it appears that the proliferative response of T lymphocytes is dissociated from the hyperactivity of the hypothalamic–pituitary–adrenocortical (HPA) axis. This is supported by the finding that the administration of CRF, with the ensuing hypersecretion of ACTH and cortisol, did not suppress the proliferative response of the T lymphocytes; this finding is important as the response of T lymphocytes to mitogen stimulation gives more information regarding the plasticity of the immune system than the static counts of lymphocytes or their subsets. The lack of change in the proliferative response of T lymphocytes in patients with "pure" panic disorder would suggest that the secretion of IL-2, IL-6 and interferon would also be unchanged. However, there is evidence from other studies that female patients with panic disorder have a slight increase in the serum concentrations of IL-2 but other investigators have shown that IL-1 alpha and IL-1 beta were also unchanged when compared with age- and gender-matched controls. It is possible that the differences between the study in which only female patients were involved and the Brambilla study, in which an equal number of males and female patients were investigated, could be a reflection of the gender differences.

The potent antipanic benzodiazepine alprazolam differs in its effect on the immune system of humans and rodents. Thus in patients with panic disorder, therapeutically effective doses of alprazolam have no effect on the proliferative response of T lymphocytes. By contrast, in experimental animals, low doses of the drug have been shown to enhance the immune function, while high doses (greater than those used therapeutically) have an immunosuppressive effect. These differences are probably related to the species specificity and the duration of alprazolam administration; it again emphasizes the difficulty in extrapolating from results obtained from immune changes in animals to those obtained from patients. Despite the apparent lack of effect of alprazolam on T-cell proliferation in patients with "pure" panic disorder, there is evidence from clinical studies that alprazolam attenuates the hypersecretion of ACTH and growth hormone in these patients and normalizes the blunted dexamethasone suppression test (DST) response.

There is evidence that the circulating lymphocyte surface markers seen in patients suffering from panic disorder differ from these found in patients with other psychiatric disorders. Thus patients with panic disorder were found to have increased numbers of NK cells (CD16 cell markers), B lymphocytes (CD19 markers), human lymphocyte antigen presenting cells (HLA-DR cells) and CD19 surface markers (B lymphocytes with HLA-DR markers on their surface). This pattern of lymphocyte phenotypic markers is not present in depressed patients (nor in those with comorbid panic disorder), in bipolar patients or schizophrenic patients, but such changes have been reported in normal subjects who have been exposed to severe acute psychological stress.

The concentration of some immunoglublins has been shown to change in response to anxiety. Thus salivary IgA concentrations have been shown to decrease in anxious nurses and dental students relative to their non-anxious colleagues. However, somewhat surprisingly patients with "pure" panic disorder show a significant increase in serum IgA concentration relative to a control population; concentrations of IgG, IgM and IgE were unchanged. While the precise relevance of this finding is uncertain, it would appear that patients with panic disorder differ from those with acute anxiety or major depression in this aspect of immune dysfunction. Nevertheless, a major problem in interpreting the data relating to the immune changes associated with panic disorder is the paucity of the studies, the heterogeneity of the patients studied and the differences in the method used to assess the immune parameters.

IMMUNE CHANGES ASSOCIATED WITH OBSESSIVE COMPULSIVE DISORDER

Obsessive compulsive disorder (OCD) is an anxiety disorder characterized by recurrent obsession and/or compulsions which cause marked distress and interfere with the daily life of the patient; OCD is commonly associated with depression and anxiety. Unlike the other subtypes of anxiety disorder, there is evidence of a neurological deficit in OCD associated with a dysfunction of the central serotonergic system, particularly in the region of the basal ganglia. While there have been a number of studies devoted to an examination of the endocrine axis in OCD, little attention has been paid to changes in immune function in this condition. However, there is evidence of serum antibodies against somatostatin-14 and prodynorphin 209-240 in some patients with OCD, which suggests that there is an underlying autoimmune mechanism in some patients.

T-helper cells play a major role in the pathogenesis of some autoimmune diseases. This leads to excessive IL-2 release from the activated T-helper cells which could result in the activation of B cells and autoantibody production. However, in a group of 11 non-depressed patients with a history of OCD, no changes in the *in vitro* synthesis of IL-1 beta, IL-2 and IL-3 like activity could be detected. Furthermore, effective treatment of the patients with clomipramine did not affect the basal cytokine concentrations. Other studies have also shown that the basal concentrations of IL-1 beta, IL-6 and IL-6 (IL-6R) receptor were unchanged in patients with OCD but there was a correlation between IL-6 and IL-6R and the severity of the compulsive symptoms of the disorder. It is, of course, possible that cytokine synthesis *in vivo* is altered in these patients. Clearly there are fundamental differences in the immune profiles of patients with OCD and those with major depression; clomipramine has been found largely to normalize the effective synthesis of proinflammatory cytokines in depression.

Despite the apparent lack of change in serum IL-1, IL-2 and IL-3 like activity in adult patients with OCD, there is evidence that children with the disorder have an abnormality in cell-mediated (Th1) cytokines, but not humoral (Th2) cytokines in the cerebrospinal fluid (CSF). Thus the concentrations of IL-2, IFN-γ and TNF-β were slightly raised in the CSF of children with OCD but no change could be detected in the type 2 cytokines (IL-4, IL-5, IL-10) and TNF-α. It has been postulated that infection with *Streptococcus pyogenes* may be involved in the pathogeneisis of OCD in some children; an increased prevalence in the genetic marker associated with rheumatic fever in children with OCD has also been detected, which may account for the fact that symptoms of OCD may occur transiently in children with Sydenham's chorea, a varient of rheumatic fever. It would appear that there are a number of known immunogens associated with *S. pyogenes* that induce an immune response associated primarily with an increase in Th1 cytokines.

The results of this study serve to emphasize the importance of determining cytokine concentrations not only in the serum but also in the CSF in order to gain an insight into the immune changes that are coincidentally, or possibly causally, related to OCD.

IMMUNE CHANGES ASSOCIATED WITH POST-TRAUMATIC STRESS DISORDER (PTSD)

A vast literature is available on the symptoms that arise following combat trauma, rape, kidnapping, natural disasters, accidents and imprisonment. Such studies have shown that the traumatic response is biphasic in that hypermnesia, hyperreactivity to external stimuli and re-experiencing of the trauma coexist with psychic numbing, avoidance, amnesia and anhedonia. In many patients with PTSD, the symptoms decrease with time, but they may presist for years in others. It is not surprising to find that the intense stress that occurs in patients who are exposed to a traumatic event is accompanied by the release of cortisol, adrenaline and noradrenaline, vasopressin, oxytocin and endogenous opioids. While acute stress is known to activate the HPA axis and increase the secretion of glucocorticoids, animals (including humans) adapt to chronic stress by activating the negative feedback loop. However, patients with PTSD often fail to show this adaptive response. Thus there is evidence of a chronic increase in the activity of the sympathetic nervous sytem even though some studies have shown that some PTSD patients have a lower cortisol excretion and an increased density of lymphocyte glucocorticoid receptors. With regard to the changes in endogenous opioid concentrations in such patients, it has been shown that even two decades after the original trauma, PTSD patients develop opioid-mediated analgesia in response to a traumatic stimulus. The increase in endogenous opioids appears to be responsible for the blunting of the emotional response to the traumatic stimulus. From such studies it would appear that PTSD is associated with a maladaptive response to traumatic stimuli which clearly differs from the changes seen following exposure to a chronic stress or that occur in the other anxiety disorders.

Despite the numerous studies of changes in the endocrine system in patients with PTSD, few studies have investigated immune function in such patients. There is evidence of a higher frequency of delayed-type hypersensitivity response to numerous antigens in Vietnam combat veterans with

PTSD compared to those veterans without combat exposure or to civilians. It would be anticipated that the higher basal glucocorticoid receptor density on lymphocytes, and increased down-regulation of these receptors following dexamethasone administration, would have a major impact on cellular immunity. However, while some studies have found that NK cell activity in Vietnam combat PTSD patients did not differ from age-matched alcohol and drug abuse controls, others have shown that the activity of the NK cells is increased.

A major problem in interpreting the results of studies of changes in the immune system relates to the high frequency of comorbidity of this condition, depression, alcohol and drug abuse being frequently associated with PTSD. Alcoholism and depression appear to be additive in their negative impact on NK cell cytotoxicity. Furthermore, the delayed-type hypersensitivity response is elevated in PTSD but reduced in depressed patients, which emphasizes the difficulty in assessing the relationship between the symptoms of PTSD and the changes in immune competence. Nevertheless, preliminary studies suggest that the chronic effects of PTSD may differ from those occurring immediately following a traumatic event. Studies of populations immediately following natural disasters, such as earthquakes or hurricanes, suggest that the activity of NK cells is reduced. Clearly, more detailed studies are urgently required to assess fully the changes in cellular and humoral immunity that are associated with PTSD.

SUMMARY AND CONCLUSION

Peripheral benzodiazepine receptors occur on circulating lymphocytes that appear to modulate the humoral immune response and enhance the synthesis of IL-1 and TNF-α. In addition, *in vitro* studies show that these receptors stimulate monocyte chemotaxis. Patients with generalized anxiety disorder have a reduced density of peripheral benzodiazepine receptors on lymphocytes; treatment with benzodiazepines largely normalizes the density of these receptors. In the brain, the peripheral benzodiazepine receptors stimulate steroidogenesis. The resulting neurosteroids have an affinity for the GABA-A receptors, which could account for their anxiolytic and stress-reducing effects.

Panic disorder is associated with hyperactivity of the HPA axis, yet the proliferative response of T lymphocytes is unchanged. Patients with panic disorder may be distinguished from those with depression with respect to the increase in the number of NK cells, B lymphocytes and human lymphocyte antigen presenting cells found in those with panic disorder. These changes appear to be related to the effects of severe, acute stress. With respect to humoral immunity, the IgA concentration is raised in those with panic disorder.

Patients with *obsessive compulsive disorder* show an abnormality in humoral immunity; antibodies against somatostatin and prodynorphin are raised but no changes in the *in vitro* synthesis of IL-1, IL-2 and IL-3 like acivity are apparent. However, there is evidence from the analysis of the CSF of children with OCD that the concentrations of IL-2, IFN-γ and TNF-β are raised, which suggests a disorder in type I (cell-mediated) immunity in this subgroup of patients. Finally, patients with *post-traumatic stress disorder* appear to have a higher frequency of delayed-type hypersensitivity responses to numerous antigens when compared to non-traumatized control subjects. There is some evidence that NK cell activity is increased in some patients with this disorder but other studies have failed to replicate this finding; the activity of NK cells is reduced in recently traumatized patients.

The evidence suggesting that different subtypes of anxiety are associated with different immune profiles requires more extensive studies on homogeneous populations of patients using the same standard methods for determining the same parameters of cellular and humoral immunity. Until this is done, no firm conclusion can be drawn regarding the possible importance of changes in immune function to the aetiology of these disorders.

In attempting to relate immune changes to the psychopathology of different types of anxiety disorders, an additional problem relates to the role that the glucocorticoids and sympathetic system may play in activating or inhibiting cellular immunity. All anxiety disorders are associated with an over-activation of the sympathetic system which is anatomically connected to the major immune organs and the pituitary–adrenal axis. Thus many of the changes in immune function could be a consequence of the increased activity of the sympathetic system and the pituitary–adrenal axis.

BILBIOGRAPHY

Brambilla, F., Bellodi, L., Perna, G., Battaglia, M. et al. (1992) Psychoimmuno-endocrine aspects of panic disorder. *Neuropsychobiology* **26**: 12–22.

Ferrarese, C., Appollonio, I., Bianchi, G., Frigo, M. et al. (1993) Benzodiazepine receptors and diazepam binding inhibitor: a possible link between stress, anxiety and the immune system. *Psychoneuroendocrinology* **B18**: 3–22.

Laudenslager, M. L., Aasal, R., Adler, L., Berger, C. H. et al. (1998) Elevated cytotoxicity in combat veterans with long term post traumatic stress disorder: Preliminary observations. *Brain, Behavior, and Immunity* **12**: 74–79.

Mittleman, B. B., Catellanos, F. X., Jacobsen, L. K. et al. (1997) Cerebrospinal fluid cytokines in pediatric neuropsychiatric disease. *Journal of Immunology* **159**: 2994–2999.

Rapaport, M. H. (1998) Circulating lymphocyte phenotypic surface markers in anxiety disorder patients and normal volunteers. *Biological Psychiatry* **43**: 458–463.

Weizman, R., Laor, N., Barber, Y. et al. (1996) Cytokine production in obsessive compulsive disorder. *Biological Psychiatry* **40**: 908–912.

8 Polyunsaturated Fatty Acids, the Immune System and Psychiatric Disorders

ESSENTIAL FATTY ACIDS

The importance of essential dietary, polyunsaturated fatty acids, particularly the ω-6 fatty acids linoleic and arachidonic acids, has been known since the pioneering studies of George and Mildred who showed in 1929 that young rats when fed on a fat-free diet failed to grow, developed a scaly dermatitis and were largely sterile. More recently, it has been shown that the other main group of dietary polyunsaturated fatty acids, namely the ω-3 compounds exemplified by eicosapentaenoic and docosahexanoic acids, when deficient in the diet produce malfunction in the brain and the visual system. This outline of the pathways leading to the synthesis of the ω-3 and ω-6 fatty acids in the brain is shown in Figure 8.1.

Diets deficient in ω-3 fatty acids result in defects in learning, lowered visual activity thresholds and abnormal electroretinograms in rodents, monkeys and human infants. It is now known that the rod outer segments of photoreceptors in the retina contain a high concentration of the ω-3 docosahexanoic acid. A high concentration of this fatty acid is also found in the synaptic membranes. Indeed, there is now considerable evidence to show that polyunsaturated fatty acids of both the ω-3 and ω-6 series are crucial to the normal functioning of excitable membranes in both the retina and brain.

The term "eicosanoid" was proposed by Carey in 1980 to denote a series of oxygenated compounds that had been derived from 20-carbon polyunsaturated fatty acids. The major precursor of the eicosanoids is arachidonic acid and this can give rise to a number of different oxygenated products such as the prostaglandins, prostacyclins and leucotrienes. The main pathways are illustrated in Figure 8.2.

Fatty acids of the ω-3 series, such as eicosapentaenoic acid and docosahexanoic acid, are important constituents of fish oils, whereas the ω-6 fatty acids are primarily found in vegetable oils. Thus the ω-3 and ω-6 fatty acids would appear to fulfil different physiological functions, the former being associated with vision and synaptic plasticity, while the latter, through the synthesis of prostaglandins of the E series, appear to function as second messengers and modulators of synaptic transmission. In addition, there is ample evidence to

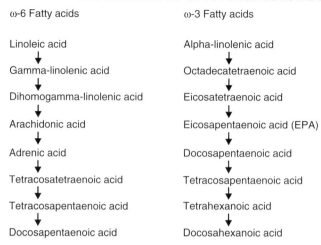

Figure 8.1 Diagramatic representation of the pathways leading to the synthesis of ω-3 and ω-6 polyunsaturated fatty acids in the brain. Summary of the synthesis of the essential polyunsaturated fatty acids of the ω-3 and ω-6 series from their dietary precursors linoleic acid (from vegetable sources) and alpha-linolenic acid (from fish oil). Functionally, arachidonic and docosahexanoic acids are the most important members of the ω-6 and ω-3 series respectively. Dihomogamma-linolenic and eicosapentaenoic acids are important as cell signalling and enzyme regulating molecules in addition to their role as precursors of other eicosanoids.

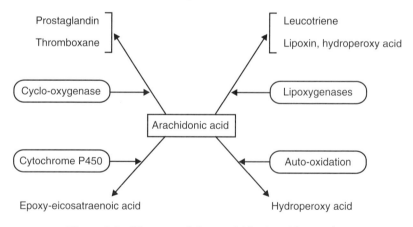

Figure 8.2 Diagram of the arachidonic acid cascade.

show that inflammatory changes in the brain and non-nervous tissue involve the intervention of several products of the arachidonic acid pathway (such as the prostaglandins, thromboxanes, leucotrienes) as well as the interferons and proinflammatory cytokines. These mediators act in concert to amplify the inflammatory response and of these, the prostaglandins of the E series appear to play a particularly important role in the inflammatory process. This is shown by their detection in the inflammatory exudate and also by the efficacy of cyclo-oxygenase inhibitors such as indomethacin and aspirin to inhibit the inflammatory response. Of the other arachidonic acid products that play a role in the inflammatory response, leucotriene B4 has been shown to possess potent chemotactic and degranulating effects on polymorphonuclear leucocytes and to cause the accumulation of these immune cells at the site of inflammation in the brain tissue. Other leucotrienes (for example, the leucotrienes C4, D4 and E4) are synthesized by macrophages and eosinophils and functions in a similar manner to leucotriene B4; the net effect of the increased concentrations of prostaglandins and leucotrienes is to enhance the inflammatory response.

Should brain ischaemia occur, the activation of phospholipases and lipases results in the generation of free fatty acids, particularly arachidonic acid, and the inflammatory response. As a consequence of the release of the vasoconstrictor thromboxanes and vasodilator prostacyclins, haemostasis and the integrity of the vascular system is affected. This leads to alterations in the microcirculation. In addition, free radicals are produced by the action of hydroperoxidase products that arise when prostaglandin G2 is converted to prostaglandin H2. These free radicals can cause intracellular damage and may ultimately be responsible for the brain destruction that arises during ischaemic injury. This situation is further exacerbated by the increased production of fatty acid hydroperoxides.

EICOSANOIDS, PROINFLAMMATORY CYTOKINES AND INFLAMMATORY PROCESSES

The interrelationship between the cytokines and the eicosanoids can be summarized as shown in Figure 8.3. From this diagram, it can be seen that the ω-3 and ω-6 fatty acids have antagonistic effects upon the inflammatory response, the former decreasing the formation and release of proinflammatory cytokines, while the latter enhance the inflammatory response largely due to the increased synthesis of prostaglandins.

Evidence for this view is provided by studies in animals in which the proinflammatory cytokine interleukin-1 (IL-1) is shown to cause anorexia. This effect of IL-1 is abolished by pretreatment with ω-3 polyunsaturated fatty acids such as eicosapentaenoic acid (EPA); EPA is the principal active metabolite of alpha-linolenic acid in the ω-3 series of fatty acids. In humans, a dietary supplement of fish oil rich in ω-3 polyunsaturated fatty acids suppresses the ability of mononuclear cells to synthesize both IL-1 and tumour necrosis factor alpha (TNF-α). Other clinical studies have also shown that ω-3 fatty acids can attenuate the symptoms of rheumatoid arthritis, an effect that may be attributed to the decrease in the synthesis of prostaglandins from arachidonic acid and a reduction in proinflammatory cytokines.

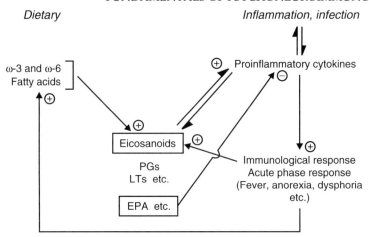

Figure 8.3 Relationship between cytokines and eicosanoids. PGs, prostaglandins; LTs, leucotrienes; EPA, eicosapentaenoic acid.

Eicosanoids such as leucotriene B4, prostaglandin E2 (PGE2) and thromboxane B2 are known to be contributory factors in the development of inflammatory and artherosclerotic diseases. It can therefore be hypothesized that feeding diets that are enriched with ω-3 polyunsaturated fatty acids should reduce the severity of such diseases. Epidemiological, clinical and experimental studies support this hypothesis. For example, Greenland Eskimos who consume diets that are enriched with fish oil have a low incidence of atherosclerosis, autoimmune and inflammatory diseases when compared to European populations which consume a varied diet. In clinical studies of patients with psoriasis, a common inflammatory disease of the skin, it has been shown that feeding fish oil supplements reduces the symptoms of the disease, an effect that was correlated with a decrease in the synthesis of proinflammatory cytokines and a reduction in arachidonic acid derived eicosanoids. Other clinical studies have shown that dietary supplementation with fish oil has a modest, but beneficial effect on inflammatory bowel disease, particularly ulcerative colitis, diseases in which IL-1 and the eicosanoids (particularly leucotriene B4) have been implicated.

It would appear from both clinical and experimental studies that in the case of inflammatory diseases, ω-3 polyunsaturated fatty acids have a beneficial effect. However, in those with a compromised immune status, or the elderly, a reduction in cytokine or eicosanoid synthesis could lead to an impairment of host defence and normal platelet aggregation. It is known that an increase in ω-3 fatty acids in the diet decreases IL-2 synthesis, T-cell mitogen induced proliferation and delayed hypersensitivity skin responses. There is clinical evidence that dietary supplements of fish oil in elderly women cause a significant reduction in IL-2 synthesis and T-cell-mediated function.

In animal studies, feeding fish oil was found to inhibit the ability of assessory cells in the mouse to present antigens to T-helper cells. These animals also had a reduced ability to destroy mastocytoma cells upon stimulation with lipopolysaccaride or interferon (IFN) gamma, which may be a consequence of the reduction in the number of natural killer (NK) cells that also occurred in these animals following the feeding of a high fish oil diet.

Thus the effect of ω-3 polyunsaturated fatty acids on resistance to infectious diseases appears to vary depending on the nature of the infectious agent, the age of the subject and the mechanism involved in the pathogenesis of the disease. Clearly, further studies are required to determine the clinical implications of dietary supplementation with fish oil on host defence mechanisms in humans. It should be emphasized that the mechanism whereby ω-3 fatty acids suppress the synthesis of proinflammatory cytokines is still unknown.

Mention has already been made of the adverse effects of free radicals produced by the oxidation of ω-3 fatty acids. Without adequate antioxidant protection (for example, by vitamin E) ω-3 fatty acids such as eicosapentaenoic and docosahexanoic acids may potentiate the oxidation of neuronal membranes which can result in cell death. Free radicals have been implicated in stroke, emphysema, cataract and cancer. The high incidence of depression that occurs following a stroke is pertinent not only to the excessive production of free radicals that could arise following the administration of eicosanoids in the absence of an antioxidant, but also to the macrophage theory of depression. It is well established that both monocytes and microglia rapidly infiltrate the damaged tissue following experimentally induced stroke. IL-1 would appear to be the primary cytokine involved in the pathological changes that subsequently occur. This would support the hypothesis that depression following stroke is caused by an increase in proinflammatory cytokines within the brain. Thus the addition of ω-3 polyunsaturated fatty acids to the diet should not always be seen as being beneficial to health or as a positive way to reduce the harmful effects of inflammatory cytokines.

In summary, the ω-3 polyunsaturated fatty acids reduce the synthesis of proinflammatory cytokines and lipid mediators (such as the leucotrienes and thromboxanes), which contributes to the anti-inflammatory and anti-atherosclerotic effects of fish oil. However, such beneficial effects may be counteracted by an increase in free radical formation and lipid peroxidation in the absence of adequate antioxidant protection. Therefore, the potentially advantageous effects of dietary ω-3 fatty acids on the immune system may be offset by the deleterious consequences of free radical formation, lipid peroxidation and decreased T-cell-mediated immunity.

EICOSANOIDS, PROINFLAMMATORY CYTOKINES AND DEPRESSION

Epidemiological studies show that the incidence of depression, coronary heart disease and rheumatoid arthritis is significantly lower in Japan than in the USA and most European countries. One possible explanation for this observation relates to the high dietary intake of fish oil in Japan which leads to a reduction in proinflammatory cytokine synthesis. This reduction in cytokine activity could account for the reduced incidence not only of heart disease and arthritis but also of depression.

The precise mechanism whereby ω-3 fatty acids from fish oil may be protective against depression is uncertain. It is known that changes in the cholesterol and phospholipid content of neuronal membranes result in an altered membrane microviscosity and consequently, in the various neurotransmitter systems that have been implicated in depression. In patients with major depression, it has been shown that there is a positive relationship between the severity of depression and the ratio of arachidonic (an ω-6 fatty acid) to eicosapentaenic acid (an ω-3 fatty acid) in both serum phospholipids and erythrocyte membranes. Since the polyunsaturated fatty acids are either precursors of eicosanoids, or affect the synthesis of eicosanoids, they have fundamental effects on inflammatory processes. In those individuals consuming a conventional European type of diet, the most abundant eicosanoid precursor in neuronal and erythrocyte membranes is arachidonic acid from which the inflammatory mediators PGE2 and leucotriene B4 are derived.

There is evidence to show that eicosapentaenoic and docosahexanoic acids, major components of fish oil, inhibit the formation of PGE2. Thus the increased ratio of ω-6 to ω-3 polyunsaturated fatty acids reported to occur in patients with severe depression suggests that the changes in fatty acid composition may be related to immune (or inflammatory) changes in these patients.

In clinical studies, there is evidence that fish oil reduces the synthesis of IL-1, IL-2, IL-6, TNF-α and also decreases the expression of IL-2 receptors (CD25) and suppresses monocyte proliferation. Conversely, diets rich in the ω-6 fatty acid linoleic acid from corn oil increase the synthesis of proinflammatory cytokines. An additional adverse effect on the ω-3 to ω-6 fatty acid ratio could arise as a consequence of the anorexia and weight loss that is characteristic of major depression. Thus it has been shown that, in such patients, there is a relative increase in some of the ω-6 fatty acids (particularly arachidonic acid), which could result in a further increase in proinflammatory cytokines and a reduction in ω-3 fatty acids. These changes in the fatty acid composition in depressed patients appear to be largely confined to the plasma cholesteryl ester fraction rather than the plasma phospholipids. Furthermore, no changes could be found in the composition of saturated or monosaturated fatty acids in depressed patients. These results therefore suggest that a long-term dietary deficiency of ω-3 fatty acids, or abnormal metabolism of such fatty acids, possibly due to increased oxidation or decreased desaturation of the ω-3 fatty acids, may be associated with the psychopathology of depression.

Undoubtedly the relationship between the polyunsaturated fatty acids, the changes in the inflammatory markers and the consequent symptoms of depression are extremely complex. For example, it is known that some cytokines can stimulate lipid synthesis in the liver, which leads to a sustained rise in plasma triglycerides and a reduction in plasma cholesterol. Such changes could contribute to the increase in coronary heart disease and suicidal behaviour of patients with severe depression; several studies have independently shown that a low serum cholesterol concentration is correlated with increased suicidal behaviour. Furthermore, cytokines can significantly affect the metabolism of phospholipids. Thus IL-1 and TNF-α activate the enzyme phospholipase A2, thereby leading to a reduction in the arachidonic acid content of cellular phospholipids, while INF-α increases the uptake and turnover of arachidonic acid macrophages. Such cytokine-induced changes in lipid metabolism appear to be part of the increased acute phase response which occurs in patients with major depression.

The outcome of such changes would therefore contribute to the inflammatory condition in the brain which is the basis of the macrophage theory of depression. If this theory is credible, it follows that increasing the dietary intake of ω-3 polyunsaturated fatty acids (together with vitamin E as an antioxidant) should lead to a reduction in the synthesis of IL-1, IL-2, IL-6 and in PGE2 and an attenuation of the symptoms of depression.

EICOSANOIDS, CYTOKINES AND SCHIZOPHRENIA

The hypothesis that increased synthesis of IL-2 plays a pivotal role in the pathogenesis of schizophrenia is supported by the observation that this cytokine can dose dependently provoke schizophrenic symptoms in otherwise psychiatrically normal subjects. The symptoms provoked by IL-2 included delusions and severe cognitive impairment; some changes also occurred in the mood of the subjects.

In addition to the changes in IL-2, there is also evidence from other parameters of activation of the immune system in patients with schizophrenia. These changes have been discussed in detail elsewhere (see Chapter 6), but include increased CD4+ T lymphocytes, CD5+ B lymphocytes and decreased IgG immunoglobulins and NK cell activity.

A major difficulty in the interpretation of the immune changes relates to the confounding effects of neuroleptic medication. For example, there is evidence that neuroleptics suppress mitogen-stimulated IL-2 synthesis *in vitro*. Even when patients have been medication free for several weeks, erroneous results may be obtained because of the duration of action of the active metabolites of some of the phenothiazine neuroleptics. Active metabolites are excreted in some cases for up to 60 days after cessation of treatment. Nevertheless, there is evidence that the synthesis of IL-2 from mitogen-stimulated lymphocytes is elevated in neuroleptic-free schizophrenic patients and is inversely correlated with the bizarre behaviour and formal thought disorder subscales of the Scales for Assessment of Positive Symptoms. However, there is also evidence that the synthesis of IL-2 from stimulated lymphocytes is reduced in patients suffering from paranoid schizophrenia and these changes appear to be inversely related to the negative symptoms of the disorder. The decrease in the *in vitro* synthesis of IL-2 by the lymphocytes has been interpreted as an exhaustion effect caused by the increased synthesis of the cytokine by the cells.

Increased soluble IL-2 receptor concentrations have been widely reported to occur in the serum of patients with schizophrenia, but there is some evidence that the increase in the IL-2 receptor may be a consequence of neuroleptic medication. In addition to the changes in IL-2, there is also evidence that the concentration of IL-6 is raised in the serum of schizophrenic patients and of an increase in the soluble IL-6 receptor in patients with paranoid schizophrenia.

Unlike depression, where there is now substantial clinical and experimental evidence to suggest that a relative deficiency of ω-3 polyunsaturated fatty acids contributes to the immunological abnormalities, there is only very limited information available to link the immune disorder found in schizophrenic patients with disordered essential fatty acid metabolism. There is clinical evidence to show that the erythrocyte membrane of schizophrenic patients contains reduced concentrations of arachidonic and docosahexanoic acids and that these changes may be a consequence of an increase in the rate of oxidation of these fatty acids rather than due to a dietary deficiency of ω-3, and ω-6 fatty acid precursors. The atypical neuroleptic clozapine has been shown to increase the concentration of these fatty acids in the erythrocyte membranes of schizophrenic patients.

In contrast to depression, where there is substantial evidence to suggest that increased macrophage activity leading to the excessive secretion of proinflammatory cytokines may be involved in the pathology of the condition, in schizophrenia it would appear that activation of the IL-2 forming lymphocytes, rather than an inflammatory response, could form the pathological basis. This view is supported by epidemiological studies in which the incidence of arthritis and inflammatory disease is reported to be lower in schizophrenic subjects than in a non-schizophrenic population. These patients also show a greater resistance to pain (possibly related to a reduction in the synthesis of PGE2 from arachidonic acid) and an improvement in the positive symptoms in response to fever.

In regard to the effect of dietary fatty acids on the symptoms of schizo-phrenia, it has been shown in a randomized study of treatment-resistant patients that eicosapentaenoic acid produces a significant reduction in the symptoms. It is not known if this beneficial effect is associated with a reduc-tion in the serum IL-2 and IL-6 concentrations but, as mentioned above, there is evidence that ω-3 polyunsaturated fatty acids reduce the synthesis of these cytokines.

To date there have been a few experimental studies relating changes in dietary fatty acid intake to immune function and behaviour. Nevertheless, there is evidence that in rats chronic dietary alpha-linolenic acid deficiency profoundly impedes learning and memory. In addition, the concentration of dopamine, and the density of dopamine D2 receptors, is decreased in ω-3 deficient animals, while the density of serotonin 5-HT2 receptors is in-creased in the frontal cortex. A finding of relevance to the symptoms of schizophrenia relates to the increase in distractibility shown by the alpha-linolenic acid deficient rats. Clearly this is an area of research which requires much more attention, particularly in the light of the preliminary clinical studies showing that ω-3 polyunsaturated fatty acids may have a beneficial effect on the treatment of schizophrenia, an action which may be related to an attenuation of the increased IL-2 and IL-6 concentrations that correlate with some of the positive symptoms of the disorder.

SUMMARY

There is convincing clinical and experimental evidence that dietary ω-3 and ω-6 polyunsaturated fatty acids influence cytokines produced by mac-rophages and lymphocytes. The ω-6 fatty acids, such as arachidonic acid, appear to be present in a relatively higher concentration than the ω-3 fatty acids, such as eicosapentaenoic acid, in patients with depression. Mac-rophage activity is possibly increased in these patients leading to an over-production of proinflammatory cytokines which, together with increased PGE2 synthesized from arachidonic acid, forms the basis of the mac-rophage theory of depression. ω-3 fatty acids, such as eicosapentaenoic and docosahexanoic acids, attenuate the actions of these proinflammatory cytokines.

In schizophrenia, there appears to be an overexpression of IL-2 and IL-6; the erythrocyte membranes of schizophrenic patients have reduced con-centrations of arachidonic acid and docosahexanoic acid. There is evidence that ω-3 fatty acids can attenuate the synthesis of these cytokines while preliminary studies suggest that eicosapentaenoic acid improves the symp-toms of treatment-resistant schizophrenic patients. Whether the immune changes are coincidentally or causally related to the clinical effects of the ω-3 fatty acids is presently unknown.

BIBLIOGRAPHY

Horrobin, D. F. (1998) The membrane phosopholipid hypothesis as a biochemical basis for the neurodevelopmental concept of schizophrenia. *Schizophrenia Research* **30**: 193–208.

Maes, M. Smith, R. S., Christophe, A. et al. (1996) Fatty acid composition in major depression: decreased omega 3 fractions in cholesteryl esters and increased C20:4W6/C20:W3 ratio in cholesteryl esters and phospholipids. *Journal of Affective Disorders* **38**: 35–46.

Meydani, S. N. (1996) Effect of (ω-3) polyunsaturated fatty acids on cytokine production and their biologic function. *Nutrition* **12**: S8–S14.

Müller, N. and Ackenheil, M. (1998) Psychoneuroimmunology and the cytokine action in the CNS: implications for psychiatric disorders. *Progress in Neuro-Psychopharmacology and Biological Psychiatry* **22**: 1–30.

O'Donnell, M. C., Catts, S. V., Ward, P. B. et al. (1996) Increased production of interleukin 2, but not soluble interleukin 2 receptors in medicated patients with schizophrenia and schizophreniform disorder. *Psychiatry Research* **65**: 171–178.

Smith, R. S. (1991) The macrophage theory of depression. *Medical Hypothesis* **35**: 298–306.

Yehuda, S. and Mostofsky, D. I. (Eds) (1997)*Handbook of Essential Fatty Acid Biology: Biochemistry, Physiology and Behavioural Neurobiology*. Humana Press, Totowa, NJ.

9 Psychoneuroimmunology of Alzheimer's Disease and the Dementias

Alzheimer's disease (AD), previously referred to as dementia of the Alzheimer type (DAT), is a neurodegenerative disease with cognitive impairments in memory, judgement, visuospatial function, planning, concept formation and language. AD is also accompanied by non-cognitive symptoms, such as disturbances in behaviour, mood, perception and sleep. It has been associated with many impairments in neurotransmission, endocrine and immune functions. The cognitive defect in this disease has been linked to a cholinergic defect together with atrophy of the cortex and limbic system; these brain regions contain a high density of neurofibrillary tangles and senile plaques. In recent years, a defect in the immune system has been postulated as a cause of the illness. It is thought that during immune ageing, populations of activated, autoreactive T cells, B cells and monocytes (macrophages) may cross the blood–brain barrier (BBB) to initiate overactivation of brain microglia. These hyperactive microglia, in turn, may induce inflammatory or neurotoxic processes in the brain, which may cause defects in neurotransmitter synthesis and metabolism, and the development of neurofibrillary tangles, amyloid protein and antibody accumulation and oxidative damage to the neurons.

IMMUNE ABNORMALITIES IN AD

Recent studies show that patients with AD or DAT have both cellular and humoral immune dysfunction, affecting both the brain and periphery. Immune ageing, especially thymus ageing-induced changes in lymphocyte functions, may be the cause of immune abnormalities.

PERIPHERAL IMMUNE CHANGES IN AD

Ageing leads to a decrease of immune function, particularly of T lymphocytes. In healthy elderly subjects, T cells are more immature, while the functioning of CD4+ and CD8+ cells and lymphocyte numbers are decreased. Decreased mitogen-induced lymphocyte proliferation and production of IL-2 have also been reported. Normal ageing is also accompanied by a decrease in the activity of phagocytic cells such as polymorphonuclear neutrophils (PMNs) and monocytes, which are of importance in the defence against invasive agents. Diminished neutrophil and monocyte phagocytosis, and natural killer (NK) cell activity, has been reported in healthy elderly subjects. However, the production of cytokines by peripheral blood cells, e.g. interleukin-1 (IL-1) and IL-6, is not consistently altered in elderly persons. Nevertheless, many studies have demonstrated that compared to young people, some healthy elderly subjects show a significantly higher incidence of antoantibodies and higher serum concentration of IL-2R, and increased lymphocyte subsets CD8+ and CD28–. These changes indicate that an autoimmune disorder may be associated with the pathological changes which characterize the disease.

Reviewing the literature over the past ten years, there seems to be no direct causal relationship between normal immune ageing and AD. In AD patients, an autoimmune-like phenomenon is quite obvious. Thus AD patients show a reduced number of lymphocytes, but increased mitogen-stimulated lymphocyte proliferation, occasional elevated neutrophil phagocytosis and superoxide release, and increased production of the pro-inflammatory cytokines, IL-1, IL-2, IL-6 and tumour necrosis factor (TNF). Both increased and decreased NK cell cytotoxicity has also been reported in these patients. Brain and serum concentrations of positive acute phase proteins and antibodies (IgG) are also increased in AD patients. Compared to healthy elderly subjects, CD4+, CD8+ and HLA-DR markers are further increased in AD patients. Lymphocyte responses to the stimulation of amyloid beta protein are also changed in AD patients. Thus when lymphocytes from young, normal elderly and AD patients were stimulated with this protein, lymphocyte proliferation and IL-2 receptor expression were increased in young and normal elderly donors, but not in AD patients. These findings indicate that autoimmune responses may be present in AD patients but not in normal elderly people.

CENTRAL IMMUNE ABNORMALITIES IN AD PATIENTS

Evidence of an increase in the inflammatory response has also been found in the central nervous system (CNS) of AD patients. As discussed in Chapter 2, the complement system is an important factor for initiating inflammation and opsonization, and B-cell activation. In vitro studies have demonstrated that astrocytes and glial cells in the brain are capable of expressing complement proteins. During inflammatory and degenerative diseases of the brain, the expression and production of complements are increased, which is regulated by both proinflammatory and anti-inflammatory cytokines. Moreover, complement-induced activation of B cells may increase the production of antibodies in the brain, which may result in brain tissue damage. When brain tissue from AD patients was stained immunohistochemically by anti-bodies to components of the classical complement pathway, it was found that antibodies to C1q, C3d and C4d stained senile plaques, dystrophic neuritis and tangled neurons. This suggests that there is a dysfunction in the complement system in these AD markers.

In the cerebrospinal fluid (CSF) of AD patients, the concentrations of TNF-α, IL-1β and IL-6 are increased. A marked increase in IL-1 concentrations has also been reported in the brain tissue and is positively correlated with mental deterioration and negatively correlated with mental performance. Experimental studies have also shown that IL-1 may directly cause AD. Thus, systemic administration of IL-1β has been found to largely reduce extracellular acetylcholine (ACh) concentrations in the hippocampus, which could account for the cholinergic defect in AD patients. In addition, following the incubation of IL-1 with brain slices, the expression of the beta-amyloid precursor protein (APP) gene is increased. While it is still unclear how immune changes in the periphery cause immune abnormalities in the CNS, it seems possible that increased permeability of the blood–cerebrospinal fluid barrier (BCB) may be one of the reasons. In support of this, a BCB leakage and an elevation in IgG in the CSF have been reported in some AD patients.

NEUROTRANSMITTER CHANGES IN AD

CHANGES IN BRAIN NEUROTRANSMITTERS

AD is associated with extensive changes in many neurotransmitter systems. Postmortem biochemical studies have consistently reported that AD is associated with a marked reduction in the enzyme choline acetyltransferase (ChAT), which synthesizes choline to ACh in the cortex and several other brain regions. In the cortical area, a severe deficiency in ACh synthesis and uptake, and an increase in the ratio of ACh synthesis to ChAT, have been found in AD patients. In the temporal and frontal cortex, noradrenaline (NA) concentration and uptake are greatly reduced in both biopsy and autopsy samples from patients with AD. Noradrenaline turnover, as measured by the ratio of the metabolite 3-methoxy-4-hydroxy-phenylglycol (MHPG) to NA, is increased in the frontal cortex of these patients. Serotonin (5-HT) is also impaired in AD patients; changes include a decrease in 5-HT release and synthesis, but increases in 5-hydroxyindole-acetic acid (5-HIAA) and serotonin turnover (5-HIAA to 5-HT). These changes may be due to the loss of neurons and presynaptic terminals. Similarly in the hippocampus, a decrease in ChAT activity, together with reduced synaptosomal choline uptake, may indicate that a major deficit occurs in the cholinergic pathway in this area. There is also evidence of reduced NA, MHPG and 5-HT and reduced activity of dopamine-β-hydroxylase in the hippocampus of AD patients. In addition, it has been reported that a close relationship exists between a reduction in the concentration of the dopamine metabolite homovanillic acid (HVA) in the neostriatum and cerebrospinal fluid, and the degree of cognitive impairment in AD patients.

The histamine content has also been found to be reduced in the hypothalamus, hippocampus and temporal cortex of AD brains when compared to normal ageing controls. This decrease in brain histamine may contribute to the cognitive decline in AD either directly or undirectly through the cholinergic system.

INHIBITORY AND EXCITATORY NEUROTRANSMITTERS

There are no consistent findings regarding changes in the concentrations of the inhibitory neurotransmitters gamma-aminobutyric acid (GABA), glycine and taurine. There is accumulating evidence that glutamate is the principal transmitter of the corticocortical association fibres and the major hippocampal pathway. Histological studies show that these pathways degenerate quite early in AD as indicated by a positive association between glutamate binding in the striatum and the density of tangles in the temporal cortex.

The accumulation of β-amyloid protein is a diagnostic feature of AD. The relationship between this protein and neurotransmitters has been studied and it has been shown that the continuous infusion of β-amyloid protein into rat cerebral ventricle impairs learning ability and decreases ChAT activity. Neurotransmitters in cholinergic and dopaminergic neuronal systems were also studied by *in vivo* brain microdialysis. ACh and DA release induced by high-potassium stimulation was decreased in several brain regions of β-amyloid protein-infused rats compared with vehicle-infused rats. These results suggest that the release of the two transmitters was decreased by β-amyloid protein and that learning deficits observed in the β-amyloid protein-infused rats are partly due to impairment in the release of these neurotransmitters.

ENDOCRINE CHANGES IN AD

THE HYPOTHALAMIC–PITUITARY–ADRENOCORTICAL AXIS AND HYPERCORTISOLISM IN AD

In both AD patients and animal models of dementia, it is apparent that the hippocampus is damaged, particularly in the CA1 region. This brain region plays an important role in the regulation of the function of the HPA axis, especially for feedback. In AD patients, it has been shown that the degree of hippocampal damage paralleled the magnitude of hypercortisolism. Thus, loss of hippocampal neurons and changes in corticosteroid receptors may be related to the disorder of the HPA axis. In the hippocampus of an animal model of dementia, the glucocorticoid receptors exhibit a higher affinity for corticosteroids and are more resistant to "down-regulation" by glucocorticoids. This may account for the higher basal concentration of cortisol over 24 hours in patients with AD compared to their elderly controls.

Combined dexamethasone (DEX) suppression and corticotrophin-releasing factor (CRF) stimulation tests showed that cortisol secretion after DEX pretreatment and before CRF stimulation was increased in AD patients compared with healthy elderly controls. Furthermore, 21% of this group were DEX non-suppressors. None of the healthy controls escaped DEX-induced suppression of cortisol. However, following CRF administration, AD patients released significantly less cortisol and ACTH than the elderly controls. These findings have led to the hypothesis that chronically increased glucocorticoid concentrations might promote the loss of hippocampal neurons in later life.

In a study on the hypothalamic–pituitary–somatotrophic (HPS) and the HPA systems in early-onset AD, 10 drug-naive patients and matched controls were given 50 μg growth hormone releasing hormone (GHRH) at 9 a.m. and 100 μg CRF at 6 p.m. as an intravenous bolus dose. Compared with controls, patients with AD showed attenuated GHRH-induced growth hormone (GH) responses and decreased ACTH, but normal cortisol secretion following CRF. GH responses to GHRH were negatively correlated with plasma insulin-like growth factor (IGF-I) concentrations and the severity of dementia. A positive correlation was also found between GHRH-evoked GH release and ACTH responses to CRF. These results suggest that a pathological lesion occurs at the level of the pituitary or the hypothalamus, possible involving a cholinergic, monoaminergic or peptidergic imbalance in AD, and supports the view that altered HPS and HPA secretary dynamics in AD are related to the underlying brain dysfunction.

However, the CRF changes in AD are different from those in depressive disorders or the responses of exposure to stress; CRF synthesis appears to be reduced, or the metabolism increased, in these patients. It has been found that CRF immunoreactivity (IR) is dramatically reduced in the frontal, parietal and temporal cerebral cortex of patients with AD. CRF receptors are increased, while CRF-binding protein is unchanged. Cognitive impairment in AD patients is associated with a lower CSF concentration of CRF. In animal models of dementia, rats treated with CRF or a CRF receptor agonist show an improvement in learning and memory, such as spatial learning in the Morris water maze. However, these treatments also cause anxiety and stress responses.

The mechanism whereby CRF is involved in AD is unclear. Increased CRF-IR has been found in the paraventricular nucleus of the hypothalamus of some AD patients. This finding may correlate with the increased hypothalamic–pituitary–adrenal activity in AD, while the decrease in CRF content in other brain areas may be related to selective degeneration of intrinsic cortical CRF neurons.

OTHER HORMONE CHANGES IN AD PATIENTS

AD has been associated with a decline in ovarian hormone function in postmenopausal women. Many studies suggest that oestrogens play an important role in the expression of AD. Thus, the incidence of AD is reduced by 50% in postmenopausal women taking oestrogen replacement, while oestrogen treatment has also been shown to markedly improve cognitive performance in women with AD. The mechanisms whereby oestrogens affect neuronal function in AD include increasing regional blood flow, increasing glucose transport and reducing the concentration of the neurotoxic form of β-amyloid. For these reasons, oestrogens have been found to significantly improve the performance of AD patients in verbal IQ, comprehension, memory, communication and self-care.

The synthesis of other neuroendocrine peptides, such as thyrotrophin-releasing hormone (TRH), gonadotrophin-releasing hormone, somatostatin and GHRH, all decrease with age. Administration of high doses of TRH was shown to significantly increase arousal and improve memory. A decrease in the concentration of somatostatin in the cortex of AD patients may be the result of neuron loss in the area.

IMMUNE, ENDOCRINE AND NEUROTRANSMITTER CHANGES IN PARKINSON'S DISEASE AND HUNTINGTON'S DISEASE

IMMUNOLOGICAL CHANGES IN PARKINSON'S DISEASE

Both peripheral and central immunological disturbances have been reported in Parkinson's disease (PD). There could be two possibilities for these disturbances. It is possible that changes in immune system are responsible for autodestruction of neurons in PD. Alternative and adverse changes in the peripheral immune system cause neuronal damage by activating astrocytes, increasing microglia proliferation and thereby enhancing cytokine production. There is also some evidence that infections in childhood may predispose to the risk of PD later in life.

With regard to the immune system, there is no significant differene in the lymphocyte subset of CD4+, CD19+ and CD8+ and CD4+/CD8+ ratio between PD patients and their age- and sex-matched controls. Many immune changes in PD patients are similar to those occurring in ageing controls. However, some of these changes may become exaggerated. For example, it has been reported that mitogen-induced lymphocyte proliferation in PD patients is similar to controls, but when IL-1 is used to stimulate thymocyte proliferation, as an IL-1 activity index, a significant decrease in IL-1 activity was found in PD patients in comparison to controls. PD patients also show much higher serum concentrations of IgG, but lower concentrations of IgM and IgA. These changes cannot be attributed to the ageing process alone.

This finding may suggest a potential role for dopamine (DA) in the regulation of some immune functions. Thus experimental studies have deomonstrated that intraperitoneal administration of DA or its precursor L-DOPA suppresses lymphocyte response and cytotoxic T-cell generation in the mouse. Conversely, in PD patients with a lesion of the dopaminergic system, the total number of leucocytes and neutrophils is greatly increased. While no difference was found for IL-2R, IL-6, interferon gamma (IFN-γ) production, the release of IL-2 was significantly decreased in PD patients.

There are some differences between AD and PD with regard to their aetiology and therefore it is not surprising that there are immunological differences. For example, in postmortem hippocampal samples, ChAT activity is reduced (58%) in AD patients, but not in the brain samples from PD patients. Furthermore, in the hippocampus, marked elevations in IL-1β, IL-2 and IL-3 concentrations have been reported in AD patients, but not in PD patients. In addition, IL-1 and IL-2 affinity to their receptors are enhanced in AD patients, while in the PD hippocampus, a selective enhancement in IL-2 binding is apparent. In AD patients, a well-established increase in IL-1β and IL-1 receptor activation has been found. This then stimulates amyloid protein accumulation and decreases ChAT activity. However, these changes have only been found in the hippocampus of PD patients when there is a dementia associated with the disease. In the brain and CSF of PD patients, TNF-α concentrations have been found to be significantly higher than in controls. Moreover, IL-1 and IL-6 are also increased in striatal regions of PD patients. In PD patients, many other autoimmune responses also occur. For example, antibodies to dopaminergic neurons have been detected in the CSF of patients with PD, while the presence of large numbers of HLA-DR+ microglia have been demonstrated in the substantia nigra of these patients. It is known that HLA-DR antigens, a T-cell activation marker, play an important role in the induction and regulation of autoimmune processes.

ENDOCRINE CHANGES IN PARKINSON'S DISEASE

Abnormalities in the HPA axis have also been found in patients with PD. For example, the nocturnal secretion of GH, ACTH and cortisol is significantly lower, while the prolactin (PRL) release peak is higher in PD patients than in normal subjects. Furthermore, PD patients have much higher total plasma cortisol secretion over a 24 hour period than normal controls. These changes may be due to abnormalities of intrinsic cortical neurons or to a dysfunction in CRF containing neurons that innervate the cortex. Similarly in AD, a decrease in CRF neurons has been reported to occur in the frontal, temporal and occipital poles of the neocortex, but not in the hippocampus. Moreover, reductions in opioidergic immunoreactivity in AD have been correlated with reductions in the activity of ChAT.

In postmenopausal women with PD, the basal luteinizing hormone (LH) secretion is significantly lower than in normal women. Following oestrogen administration, the plasma concentration of LH is decreased in control subjects, but not in women with PD. After infusion with naloxone for 20 days, LH secretion is enhanced in normal women, but not in women with PD. This suggests that the deficiency in DA and the opioid system may be the cause of an abnormal regulation of LH secretion in women with PD.

In addition to malfunctioning dopaminergic and probably noradrenergic systems, there is also evidence of a defect in GABAergic function in PD patients. Thus, baclofen, a GABA-B receptor agonist, produces a threefold increase in GH in control subjects, but has little effect on GH secretion in patients with PD.

NEUROTRANSMITTER CHANGES IN PARKINSON'S DISEASE

Degenerative diseases of the nervous system have a predilection for specific cell populations and neurotransmitters. AD involves many neuronal populations but appears mainly to affect the cholinergic system in the forebrain. Parkinson's disease has a more marked predilection for the dopaminergic neurons of the substantia nigra. Indeed, striatal DA deficiency is the marker of primary neurochemical abnormality in PD. Reduction in DA concentration and loss of DA neurons have also been found in the substantia nigra, mesencephalic central grey matter and the hippocampus. In the whole hypothalamus of autopsied brain of patients with PD, the concentrations of NA, DA and 5-HT are greatly decreased, while the 5-HIAA/5-HT ratio is increased compared to control subjects. At the subregional level, the most consistently affected area is the intermediate subdivision of the hypothalamus where all three monoamines are significantly reduced. In this region, the DA metabolites, dihydroxyphenylacetic acid (DOPAC) and 3-methoxy-tyramine (3-MT), are also significantly decreased.

IMMUNE ENDOCRINE AND NEUROTRANSMITTER CHANGES IN HUNTINGTON'S DISEASE

Huntington's disease (HD) is an inherited disease of the CNS. It is characterized by progressive involuntary movements and dementia. Neuronal and glial loss has been found in the caudate nucleus and putamen and in layers III, IV and VI of the cerebral cortex. There is also atrophy of the basal ganglia in all areas, including the pallidum and limbic regions. Degeneration in these areas may cause cognitive problems.

Neurotransmitters are also changed in this illness. In postmortem samples of patients with HD, significant decreases in GABA and glutamate concentrations and increases in HVA and 5-HIAA have been found in the frontal and temporal cortex. The NA concentration is reduced only in the temporal cortex, while 5-HT is increased in both regions. In the striatum, concentrations of GABA and glutamate and the activity of ChAT are also dramatically reduced, while somatostatin and neuropeptide Y (NPY) concentration are increased.

Brain damage and neurotransmitter abnormalities also cause abnormalities in the limbic–hypothalamic–pituitary–adrenal axis (LHPA). CRF release is regulated by many "classical" neurotransmitters and negative feedback loops. GABA is the major inhibitory neurotransmitter on CRF neurons, while other neurotransmitters (e.g. glutamate) may exert an excitatory action. An impairment in the functional integrity of the LHPA has been demonstrated in this illness. Basal ACTH and cortisol is higher in HD patients compared to controls. After a CRF challenge, similar increases in ACTH and cortisol secretion occur in both groups. Following the dexamethasone suppression test (DST) the plasma cortisol concentration is 57% lower in patients with HD than in controls.

The pathophysiology of hyperactive CRF neurons in HD might be partly due to an abnormality in GABAergic neurotransmission frequently found in HD. In experimental studies it has been demonstrated that intracerebroventricular administration of GABA antagonists to animals results in elevated basal concentrations of ACTH and cortisol. In patients with HD who then develop depression, CRF concentrations in the CSF are markedly increased, which may result in hyperactivity of the HPA axis.

So far, there have been limited studies of immune changes in Huntington's disease. No significant differences have been reported in the percentage of B-cell and T-cell subsets (CD4+, CD8+ and DR+ cells) between patients with HD and controls, but lymphocyte proliferation and IL-1 release from leucocytes are significantly reduced in HD patients. Other studies have shown that the HLA-DR marker on T cells is normal, but the CAG repeat gene is abnormally expanded in the lymphocytes and brain of these patients. However, as with AD and PD, the relationship between neurotransmission, endocrine and immune changes in HD is unclear.

GENETIC FACTORS AND THEIR ROLE IN THE AETIOLOGY OF THE DEMENTIAS—LINK TO THE IMMUNE CHANGES

Although the cause of AD still remains elusive, intensive efforts have been made to find the major risk factors associated with this disorder. In recent years, AD has been studied from many aspects including genetics, immune disorders, viral infection, toxic effects, environmental factors and head trauma.

GENETIC HYPOTHESIS OF AD

Genetic factors in the aetiology of AD have been intensively investigated. A significant association has been identified between a family history of dementia and AD. Reports on seven large kindred studies have shown that AD appears to have been inherited as an autosomal dominant disorder over several generations. The fact that onset is consistently early in all affected relatives suggests that special factors control age of onset in these kindreds. There are also many reported families in whom the incidence of the disease over at least two generations is compatible with autosomal dominant inheritance. These investigations suggest that a substantial proportion of cases, at least those of early onset, may have a genetic aetiology and be transmitted in this manner.

Several genetic studies found a linkage between chromosome 21 and AD in some families with primarily early-onset AD. At least 50% of offspring in these families develop AD. That this is due to genetic causes is made plausible by the discovery of a familial pattern gene on chromosome 21. Familial AD does not differ from other cases of AD clinically or pathologically. The locus of this gene on chromosome 21 also explains the association of AD with Down's syndrome. However, approximately 50–60% of AD cases were reported not to show any familial aggregation, suggesting that other factors must be involved in this illness.

THE IMMUNE HYPOTHESIS

In the 1980s, immunological factors were linked to AD because senile plaques are largely composed of β-amyloid and located in immune-competent cells (i.e. the microglia). Since then more and more immunological impairments have been found in AD patients. For example, an association between a family history of AD and immune diseases such as lymphoma, lymphosarcoma, Hodgkin's disease and other immune disorders has been reported. A high incidence of certain types of cancer was also found in patients with Down's syndrome and among relatives of people who have AD. However, not all studies have established an increased occurrence of allergies and cancers. It would appear, however, that there is a negative correlation between occurrence of rheumatoid arthritis and AD.

It is now well known that viral infection may affect brain functions, leading to behavioural and intellectual disturbances by causing proinflammatory cytokine secretions. Dementia has been associated with postencephaltic Parkinson's disease that is thought to be a late sequel of influenza. It has also been hypothesized that viral protein participates in the formation of the paired helical filaments based on the observation that microtubules are involved in the replication cycle of viruses. It has been shown that herpes simplex virus frequently occurs in many human trigeminal ganglia and lifelong lymphocytic infiltrations are present even in the absence of any pathological changes in the sensory neurons. These lymphocytic infiltrations may represent a histological marker of latent herpes virus, which, when activated, is well established as the ganglionic source of recurrent herpes labialis. This suggests that reaction of the same virus centripetally may damage the ageing brain.

Previous chapters have discussed how viral or bacterial infections, or tissue damage (such as head trauma), trigger the secretion of proinflammatory cytokines. Indeed, increases in these cytokines or cytokine receptors have been reported in the brain of AD patients. It has been reported that peripheral administration of proinflammatory cytokines, or virus and bacteria challenge, could induce IL-1 and IL-6 mRNA expression and increase cytokine production from glial and astrocyte cells in the CNS. IL-1 and IL-6 then further trigger an inflammatory cascade within the brain. These changes include activation of the complement system, increase in positive acute phase proteins and antibodies, accumulation of β-amyloid proteins and stimulation of other inflammatory cytokines. Finally, such changes disturb neurotransmission by causing damage to membrane structure, G-protein link between the receptors and their second messengers and changing calcium flux, which then cause neuron death.

These immune changes may be genetically linked. Thus, genetically induced early immune ageing may result in some types of autoimmune disorder. Autoimmune diseases are highly associated with family history. For example, the timing of thymus ageing is genetically related. It has been shown that thymus ageing impairs T-lymphocyte function and alters the balance between T-cell subsets and T and B cells, which increases the production of inflammatory cytokines and antibodies. Furthermore, the sensitivity of the immune system in response to adverse events (such as viral or bacterial infection, tissue damage, allergen factors, and physical or psychological stress) may be influenced by the genetically linked changes. In addition, non-genetic factors, such as the environment, are also of importance in the aetiology of AD.

EFFECTS OF ANTI-DEMENTIA DRUGS ON THE IMMUNE SYSTEM

As discussed previously, if AD results from abnormal immune ageing, treatment with anti-dementia drugs should attenuate such changes. Similarly, anti-inflammatory drugs should have beneficial effects in the treatment of dementia. Despite the relative paucity of data, there is some evidence to support the hypothesis that some anti-dementia and anti-inflammatory drugs have a neuroprotective action in AD.

EVIDENCE THAT ANTI-DEMENTIA DRUGS AFFECT INFLAMMATORY RESPONSES

As mentioned previously, a reduction in NK cell activity has been reported in healthy elderly subjects and AD patients. Thus, the effect on the immune system of the muscarinic cholinergic agonist, arecoline, which also stimulates the secretion of CRF and ACTH, has been investigated in rats. In this study, it was demonstrated that peripherally administered arecoline or ACTH can increase activity of pre-activated NK cells. Furthermore, central administration of a low dose of arecoline (that has no effect on peripheral immune functions) can also induce a significant increase in the activity of pre-activated NK cells. Finally, it has been shown that the pairing of a novel odour (camphor) with administration of arecoline can be used to alter NK cell activity, and indirectly that aspects of cellular immunity can be conditioned. However, the effects of arecoline on the immune system are complex as arecoline has also been shown to suppress some immune functions. For example, the effect of this drug on delayed-type hypersensitivity (DTH) reactions to sheep red blood cells (SRBC) has been evaluated in mice, and it was shown to suppress DTH reactions. However, arecoline treatment did not appreciably alter the host resistance to endotoxin shock.

In vitro experiments revealed both dose-dependent and time-dependent cytotoxic effects of arecoline when spleen cells were incubated with varying concentrations of arecoline. Concomitant exposure of arecoline at concentrations of 10^{-6}–10^{-4} M with concanavalin A (Con A) markedly suppressed both [^{3}H]-thymidine incorporation and IL-2 production by splenic cells. In the same experiment, it was found that the administration of arecoline following SRBC immunization also exerted dose-dependent suppression of the primary antibody response. Similarly, when treated 12 h after immunization, a significant reduction in response was observed, while moderate suppression of antibody response was noticed at the dose level of 10 mg/kg. These studies suggest that arecoline suppresses thymus-dependent immune responses and some aspects of non-specific resistance.

Another anti-dementia drug, 9-amino-1,2,3,4-tetrahydroacridine (THA), has been shown to suppress NK cell maximal cytotoxic potential and NK-mediated activity and cytolysis. Increased proinflammatory cytokines are one of the immune markers for AD. Cytidine-5-diphosphate (CDP)-choline is a choline donor involved in the biosynthesis of acetycholine and in brain phospholipid metabolism. This drug has been used to treat dementia and conditions involving age-related cognitive disturbances. The effect of CDP-choline on the serum concentration of IL-1β has been studied in patients with early-onset AD, late-onset AD and multi-infarct dementia. Compared to normal controls, all patients with dementia were shown to have an increased serum IL-1β concentration, which was marked in early-onset AD. After CDP-choline treatment for three months, IL-1β concentration in the three groups of patients all returned to normal levels accompanied by a significant improvement in mental performance. In other studies increases in the blood concentrations of IL-1β and histamine have been reported in early-onset AD patients. CDP treatment has been found to reduce not only IL-1β concentration but also blood histamine concentrations, which are positively correlated with improvement in cognitive performance in these patients. Such findings suggest some anti-dementia drugs have anti-inflammatory effects which could be relevant to their therapeutic activity.

EFFECTS OF ANTI-INFLAMMATORY DRUGS ON AD MARKERS

The idea that anti-inflammatory therapy may be useful in the treatment of AD is based on the finding that a lower than expected prevalence of delayed-onset AD occurs in patients using anti-inflammatory drugs for the treatment of arthritis and related conditions. However, there are few studies that demonstrate the direct effect of anti-inflammatory treatment on AD. Recent findings from the study of postmortem brains show there is no significant difference in the presence of senile plaques, neurofibrillary tangles and amyloid protein accumulation between patients treated with non-steroidal anti-inflammatory drugs and patients without this treatment. However, even though the presence of senile plaques correlates positively with the number of CR/43+ microglia in both groups of patients, a history of anti-inflammatory treatment was associated with far fewer (one third) activated microglial cells than in patients without such treatments. This result suggests that anti-inflammatory drugs may suppress microglial activity and thereby exert some neuroprotective actions.

IS ALZHEIMER'S DISEASE AN AUTOIMMUNE DISEASE?

Immune factors such as cellular immunity, autoimmunity and inflammation may play a pathogenic role in AD. It has been proposed that AD is a heterogeneous disease that may be partly immunological in origin. In addition to possible proinflammatory cytokines being involved, autoimmune processes may also play a role in predisposing the patients to AD.

T-LYMPHOCYTE ACTIVATION AND NEUROAUTOIMMUNITY

The term "neuroautoimmunity" refers to an autoimmune response specifically directed against the brain. This may be relevant to a neurodegenerative disease such as AD. Neuroautoimmunity has three key characteristics: (i) a blood-borne acute phase response leads to a chronic disease in the brain; (ii) activated lymphocytes and macrophages directly, through cell-mediated immunity or through the activation of microglial cells and astrocytes, induce target cell cytotoxicity; and (iii) glia activation leads to non-specific inflammatory damage; but brain-specific autoantibodies are responsible for directly cell-mediated immunity to initiate neuron-specific neurodegeneration.

As mentioned earlier, T-cell mitogen-induced proliferation is largely increased in AD patients. Within the CD4+ cell populations, there is a decrease in CD4CD45R+, but an increase in CD4CD45–, IL-2R and HLA-DR+ activated T cells. These changes, together with an increase in IL-2 production, indicate that T-cell activation occurs in AD. An increase in CD8+ subset and a decrease in CD4+ in AD suggest that a dysregulation of T-helper/T-suppressor cells occurs. Moreover, an increase in soluble CD8 and S100 protein (protein produced by macrophages), which implies an activation of CD8+ T cells, has also been found in the blood of patients with AD.

INFLAMMATORY RESPONSES IN AD

Inflammatory processes are initiated by activated macrophage and T lymphocytes. These cells then produce cytokines to induce further inflammatory responses, including the acute phase response (increased total leucocyte and neutrophil number, stimulated B cell to produce antibodies and increase positive acute phase proteins). The number of neutrophils has been found to be increased in the blood of AD patients. Many other inflammatory markers, such as MHC class I and II antigens, leucocyte antigens, inflammatory cytokines IL-1, IL-6, TNF and IL-2, and their receptors, have all been localized in the brain of patients with AD. Several studies have shown that cytokines can alter the fluidity of neuronal membranes, and also alter the structure of myelin, which may affect neurotransmitter release and transport. Activated T cells and macrophages can also change the permeability of the BBB and allow cytokines and antibodies to gain access to the brain. As evidence for the increase in BBB permeability, it has been shown that AD patients have increased acute phase proteins (alpha-1-antitrypsin and alpha-2-globulin) and complement proteins (C3, C4 and properdin factor B) in both their brain and blood. Furthermore, β-amyloid protein can induce activation of the complement system, which further supports the hypothesis that an inflammatory response occurs in AD.

BRAIN AUTOANTIBODIES IN AD

There is ample evidence from different groups of researchers throughout the world that organ-specific brain autoantibodies exist in the serum and also in the CSF of AD patients. These take the form of antibrain antibodies, anticholine cell and anti-pituitary cell antibodies, anti-myelin basic protein, anti-microglial cells, anti-astrocytes and anti-β-amyloid protein. As mentioned previously, brain tissue or CSF samples (which may contain macrophages and proteins) from AD patients stained microglial cells surrounding senile plaques in postmortem AD brain. Furthermore, focal staining of senile plaque cores, neuronal perikarya and astrocytes has been reported in AD brain autopsies. IgG immunoreactivity has also been located in the senile plaques of AD brain. After finding antibodies in senile plaques, it is important to find autoantibodies and/or C1q in the senile plaques because immune complexes contain antigens, antibodies and C1q. Fortunately, some researchers have recently located C1q with β-amyloid protein in the senile plaques. This finding combined with the finding of antibodies to β-amyloid proteins suggests that β-amyloid protein is the antigen.

Many experiments on animals, from the aspect of neurotransmitters, AD markers and immune functions, have also demonstrated that autoimmune disorders may be involved in AD. For example, in the autoimmune dementia model in rats, IgG accumulation occurs in the septum, hippocampus and entorhinal cortex. This is accompanied by a marked reduction in the density of the cholinergic neurons; there is an inverse correlation between IgG accumulation and the density of cholinergic neurons. These animals also show significant cognitive deficits.

In conclusion these findings strongly suggest that an autoimmune disorder may be a cause of AD. The possible contributing factors in autoimmune diseases are summarized (Figure 9.1); over-production of inflammatory cytokines may cause hypersecretion of cortisol and other hormonal changes which predispose to the neuronal death that characterizes the disease.

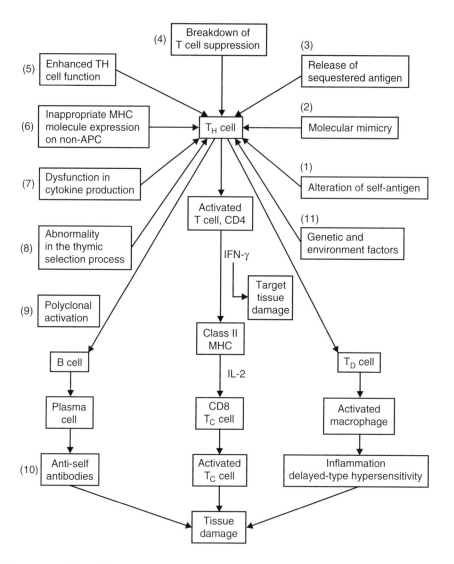

Figure 9.1 Possible contributing factors in autoimmune diseases (adapted from Elgert, 1996). (1) Alteration of self-antigens by chemicals or virus. (2) Cross-reactive antibody production. (3) Exposure to sequestered self-antigens. (4) decrease in CD8+ regulatory T-cell number or function. (5) Enhance TH (CD4+) function. (6) In appropriate class II MHC molecule expression. (7) Dysfunction in cytokine production. (8) Thymic defects. (9) Polyclonal B-cell activation. (10) Disruption of idiotypic antibody network. (11) Genetic and environment factors.

BIBLIOGRAPHY

Araujo, D. M. and Lapchak, P. A. (1994) Induction of immune system mediators in the hippocampal formation in Alzheimer's and Parkinson's diseases: selective effects on specific interleukins and interleukin receptors. *Neuroscience* **61**: 745–754.

Cacabelos, R., Caamano, J., Gomez, M. J., Fernandez-Novoa, L., Franco-Maside, A. and Alvarez, X. A. (1996) Therapeutic effects of CDP-choline in Alzheimer's disease. *Annals of the New York Academy of Sciences* **777**: 399–403.

De Greef, G. E., Van Staalduinen, G. J., Van Doornick, H., Van Tol, M. J. and Hijmans, W. (1992) Age-related changes of the antigen-specific antibody formation in vitro and PHA-induced T-cell proliferation in individuals who met the health criteria of the Senieur protocol. *Mechanisms of Ageing and Development* **66**: 1–14.

De Souza, E. B. (1995) Corticotropin-releasing factor receptors: physiology, pharmacology, biochemistry and role in central nervous system and immune disorders. *Psychoneuroendocrinology* **20**: 789–819.

Dubovik, V., Faigon, M., Eldont, J. and Michaelson, D. M. (1993) Decreased density of forebrain cholinergic neurons in experimental autoimmune dementia. *Neuroscience* **56**: 75–82.

Elgert, K. D. (1996) *Immunology: Understanding the Immune System*. Wiley-Liss, New York.

Fiszer, U., Fredrikson, S. and Czlonkowska, A. (1996) Humoral response to hsp 65 and hsp 70 in cerebrospinal fluid in Parkinson's disease. *Journal of the Neurological Sciences* **139**: 66–70.

Francis, P. T., Cross, A. J. and Bownen, M. D. (1994) Neurotransmitters and neuropeptides. In Terry, R. D., Katzman, R. and Bick, K. L. (Eds) *Alzheimer's Disease*, pp. 247–261. Raven Press, New York.

Heuser, I. J. E., Chase, T. N. and Mouradian, M. M. (1991) The limbic-hypothalamic–pituitary–adrenal axis in Huntington's disease. *Biological Psychiatry* **30**: 943–952.

Kay, D. W. K. (1989) Genetics, Alzheimer's disease and senile dementia. *British Journal of Psychiatry*; **154**: 311–320.

Kuhn, W. and Muller, T. (1995) Neuroimmune mechanisms of Parkinson's disease. *Journal of Neural Transmission* (Suppl) **46**: 229–233.

Li, G., Shen, Y. C., Li, Y. T., Chen, C. H., Zhau, Y. W. and Silverman, J. M. (1992) A case-control study of Alzheimer's disease in China. *Neurology* **42**: 1481–1488.

Rocca, W. A. (1987) The etiology of Alzheimer's disease: epodemiologic contributions with emphasis on the genetic hypothesis. *Journal of Neural Transmission* **24**: 3–12.

Singh, V. K. (1994) Studies of neuroimmune markers in Alzheimer's disease. *Molecular Neurobiology* **9**: 73–81.

Singh, V. K. Neuroautoimmunity pathogenic implication for Alzheimer's disease. Gerontology 1997; **43**: 79–94.

Song, C., Vandewoude, M., Stevens, W. et al. (1999) Alteration in immune functions during normal ageing and Alzheimer's disease. *Psychiatry Research* **85**: 71–80.

utoimmune Diseases

INTRODUCTION

A fundamental feature of the immune system lies in its ability to discriminate between tissues that are natural components of the organism and those that are not, in other words to distinguish between "self" and "non-self". This form of immunological tolerance arises because the immune system becomes unresponsive to antigens ("self antigens") that may be in the circulation and tissues. If, however, the mechanism of immunological tolerance breaks down, an autoimmune disease occurs.

The incidence of autoimmune disease is relatively low (5–7% of the population), which suggests that the recognition of "self-antigen" is a normal function of the immune system. Immune responses to "self antigens" appear to be regulated by a specific set of T and B cells. Regulated production of autoantibodies by B cells is consistent with normal health but the unregulated production of autoantibodies to "self antigens" may lead to abnormal autoimmunity. Similarly, autoreactive T cells, when they become unregulated, can cause tissue destruction. Thus autoimmmune diseases may be characterized by abnormal or excessive "anti-self" immune responses that are harmful to the host.

CRITERIA FOR IDENTIFYING AN AUTOIMMUNE DISEASE

There are four main criteria that have been used to establish the presence of an autoimmune disease. The first is by obtaining direct proof of transferring autoantibodies or "self-reactive" lymphocytes to another individual and thereby reproducing the disease. For ethical reasons such studies are not possible in humans but there is evidence that abnormal antibodies may be transferred transplacentally from the mother to the foetus to cause neonatal myasthenia gravis. Indirect evidence can be obtained by identifying the target antigen in humans, isolating the homologous antigen in an animal model, and then reproducing the disease in the experimental animal by administering the offending antigen. Using this approach, myasthenia gravis has been produced with antigens against the acetylcholine receptor. The third approach is based on isolating self-reactive autoantibodies or T cells from the target organism. For example, cytotoxic T cells have been found in the thyroid gland of patients with Graves' disease. The final criterion used to identify an autoimmune disease is based on circumstantial evidence. This involves an assessment of the familial tendency, lymphocyte infiltration and clinical improvement following the use of immunosuppressive drugs.

AETIOLOGY OF AUTOIMMUNE DISEASE

Autoimmune diseases are multifactorial involving both genetic and environmental factors. The genetic predisposition to autoimmune disease is indicated by the increased incidence in mono- and dizygotic twins and close relatives of an affected person. The pattern of inheritance is complex and is polygenic in nature. The family of genes associated with autoimmune disease that has been extensively studied involves the human major histocompatibility complex (MHC), which is not surprising considering its involvement in the shaping of the T-cell receptor. Environmental factors can also trigger autoimmune disease. Some autoantigens are protected from the immune system by a process of sequestration. The lens and uveal proteins of the eye, the chondrocyte antigens in cartilage and antigens of the spermatozoa are examples of sequestered antigens. When such antigens are introduced into the immune system, however, an autoimmune response results. Drugs have also been shown to induce a variety of organ-specific and non-organ-specific autoimmune diseases. For example, procainamide is the most common cause of drug-related systemic lupus erythematosus, a condition that has also been induced by a variety of other drugs including hydralazine, isoniazid, methyldopa, chlorpromazine and quinidine. However, with the exception of the adverse immunological reactions to penicillin, few drug-induced immune reactions have been studied in a systematic fashion. Thus investigations of specific antidrug reactions of T lymphocytes are scarce so that in most instances of drug-induced autoimmmunity it has not been proven that T-helper cells are involved in the pathogenesis of the condition, which would be postulated on theoretical grounds. It is also unclear in most cases of adverse immunological reactions that the changes are elicited by the drug or its metabolites. In contrast to the well-documented potential for some drugs to induce autoimmune side effects, little is known about the autoimmune potential of environmental chemicals. Severe scleroderma-like lesions have been reported to occur in workers exposed to vinyl chloride and quartz while such lesions, as well as systemic lupus, have been reported in women carrying silica-containing breast prostheses. A systemic lupus-like autoimmune disease can also develop in some individuals exposed to the tartrazine food additive.

PREGNANCY, IMMUNE FUNCTION AND AUTOIMMUNE DISEASES

Anecdotal evidence suggests that rheumatoid arthritis remits when the patient is pregnant but recurs during the postpartum period. Conversely autoimmune thyroiditis develops during the postpartum period while systemic lupus frequency occurs during pregnancy. Recently, a possible explanation for these occurrences has been found and relates to the changes in aspects of the immune system during pregnancy and the postpartum period.

Pregnancy is associated with a suppression of cell-mediated immune function and preservation, or enhancement of humoral immunity. It has been shown in rodents that these changes are associated with a depletion of CD4+ and CD8+ thymocytes, a reduction in B-lymphocyte precursors in the bone marrow and marked shifts in the synthesis of cytokines. While early pregnancy is associated with a marked increase in several cytokines as the condition progresses, interleukin-1 (IL-1), IL-2 and interferon gamma (IFN-γ) decline while IL-4 increases. This shift in the balance of the cytokines appears to be important to the histoincompatible foetus and thereby to avoid rejection by a cell-mediated immune attack by the mother. Furthermore, suppression of IFN-γ is essential as it is also a potent abortifacient.

These immune changes develop in parallel with an increase in plasma glucocorticoids, as well as an increase in oestrogen and progesterone concentrations. Such changes appear to be essential for the survival of the foetus as experimental studies have shown that when the oestrogen and progesterone receptors are blocked by the antagonist RU486, abortion follows. As the glucocorticoids are potent inhibitors of T-cell IFN-γ synthesis, suppressing cell-mediated immunity and enhancing humoral immune functions, it is understandable why such conditions as rheumatoid arthritis remit during pregnancy, whereas diseases such as systemic lupus, which is aggravated by the increase in humoral immune factors, increase under these conditions.

During the postpartum period, the hormonal status rapidly changes. Corticosteroids, oestrogen and progesterone decrease and cell-mediated immunity recovers. This increase in cell-mediated immune function permits autoimmune diseases such as rheumatoid arthritis to re-emerge. Furthermore, the rise in the plasma prolactin concentration during the postpartum period may play an important role in the development of autoimmune disease. Thus it has been found that rheumatoid arthritis develops particularly in nursing mothers. Nursing is associated with an elevation of prolactin and suppression of the hypothalamic–pituitary–adrenocortical (HPA) axis. It may therefore be concluded that although the precise mechanism linking changes in the endocrine and immune systems awaits elucidation, there is sufficient evidence to suggest how changes in these systems during pregnancy may impact on autoimmune processes. Preliminary evidence clearly implicates a permissive role for the glucocorticoids, prolactin and the immune system in autoimmunity. Table 10.1 summarizes the role of various hormones that facilitate the development of autoimmunity leading to autoimmune disease.

Table 10.1 Neuroendocrine abnormalities that facilitate the development of autoimmunity and autoimmune disease

1. Reduced corticosteroid concentration promotes Th1-dependent autoimmunity.
2. Resistance to the immunosuppressive effects of corticosteroids enhances Th1-dependent autoimmunity.
3. Reduced testosterone or dehydroepiandrosterone promotes both Th1 and Th2-dependent autoimmunity.
4. Excess oestrogen concentration, or increased oestrogen/androgen ratio, increases Th2-dependent autoimmunity.
5. Low oestrogen concentrations may potentiate Th1-dependent autoimmunity.
6. High prolactin concentrations may stimulate both Th1- and Th2-dependent autoimmune diseases.
7. A decrease in the activity of the sympathetic nervous system may enhance Th1-dependent autoimmunity.

ROLE OF GENDER IN THE SUSCEPTIBILITY TO AUTOIMMUNE DISEASE

There is evidence that marked gender differences occur in the incidence and prevalence of some autoimmune diseases. For example, women are four to nine times more likely to develop Graves' disease than men and rheumatoid arthritis is three times as likely to occur in women of childbearing age as in men of the same age. In the case of systemic lupus erythematosus the ratio of women to men is 10 : 1. This increased vulnerability does not apply to all types of autoimmune disease, however, as the incidence of ulcerative colitis is similar in both genders.

While gender differences occur, the role of the sex hormones may be implicated. For example, the incidence of rheumatoid arthritis is reduced by about 50% in women using oral contraceptives compared to those who do not. There are also reports that men who were exposed to the synthetic oestrogen diethylstilboestrol *in utero* have a similar incidence of the disease as women.

These observations suggest that there is sexual dimorphism in the organization of the immune system. The precise mechanism whereby this occurs is unknown but it is known that sex steroids affect thymic secretory function (via steroid receptors in thymic cells) which could then impact on the development of the immune system.

With regard to the effect of sex steroids on the immune system, it is known from experimental studies that gonadectomy enhances cell-mediated immunity and stimulates antibody synthesis; oestradiol inhibits the activities of CD8 cells while enhancing B-cell maturation and antibody synthesis, the effect on CD8 cells possibly being mediated by the inhibition of

IL-2 and other cytokines. In rodents, oestradiol has been shown to inhibit natural killer (NK) cell activity. Progesterone largely has the opposite effects to oestradiol, as do the androgens.

While the various studies implicating the sex steroids in the pathology of different autoimmune diseases have been undertaken in rodents, they do provide an insight into the reasons for the higher incidence of diseases such as rheumatoid arthritis and thyroiditis in women than in men. Clearly, this is an area of research which requires further study. In addition to the examples chosen to illustrate the immune changes that occur in these diseases, it should be emphasized that neurodegenerative diseases such as Alzheimer's disease can also be visualized as being due to an autoimmune process (Table 10.2). Evidence for this possibility is discussed elsewhere (see Chapter 9).

Table 10.2 Evidence suggesting an immune abnormality as a causal factor in Alzheimer's disease

1. Focal accumulation of abnormal proteins such as cerebrovascular and neuronal amyloid plaques, paired helical filaments and A68 proteins.
2. Focal lesions associated with neuron loss and granulovascular degeneration.
3. Focal aggregation of lytic scavenger cells, some of which contain phagocytosed amyloid protein.
4. The blood–brain barrier becomes more permeable with age thereby rendering the brain of the elderly patient more likely to attack by peripheral components of the immune system.
5. Antibrain antibodies have been identified in the sera and cerebrospinal fluid of patients with Alzheimer's disease together with complement proteins. Such factors provide the potential for an immune response once the immunocompetent cells with the appropriate surface markers and binding sites are present in the brain.
6. There is evidence that astrocytes, macrophages, activated T cells, endothelial cells and microglia are present in the brain of the patient with Alzheimer's disease.

It is self-evident that the neuroendocrine–immune network is involved in adaptation to stress and the precise function of this network varies according to the age, gender, reproductive status and various genetically determined factors together with the response to environmental stimuli. Undoubtedly the interrelationship between the immune and reproductive systems is particularly important because of their role in the development of autoimmune diseases.

MYASTHENIA GRAVIS

Myasthenia gravis is characterized by muscle weakness and fatigability, usually involving ocular, facial and bulbar musculature. If the respiratory muscles are also involved, the disease may be life-threatening. Myasthenia gravis is mediated by a T-cell-dependent polyclonal antibody that directly attacks the postsynaptic nicotinic receptors located in the neuromuscular junction. As a consequence, the nicotinic receptors cease to function and the skeletal muscles fail to contract.

The autonicotinic receptor antibodies induce their effects on the neuromuscular junction by three distinct mechanisms. The most important of these is complement-induced damage. The antibodies, once they have bound to the receptor, bind to complement. This leads to the activation of the complement cascade with the destruction of the postsynaptic membrane, flattening of the postsynaptic folds in the membrane and a reduction in the density of the nicotinic receptors.

In addition to the destruction of the receptors, autonicotinic receptor antibodies can crosslink the receptors, which are then shed or endocytosed with a reduction in the receptor number on the muscle membrane. While most antibodies are directed against portions of the nicotonic receptor that are not involved in the binding of acetylcholine to the receptor surface, some antibodies are directed at the acetylcholine binding site. When this occurs, the patient develops a sudden and severe worsening of the symptoms.

The process whereby loss of immune tolerance to the nicotinic receptor leads to myasthenia gravis is unknown. It has been hypothesized that the self antigens are structurally changed. This may occur due to changes in the activity of the thymus gland; the activity of the thymus is exceptionally high in the disease, which suggests that it may play a causal role. The thymus is the main site of development of tolerance during autogeny and may also be the cause of the loss of tolerance to the nicotinic receptors. Nicotinic receptors are expressed on the surface of the thymic epithelial cells and structural alterations in this thymic receptor are hypothesized to lead to an immune response that is cross-reactive with the nicotinic receptors in the neuromuscular junctions.

A second hypothesis suggests that cross-reactivity occurs with bacterial antigens normally found in the gastrointestinal and nicotinic receptors leading to myasthenia gravis. Some antinicotinic receptor antibodies have been detected in patients which cross-react with a herpes simplex virus glycoprotein that shows a sequence homology with a small peptide sequence in the nicotinic receptor.

GUILLAIN–BARRÉ SYNDROME

Guillain–Barré syndrome (GBS) is characterized by rapid development of weakness, often starting distally in the lower extremities and progressing to the upper extremities. The autonomic nerves are involved, the nerves and nerve roots showing a perivascular infiltrate of T cells and macrophages and segmental demyelination. GBS occurs as a sequel to infection with herpes virus, cytomegalovirus, the Epstein–Barr virus and varicella zoster.

It seems probable that GBS is an autoimmune process, perhaps caused by cross-reactions between myelin and microbial antigens. While an autoantigen is involved, the mechanism of immune mediated damage and the aetiology of the disease remain poorly understood. Macrophages appear to be ultimately responsible for the myelin destruction. Tumour necrosis factor (TNF), released from the macrophages, is known to be toxic to the oligodendrocytes, causing demyelination; presumably it shows similar toxicity to the Schwann cells. Immunoglobulins and complement are present in peripheral nerves and therefore it seems possible that the antibody binds to myelin, activates complement and then causes damage to the blood–nerve barrier. This could facilitate the entry of T cells and thereby potentiate the nerve destruction. Circulating anti-immune complexes could also increase the permeability of the blood–brain barrier.

In addition to various viruses (and more recently *Campylobacter* infection), several drugs have been reported to cause GBS. The first marketed selective serotonin reuptake inhibitor, zimelidine, was withdrawn because of the occurrence of peripheral neuropathy and GBS. Frequent reports of GBS have also been associated with the use of gangliosides which have been used in some European countries to promote nerve repair, by increasing collateral sprouting in nerve-damaged patients. It has been estimated that the risk of GBS is increased at least 200 fold following the use of ganglosides. Antimuscular antibodies have been detected in the sera of patients who develop GBS or motor-neuron-like disorders following treatment with gangliosides. Other drugs reported to be associated with the onset of GBS include organic arsenicals, captopril, corticosteroids, Fansidar (pyrimethamine with sulfadoxine), gold salts, floxacillin, penicillamine and streptokinase.

MULTIPLE SCLEROSIS

Multiple sclerosis (MS) is a disease characterized by multiple neurological deficits occurring at different times and involving different parts of the nervous system. The course of MS is often relapsing and remitting but occasionally a rapid deterioration in the condition of the patient can occur.

The clinical features of the disease include optic neuritis, brain stem dysfunction associated with nausea, vertigo and diplopia, cerebellar ataxia, spasticity with motor weakness, bladder and bowel dysfunction. Psychiatric symptoms are common and include apathy, depression, memory deficits and inappropriate behaviour. It is generally assumed that the psychiatric symptoms arise as a consequence of the enhanced release of cytokines which are responsible for the apathy, depression and memory deficits (see Chapter 5 for the role of cytokines in depression). Thus MS is generally considered to be a T-cell-mediated autoimmune disease. The lesions resemble the cellular infiltrates associated with T cells reminiscent of delayed-type hyperactivity. It is uncertain whether the autoimmune response is due to a failure of clonal deletion, sensitization by neuroantigens or following a virus infection with molecular mimicry to a neuroepitope. It would therefore appear that the evidence implicating MS as an autoimmune disease is indirect and largely based on a rodent model of experimental allergic encephalomyelitis.

Attacks of MS usually occur without warning or any obvious antecedent. Ten per cent of infectious illness in MS patients is followed by an attack, a frequency three times greater than expected. Attacks have also been precipitated by the administration of IFN-γ, a T-cell cytokine. Thus stress and infection may precipitate the attack of MS at least partly because of the release of IFN-γ from activated T cells.

Pathologically there are numerous areas of demyelination associated with inflammatory cells located in the white matter. Large lesions are formed by the coalescence of smaller ones and by the extension of myelin destruction at the margin of the lesions.

The aetiology and the pathogenesis of MS are unknown but a viral or autoimmune cause seems probable. There is, however, no association with other autoimmune diseases in MS patients. Those carrying the HLA-DRZ antigen have a fourfold increased risk of MS and it would appear that inheritance of the susceptibility to MS is polygenic.

Despite the evidence that TNF-α and IFN-γ are of pathogenic importance in MS, no effective therapies have yet been developed to impede the progress of the disease. There is some interesting preliminary data showing that the phosphodiesterase inhibitor rolipram (which was initially developed as an antidepressant) suppresses the production of these cytokines in both human and rat autoreactive T cells. This suggests that it may be possible to develop drugs that, by suppressing the cytokines causally implicated in MS, could be useful in reducing the progression of the disease.

LIMBIC ENCEPHALITIS

This is a rare syndrome that presents with predominantly psychiatric features. Severe anxiety and depression are usual in addition to a short-term memory defect and dementia. Patients may also experience hallucinations and exhibit bizarre behaviour. Neurological findings suggest a primary midbrain/brain stem lesion which could account for the symptoms of the condition, including vertigo, ataxia, nystagmus, nausea, vomiting and cranial nerve palsies. Pathological features include lymphocyte perivascular infiltration with neuronal loss, reactive microglia and astrocyte proliferation. These changes are particularly prevalent in the frontal cortex and while the lesions closely resemble those seen in herpes simplex encephalitis, no virus has been implicated in the disease. Many of the psychiatric symptoms are possibly a consequence of excessive cytokine release from the reactive microglia.

SYSTEMIC LUPUS ERYTHEMATOSUS (SLE)

Changes in the functioning of the central nervous system (CNS) are particularly common in SLE, which is a multisystem disease characterized by multiple immune abnormalities with involvement of the skin, joints, kidneys, blood, heart, lungs and the nervous system. More than 50% of SLE patients have psychiatric and neurological symptoms at some point in the course of the disease. When the CNS is involved, the most common feature is a fluctuating, acute confusional state with inattention, disorientation, disturbance of short-term memory and perceptual difficulties which may herald the onset of coma. Visual and auditory hallucinations are often present which could be confused with acute schizophrenia. Depression and anxiety may also occur in the absence of confusion. Epileptiform seizures occur in approximately 50% of patients exhibiting the psychiatric features; migraine-like headaches are common.

Pathologically, the brain shows only low grade non-inflammatory vasculopathy characterized by vessel wall thickening and intimal proliferation of small arteries which may result in scattered microinfarcts. It is possible that these changes occur as a consequence of circulating immune complexes. These pathological features do not account for the psychiatric features of the disease and therefore it is proposed that the increased release of cytokines may be responsible. In addition, antineuronal antibodies have been found in SLE patients and it is thought that they may gain access to the brain as a result of the increased permeability of the blood–brain barrier that has been damaged by the circulating immune complexes. This seems credible as there is a good correlation between the elevated CSF antineuronal antibody concentration, confusional states and seizures seen in these patients.

RHEUMATOID ARTHRITIS (RA)

RA is a common disease that affects about 3 million individuals in the United States alone. It is a systemic autoimmune disease characterized by crippling inflammation of the joints, particularly the hand, wrists and knees. Outgrowths of bone tissue form in the affected joints and cause damage to the cartilage and normal bone. These growths result in a decrease in the ability of the patient to move the affected joints. RA is particularly prominent in the female (3 : 1 female : male ratio), usually occurs in individuals of 35–45 years of age and progressively worsens over the following 10–30 years. In addition to the joints, the eyes, lungs, heart, spleen, skin, muscles and peripheral nerves may also be affected.

In RA, autoantibodies, called rheumatoid factors, are present in the plasma. Rheumatoid factors are antibodies against the Fc portion of normal self-IgG immunoglobulins. However, not all patients with RA have rheumatoid factors and not all those with rheumatoid factors have RA.

The fluid around the arthritic joints contains rheumatoid factors (either IgM or IgG) and normal IgG, which together form anti-antibody complexes. Inflammation results and the synovium becomes heavily infiltrated by plasma cells and lymphocytes. Two of the major symptoms of RA are usually synovitis and vasculitis.

The causes of the formation of rheumatoid factors are unknown. However, signs of immune activation proceeding in the affected synovium are seen when immune cells of the cultured synovium produce gammaglobulin, and the complement concentrations in the synovial fluid are depleted.

Although the aetiology of RA is poorly understood, the pathology of the condition is understood. Thus RA starts with an inflammatory reaction within the joints. Speculation about the nature of the antigenic stimulus has ranged from bacteria to mycoplasma and viruses. In addition, the severity of the inflammatory response may depend on the genetic background of the individual. Thus those with the MHC gene producing HLA-DE4 are statistically more likely to develop RA than those who lack the gene. The resulting antigen–antibody complexes are then deposited in the joints and macrophages and neutrophils enter the space around the joints by chemotactic factors. Damage to the joints is increased by the release of proteolytic enzyme released by macrophages during phagocytosis. The activated macrophages also release IL-1 which activates T and B lymphocytes, which in turn produce interferons and other mediators that favour macrophage activation and chemotaxis. This cascade of inflammatory mediators enhances the destruction of the surrounding tissue. It has been speculated that the absence of a mechanism whereby the inflammatory processes are reduced could be due to the lack of immune suppressor cells.

The immune factors that contribute to the degenerative changes in the joints of patients with RA include IL-1, IL-6 and TNF, whose concentrations have been shown to increase in the synovial fluid. The chemotactic factors which are responsible for attracting the macrophages to the inflammatory site include macrophage inflammatory protein 1 alpha, monocyte chemotactic protein-1 and a number of neutrophil chemoattractants. The concentration of IL-8 is also raised in the synovial fluid of RA patients and the increase in the concentration of anti IL-8 IgG has been shown to reflect the severity of the arthritis.

While both cellular and humoral immune mechanisms are inextricably linked to the pathogenesis of RA, there is evidence that RA may not be a single disease. For example, there is evidence of a significant association between the HLA-DW4 haplotype and the seropositive form of the disease but not between the HLA haplotype and the seronegative form. Given their diversity and the likelihood that rheumatoid factors plus complement damage the joints in only one form of RA, it seems unlikely that the same cellular and humoral factors play a role in all forms of the disease.

Studies on psychosocial factors in RA imply that such factors participate in the breakdown of tolerance to native antigens and resistance to infection through the mediation of the CNS. The precise mechanism whereby the CNS initiates or contributes to the inflammatory process is uncertain but there are several possibilities whereby this may occur. Thus axon reflexes release substance P, which is a potent vasodilator that increases vascular permeability. In addition, substance P recruits polymorphs, stimulates their phagocytic activity and degranulates most cells. Unmyelinated afferent fibres also release substance P; experimentally this peptide is also released by synovial cells in joints where it stimulates the secretion of collagenase and prostaglandin E (PGE). Finally, efferent pathways of unmyelinated fibres pass through the dorsal root ganglion; substance P is released from these neurons. In addition to substance P, other peptides may also be released at the site of inflammation and contribute to the degenerative process. These peptides include vasoactive intestinal peptide, somatostatin and calcitonin gene-related peptide, all of which are vasodilators that also affect leucocyte function.

Evidence in favour of the role of substance P and related inflammatory peptides in RA is obtained by the use of drugs such as capsaicin that reduce inflammation and joint damage in RA.

A distinguishing feature of RA is the relatively low concentrations of IL-2 and IFN-α in the synovial fluid in addition to the high concentrations of the proinflammatory cytokines. There is also evidence that the macrophages from RA patients secrete an inhibitory factor that inhibits IL-2 and IFN synthesis by lymphocytes. Thus RA may be considered a disease of macrophage activation and lymphocyte suppression.

Epidemiological studies suggest that the risk of developing schizophrenia is five times greater in the general population than in patients with RA; RA has therefore been considered to be a protection against developing schizophrenia, possibly due to the fact that the latter may be associated with an excessive secretion of causative cytokines (see Chapter 2). Conversely depression is positively associated with RA, the incidence of depression being reported to be twice as high in those with RA as in those without the disease. One possible explanation is that both depression and RA are associated with excessive macrophage activation.

The causes of the increased macrophage activation in RA and depression are unknown but there is some evidence that the fatty acid content of the diet could play a role (see Chapter 8). In Japan, for example, the incidence of both depression and RA is said to be substantially lower than in European countries or North America. This has been attributed to the high consumption of fish oil in the Japanese diet. Fish oil is rich in eicosapentaenoic acid

(EPA), a source of the anti-inflammatory form of postaglandin and the leuc-otrienes (PGE3 and LTDS). Macrophage activity is known to be reduced by fish oil; IL-1 and TNF-α concentrations have been shown to be reduced by about 50% following the consumption of fish oil for six weeks and the inflammatory response by macrophages correspondingly reduced. Such observations open up the possibility that dietary supplementation with EPA, together with docosahexanoic acid, which is a unique component of fish oil and which is concentrated in the brain, could be therapeutically beneficial to patients suffering from RA or depression. It must be emphasized, however, that the incidence of depression in Japan may be much higher than epidemiological studies suggest. This is due to the culturally based lack of recognition of depression by many Japanese psychiatrists.

In conclusion, it would appear that in addition to the proinflammatory cytokines (and IL-8) that are causally related to RA, several neuropeptides (of which substance P appears to be of importance) are also involved directly and indirectly in the inflammatory process.

Unlike many of the autoimmune diseases that affect humans, there are several acceptable animal models of the condition. These include the type II collagen arthritis model in the rat that mimics the joint lesions found in human RA, but rheumatoid factors are absent from the serum. It is of interest that changes in the environment of the animals, for example by overcrowding in some studies, have caused the lesions to develop more rapidly and severely. This suggests that, as with human RA, psychosocial factors may play a crucial role in the onset and severity of the disease.

AUTOIMMUNE THYROID DISEASE

Classical hyperthyroidism is a multisystem disease characterized by diffuse goitre with hyperthyroidism, exophthalmos and pretibial oedema. These three features may occur together or in isolation. When thyroiditis is not due to infection, it is ascribed to cell-mediated immune dysfunction. Circulating antithyroid colloid, antithyroglobulin and antithyroid microsomal antibodies are detectable in the serum of the patient. Marked lymphocytic infiltration of the thyroid gland occurs in both acute and subacute forms of thyroiditis. In Grave' disease (hyperthyroidism) a number of inhibitory and stimulatory antibodies also occur. These are the long-acting thyroid stimulator (LATS) and the thyroid-stimulating immunoglobulins (TSI). The latter bind to the thyroid follicular thyrotrophin (TSH) receptor to increase thyroid hormone synthesis by activating cyclic AMP.

Genes coding for some HLA antigens are involved in autoimmune thyroid disease. Those belonging to class I may modulate thyroid hormone action while class II antigens appear to be particularly liable to be induced on the thyroid cells. There is evidence that one or more HLA antigens may influence the severity, the presence or absence of exophthalmos and the response to antithyroid medication. Other genes that code for the T-cell receptor are also involved. Their products interact with the specific HLA antigens, DRW3 and B8 to enhance the risk, but not the severity, of the disease.

The most frequent initial symptom of Graves' disease is anxiety and "nervousness", the acute onset of the disease often occurring after a major life event (e.g. physical trauma, bereavement) but the precise mechanism whereby such events trigger thyroid dysfunction is unclear. It has been estimated that 30–50% of cases remit spontaneously.

In hyperthyroidism, the HLA-DR antigen is expressed on the surface of the thyroid cells. The lymphocyte numbers, NK cells and antigen-specific CD8 cell functions are diminished in most cases of the disease; the CD8 defect persists during the period of remission from the disease.

Circulating T cells proliferate when exposed to the microsomal antigen and thyroglobulin antibodies and then produce the cytokine migration inhibition factor. Treatment with the anti-thyroid drug methimazole is accompanied by a reduction in the number of activated CD4 cells and a transient increase in the number of activated CD8 cells. B cells bind to the anti-thyrotrophin-releasing hormone (anti-TRH) antibody; anti-idiotypic autobodies to anti-TRH have been isolated from the serum of patients with Graves' disease.

In hyperthyroidism, the thyroid gland is infiltrated with monocytes and macrophages in addition to B and T cells that comprise 80% of the total number of cells. Whereas the number of CD8 cells in the gland is reduced, activated CD4 cells are increased and the B cells in the gland secrete anti-thyroglobulin antibodies and other immunoglobulins.

In summary, it would appear that the immune pathology of hyperthyroidism remains to be fully explained. Undoubtedly the anti-thyrotrophin receptor antibody plays a central role in the pathogenesis of the disease but the source of this antibody is unknown. Experimental models of the disease have been developed that may help in elucidating its pathogenesis. Experimental autoimmune thyroiditis and hypothyroidism have been produced by the injection of thyroglobulin and adjuvant into rabbits, guinea pigs, mice and chickens. A spontaneous form of the disease has been described in monkeys and dogs. While such models have been useful in elucidating the role of CD8 and cytotoxic T cells in the pathogenesis of experimental autoimmune thyroiditis, animal models of stress-induced changes in thyroid physiology have been unhelpful in the understanding of the pathogenesis of the disease.

CONCLUSION

Normally, a reactivity of T and B cells to mature antigens occurs during the course of their development. It would appear that B cells are exposed to such antigens during an early stage of their maturation and become permanently unreactive to them on subsequent exposure. Thus under normal conditions the danger of autoimmune disease is averted. In patients with autoimmune diseases, this process does not occur, thereby rendering the patient vulnerable to the consequences of immune activation by autoantibodies. Why antigen–antibody complexes (and complement) are not cleared from the body in the case of autoimmune disease is unknown.

Another factor that appears to be a common predisposing feature of RA, SLE, hyperthyroidism and possibly type I (insulin-dependent) diabetes mellitis and irritable bowel disease is the effect of major life events (particularly bereavement and divorce). It would appear that patients with these diseases are particularly sensitive to disrupted human relationships and may have defective coping strategies. It is well established that major life events such as bereavement and divorce can lead to major changes in both cellular and humoral immunity. This has been discussed in detail elsewhere (see Chapter 2). Clearly the immunological correlates of bereavement, depression and autoimmune disease differ but such social stressors may be particularly important triggers in the development of the pathological changes in the immune system that lead to a specific immune disease. Some of the neuroendocrine factors that may contribute to the immune changes seen in autoimmune diseases are listed in Table 10.1.

It is obvious that there are many gaps in our knowledge about the cause of autoimmune disease. So far, there is an absence of a theory of autoimmunity which is complicated by the welter of contradictory data. It is evident, however, that each autoimmune disease is multifactorial.

BIBLIOGRAPHY

Aisen, P. S. and Davis, K. L. (1994) Inflammatory mechanism in Alzheimer's disease: implications for therapy. *American Journal of Psychiatry* **151**: 1105–1113.

Benjamini, E., Sunshine, G. and Leskowitz, S. (1996) *Immunology—a Short Course*, 3rd edn: Wiley-Liss, New York.

Elgert, K. D. (1996) *Immunology: Understanding the Immune System.* Wiley-Liss, New York.

Jain, K. K. (1996) *Drug Induced Neurological Disorders.* Hogrefs and Huber, Seattle.

Nakane, Y. Ohta Y., Uchino J. et al. (1988) Comparative study of affective disorders in three Asian countries. *Acta Psychiatrica Scandinavica* **78**: 698–705.

Rose, N. R. and Bona, C. (1993) Defining criteria for autoimmune diseases (Witebsky's postulates revisited). *Immunology Today* **14**: 426–430.

Theofilipoulos, A. N. (1995) The basis of autoimmunity: Part 1. Mechanism of aberrant self-recognition. Part 2. Genetic Predisposition. *Immunology Today* **16**: 90–98; 150–159.

Weiner, H. (1991) Social and psychobiological factors in autoimmune disease. In: Ader, R. Felten, D. L. and Cohen, N. (Eds) *Psychoneuroimmunology*, pp. 955–1012. Academic Press, New York.

Wilder, R. L. (1995) Neuroendocrine-immune system interactons and autoimmunity. *Annual Review of Immunology*, **13**: 307–338.

11 The Role of the Thymus Gland in Psychoneuroimmunology

It is well known that the thymus as the central lymphoid organ generates immunocompetent T lymphocytes. The bone-marrow-derived T-cell precursors undergo a complex intrathymic process of maturation, eventually leading to the migration of mature thymic lymphocytes to the T-cell-dependent areas of peripheral lymphoid organs. This differentiation process involves sequential expression of a variety of membrane markers, and rearrangements of the T-cell receptor (TCR) genes. Following migration and differentiation, most thymic lymphocytes are deleted by apoptosis during the negative selection process. Those rescued are subject to a positive selection, and then become the majority of the T cells. These key events in intrathymic T-cell differentiation are driven by the influence of the thymic microenvironment which includes a three-dimensional network comprising distinct cell types such as thymic epithelial cells, macrophages and dendritic cells. The thymic epithelium is the major component of the thymic microenvironment and has at least two functions: (i) production of polypeptides including thymic hormones and cytokines and (ii) the formation of cell–cell contact such as the interactions occurring through classical adhesion molecules.

As mentioned previously, there are a number of pathways between the central nervous system (CNS) and thymus gland. It is well known that the thymus gland is innervated by the sympathetic noradrenergic nervous system. In addition, it was found that the release of noradrenaline is subjected to negative feedback modulation via presynaptic α_2–adrenoreceptors. On the other hand, at least two neuroendocrine systems are regulated by the thymus: the hypothalamo–pituitary–gonadal (HPG) and the hypothalamic–pituitary–adrenal (HPA) axes.

It has been well established that ageing is paralleled by an increase in vulnerability to infections and an increase in the frequency of malignant tumours and autoimmune disease. The high incidence of diseases, such as vascular disease, maturity-onset diabetes, cancer, amyloidosis and senile dementia, that occur in the elderly are associated with malfunctions of the immune system. Ageing affects the immune system (i) by causing a progressive breakdown of functioning of immunocompetent cells and (ii) by clonal exhaustion of immunocompetent cells, as indicated by somatic mutations, errors in DNA replication or repair, or a malfunctioning of DNA poly-merases and related enzymes. In particular, the T-cell system-dependent immune functions appear to decline with age. This is due to the ageing of the thymus which as a consequence affects T-lymphopoiesis. The alterations in this organ during ageing have been held responsible for the decline in the immune functions of the entire T-cell system.

THE ROLE OF THYMUS AGEING AND THYMIC HORMONES

After birth, the human thymus grows only during the first year of life. During ageing, a slight but not significant decrease in thymus weight occurs in humans due to the increased portion of fat in the tissue. The most impressive change in the human thymus during ageing is the occurrence of lipomatous atrophy. The cortical areas of the thymus are depleted of lymphoid cells and the epithelial cells show cystic changes and reduction in intracellular granules. The involution of the thymus with age is characterized by a puberty-independent continuous degeneration of the thymic epithelial space. This starts in the first year of life and progresses during the first decade. Then the rate of involution is decreased. Defects of the epithelial–lymphocytic microenvironment occur even in early life and continue at a constant rate. This defect of cellular interaction may be caused by excesses of interleukin-mediated lymphocyte proliferation and/or by intrinsic impairments and cell death of epithelial cells.

Thymus ageing induces changes in the microenvironment of T cells, which also results from the reduction in production and secretion of circulating thymic hormones and lymphokines with loss of humoral and cell-mediated functions. Thymic hormones, such as the thymosins, are peptides produced and secreted by the thymus gland that influence the maturation and functioning of T cells. Lymphokines are a type of cytokine that are produced by T cells and other lymphocytes, which can affect immune response and the synthesis of cytokines.

The thymic hormones (Table 11.1), such as thymosin fraction (TF)-5 and thymosin (T)-α_1, have been used clinically for stimulating T-cell immunity associated both with the ageing process and in the treatment of some types of cancer. Thymopoietin (TP-5) is effective *in vitro* and *in vivo* in reversing the immunological effects of ageing on the generation of antibody plaque-forming cells, while thymulin and thymostimulin have been shown to repair the deficiency in the T-helper cell response in elderly humans and mice. Thymic hormones also modulate lymphokine production. Thus, TF-5, TP-1 and T-α_1 have been shown to induce and enhance interferon gamma (IFN-γ) production in both mice and humans. It has also been reported that thymic humoral factor (THF) enhances interleukin-2 (IL-2) production in nude and adult thymectomized mice. TF-5 can also markedly increase IL-2 production by human peripheral lymphocytes. In addition, TF-5 and thymic factor (TFX) have been found to regulate haemopoiesis via T-cell products and also to induce cytokines such as colony-stimulating factor. Many studies have demonstrated that the concentrations of these thymic hormones progressively decline with age and are virtually undetectable in humans older than 60 years. This decrease precedes the decline in immune function.

Table 11.1 Thymic hormones and their functions

Name	Abbreviation	Description	Functions
Thymosin fraction-5	TF-5	A 3208 molecular weight hormone	Regulating late T-cell differentiation
Thymosin-α and -β	T-α and T-β		Stimulating IFN-γ and IL-2 synthesis
Thymopoietin	TP-5	A 5562 molecular weight hormone	Regulating early T-cell differentiation and proliferation. Stimulating IFN-γ production
Thymulin	FTS	Peptide produced by thymic epithelial cells	Regulating T-cell development and response
Thymic hormone factor	THF	31 amino acid with molecular weight of 5220	Enhancing IL-2 production and T-cell functions
Thymic factor	TFX		Regulating haemopoiesis

THYMUS-INDUCED T-CELL-RELATED IMMUNE CHANGES DURING AGEING

Decreases in absolute number of T precursors in the bone marrow, spleen, lymph nodes and the blood decreases the density of T-cell surface antigens and a reduction in T-cell cytotoxity has been reported in elderly but physically healthy people. T-cell suppression of macrophage phagocytosis of syngeneic erythrocytes, delayed-type hypersensitivity (DTH) response, T-cell proliferation, regeneration and response to T-cell mitogens (phytohaemagglutinin), cortisone sensitivity of antigen-reactive lymph node lymphocytes, T-helper cell functions and T-suppressor functions are also reduced in normal ageing. However, some immune functions are increased during ageing. These include zinc suppression of mitogen response, sensitivity of T cells to prostaglandin E2 (PGE2), non-T-cell-mediated natural killer (NK) cell activity and mean cell cycle duration and G1-phase duration of peripheral blood T cells. These changes may be directly due to thymus ageing and the decline in the production of thymic hormones and lymphokines. For example, cytokine granulocyte-macrophage colony-stimulating factor (GM-CSF) is of importance as a growth factor for bone marrow stem cells which produce T cells. IL-2 modulates many lymphocyte functions including proliferation and differentiation, and the expression of some antigens, while IFN-γ is a potent inducer of null and NK cells. IFN-γ also regulates the humoral immune response which results in the activation of macrophages. This is shown by increased phagocytosis and the expression of some antigens. A decrease in NK cell cytotoxicity has been detected in ageing people. In particular, IFNs and IL-2-induced NK cell activity is significantly reduced in these subjects.

Several studies have shown that in contrast to the decline in T-cell-mediated immune functions, the functions of B cells and macrophages do not appear to decrease with age. However, it has been found that B-cell function may be reduced due to the lack of T-cell helper activity. Microenvironment changes induced by thymus ageing may affect T-cell/B-cell interactions and both T-cell and B-cell immune memory. As a consequence of thymus ageing, the cytokines produced by thymocyte and thymic epithelial cells are also decreased. This includes the influence of IL-1 on T-cell development. Nevertheless, an increase in macrophage-produced cytokines (IL-1, TNF-α and IL-6) has been reported in the blood of aged subjects, especially in those with ageing-related disorders. The mechanism involved in this change is still unclear. The autocrine and paracine actions between cytokines inside and outside the thymus may regulate cytokine production. Here authors postulate two possibilities. The first mechanism is an increase in cytokine production from other cell lines or in non-specific immunity. Thus an increase in monocyte activity, and humoral immunity such as B-cell produced antibodies, may be a dysregulation resulting from ageing of thymus-mediated specific immunity. Secondly, increased cytokines and antibodies may result from ageing-associated tissue damage, toxic accumulation and free-radical damage.

NEUROENDOCRINE–THYMUS INTERACTION

Cell-to-cell communication between the immune and the neuroendocrine system is primarily mediated by hormones, cytokines, neurotransmitters or neuropeptides. As discussed in Chapter 2, the thymus is also innervated by adrenergic and cholinergic nerves. Receptors for hormones, neurotransmitters or neuropeptides are present on T lymphocytes and thymic epithelium, while some lymphocytes and other immune cells can synthesize many types of hormone. Conversely, both thymopeptides and peripherally released hormones may pass the blood–brain barrier (BBB) and enter the brain. Thus, thymic factors may regulate immune functions and cytokine production in both the periphery and central nervous system (CNS). It has been shown that thymic hormones can act directly on pituitary cells and thereby modulate the hypophysis–thymus loop. In this way, thymic hormones can modulate the activity of the hypothalamic–pituitary axis and hormone secretions.

INFLUENCE OF THE NEUROENDOCRINE NETWORK ON THYMUS FUNCTIONS

In early experimental studies, in order to prove that the neuroendocrine system may affect the functions of the thymus, changes following the removal of endocrine glands were assessed. It was found that after removal of the thymus hypophysis or thyroid, thymus growth slowed down. Similarly, by reducing the activity of the pancreas, thymus growth is delayed. By contrast, following removal of gonads and adrenal glands, the size and growth of thymus is increased. Recent studies have shown that an increase in cortisol secretion during stress, or following the peripheral administration of cortisol, reduces the thymus weight and accelerates thymus ageing.

Compared to the measurement of thymus weight or size, detecting thymic hormone production may more directly reflect the function of the thymus. Thus it has been demonstrated that congenital hypopituitarism, experimental diabetes and thyroidectomy all result in a rapid reduction of plasma levels of thymulin, whereas removing the gonads and adrenals fails to change the circulating concentration of this thymic hormone. Thyroid hormones up-regulate thymulin secretion, even in ageing individuals, and this appears to be dependent on *de novo* thymulin synthesis since it can be prevented *in vitro* by treatment with cycloheximide. Moreover, classic pituitary hormones, such as prolactin (PRL) and growth hormone (GH), are able to enhance thymulin secretion *in vivo* in many species including humans. Conversely, deficiency in GH production in children is accompanied by low thymulin concentration. ACTH, β-endorphin and enkephalin also increase the release of this peptide. In humans, many endocrine-related disorders are associated with changes in circulating thymulin. Thus patients with hypopituitarism, type I diabetes mellitus or hypothyroidism show lower blood thymulin concentration. By contrast, hyperthyroidism is associated with higher thymulin concentrations (Figure 11.1).

INFLUENCE OF THE THYMUS ON THE NEUROENDOCRINE NETWORK

In order to study the relationship between the thymus and the neuroendocrine system, several studies were conducted on nude mice which have a

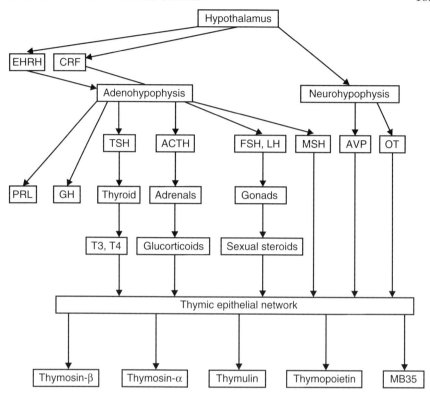

Figure 11.1 Influence of the neuroendocrine hormones on thymic endocrine activity. These interactions may occur directly on thymic epithelial cells, or via target glands that release their hormones, which in turn act upon epithelial cells. CRF, corticotrophin-releasing factor; TSH, thyroid-stimulating hormone; ACTH, adreno-corticotrophic hormone; FSH, follicle-stimulating hormone; LH, luteinizing hormone; AVP, arginine vasopressin; OT, oxytocin; PRL, prolactin; GH, growth hormone; T3, triiodothyronine; T4, thyroxine; MB35, peptide component of thymosin.

congenital absence of the thymus gland. In these mice, progressive degranulation of GH and PRL cells was observed, while the plasma concentration of PRL decreased and that of leuteinizing hormone (LH) increased. Moreover, an impairment in HPA axis function was found in the nude athymic mice. These studies showed that basal plasma ACTH concentration is significantly higher, whereas basal plasma concentration of corticosterone is unchanged. In these mice, the stress-induced release of ACTH and corticosterone is much lower than in BALB mice. In *in vitro* studies, the pituitary response to corticotrophin-releasing factor (CRF) and the adrenal response to ACTH is significantly lower in the nude athymic mouse. These findings indicate that athymic nude mice have a blunted HPA axis response to stress stimuli; this defect seems to reside at both the pituitary and adrenal levels. Thymectomy in normal adult mice also causes a reduction of thyroid hormones (T3 and T4), while in neonatal thymectomized rats it results in decreased numbers of secretory granules in acidophilic cells of the adenopituitary. In these animals, the plasma concentrations of corticosterone and ACTH are also decreased. These findings suggest that the thymus influences the adrenals via the hypophysis. With respect to thymic peptides, it has been shown that a thymosin component, thymosin-β_4, is able to stimulate LH, LH-releasing hormone and follicle-stimulating hormone (FSH) from the hypothalamus. In addition, another thymosin component, the MB-35 peptide, stimulates the production of PRL and GH. Thymopentin enhances the *in vitro* production of ACTH, β-endorphin and β-lipotrophin, but does not modulate pituitary hormone. Interestingly, thymosin-α1 is apparently able to down-regulate thyroid-stimulating hormone (TSH), ACTH and PRL secretion, but has no effect on GH synthesis. These findings suggest that different thymic hormones may play different roles in the neuroendocrine–thymic axis (Figure 11.2).

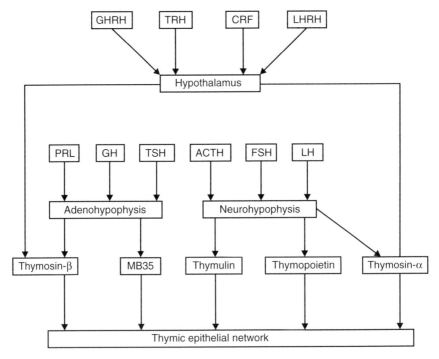

Figure 11.2   The influence of thymic hormones on the hypothalamus–pituitary axis. Thymic peptides can directly affect both pituitary and hypothalamic cells. GHRH, growth hormone-releasing hormone; TRH, thyrotrophin-releasing hormone; CRF, corticotrophin-releasing factor; LHRH, luteinizing hormone-releasing hormone; PRL, prolactin; GH, growth hormone; TSH, thyroid-stimulating hormone; FSH, follicle-stimulating hormone; LH, luteinizing hormone; MB35, peptide component of thymosin.

A reduction in the density of β-adrenoceptors in the brain and submandibular glands has also been found in mice that lack the thymus. Moreover, experimentally, it has been shown a relationship exists between thymus functions and glucocorticoids in ageing or following stress. Thus, stress exposure (footshock, isolation and novel environment) significantly reduces thymus weight and thymic hormone synthesis. Similarly, intracerebroventricular administration of CRF or systemic injection of corticosterone also causes these changes. Histological examination reveals that stress, CRF and glucocorticoids all produce changes in the structure of the thymus that are similar to those observed in ageing.

With regard to the gonads, thymectomy causes different effects on gonadal function in males and females. For example, thymectomy in male hamsters suppresses sexual function, but not in females, while in mice, thymectomy causes sterility in females but not in males. Furthermore, in both thymectomized mice and nude mice, sexual underdevelopment commonly occurs.

It is well established that neuroendocrine ageing (as indicated by a reduced activity of hypothalamic neurosecretory cells, increased hypothalamic threshold level to negative feedback, abnormalities in most endocrine glands particularly in the pituitary–adrenal axis and in thyroid hormone secretion, and reduced peripheral sensitivity to the stimulation of hormones and neurotransmitters) displays a linear progression starting early in life. The interconnection of such changes in the endocrine system with the thymus, which shows a similar age-dependent progressive deterioration, does not therefore seem to be merely coincidental. It seems likely that thymus ageing may be the first trigger eliciting these age-related changes.

EFFECTS OF THYMECTOMY ON BEHAVIOUR, BRAIN NEUROTRANSMITTERS AND MEMORY

There is evidence that the concentrations of monoamines, their metabolites and acetylcholinesterase are reduced in the ageing brain. For example, concentrations of acetylcholine (ACh), noradrenaline (NA) and dopamine (DA) have been found to be decreased, while 5-hydroxytryptamine (5-HT) concentrations may be increased or unchanged. In rodents, thymectomy may be considered to be a model of accelerated ageing for immunopharmacological studies. Thus in the rat, thymectomy-induced changes in neurotransmitter concentrations resemble those seen in the brain of ageing rats. In young adult rats, four weeks after thymectomy, the concentration of NA is reduced in the amygdala, hypothalamus and olfactory bulbs. DA is also largely decreased in the olfactory bulbs and its metabolites vanillylmandelic acid (VMA) and dihydroxyphenylacetic acid (DOPAC) are also slightly decreased in the hypothalamus and amygdala. 5-HT is markedly increased in the striatum, and its metabolite 5-hydroxyindole-acetic acid (5-HIAA) slightly increased. It would appear that the reduced concentrations of DA and NA in the hypothalamus may result in the decreased secretion of GH, ACTH and the sex hormones that characteristically occur in ageing. Mono-amine changes in the ageing brain can be reversed by the thymopeptide treatment, which suggests that these peptides help to regulate neuro-transmitter synthesis. However, in mice, thymectomy causes different monoamine changes in the hypothalamus. Increased NA and choline acetyl-transferase (ChAT) activity has been reported.

It is well established that ageing is associated with an impairment in learning and memory, which has generally been thought to result from changes in the concentrations of specific neurotransmitters. On the one hand many anti-dementia drugs facilitate neurotransmitter changes to improve learning and memory. On the other hand, thymus ageing-caused impair-ments in the CNS and the endocrine system are also well documented. However, the influence of the thymus on cognitive functions remains un-known. In clinical treatment, thymectomy is usually used for Graves' dis-ease. However, there seem to be no investigations into whether thymectomy causes any cognitive changes. In the review literature over the last 10 years, there are fewer than five papers showing the effect of thymectomy on learn-ing and memory. As mentioned above, thymectomy causes monoamine abnormalities in the brain of rats and mice. These two species also show impairment in learning and memory when they are tested in the passive avoidance apparatus or Morris water maze. In the passive avoidance test, thymectomized rats and sham operated animals do not show any dif-ferences in behaviour on day 1 and day 2. On day 3, thymectomized rats show a much shorter latency to enter the shock compartment of the appa-ratus than sham operated animals. Thymectomized rats also show a signifi-cant learning impairment in the Morris water maze, and spend much longer finding the platform on days 2 and 3. The deficit in both tests of thymec-tomized rats are largely reversed by chronic treatment with the nootropic drug piracetam and the anticholinesterase tacrine. In the hypothalamus, amygdala, striatum and olfactory bulbs, these two drug treatments also normalize thymectomy-induced neurotransmitter changes.

Thymectomized mice also show a similar impairment in conditioned learning in the passive avoidance test. In the stepdown passive avoidance test, thymectomized mice show a significant increase in total number of errors and a decrease in memory retention when compared to sham oper-ated mice. In other conditioning memory tests such as the shuttle box test and lever press test, thymectomized mice all show deterioration of learning and memory. In the Morris water maze, these animals also show spatial memory impairment. Thymectomized mice always take longer, and swim for a longer time and longer distance to reach and find the platform. These studies suggest that the thymus may play a very important role in learning and memory during ageing. If such studies are relevant to humans, it implies that thymopeptides and thymic hormone replacement may be a new direction in the development anti-ageing and anti-dementia drugs.

THYMUS FUNCTIONS AND PSYCHIATRIC OR NEUROLOGICAL DISEASES

Although numerous studies have revealed a relationship between the immune system and psychiatric diseases, such as abnormalities in cytokine production and cellular functions, the role of the thymus gland in these immune abnormalities or the relationship between the thymus and psychiatric disorders is unknown.

In the 1980s, several clinical researchers reported that psychiatric disturbances are associated with myasthenia gravis, a thymus-related autoimmune disease. An abnormality of thymus gland in the form of hyperplasia or thymoma may account for the observation that thymectomy is beneficial in the treatment of this disease. However, although about 40% of patients (or 57% of female patients) showed anxiety, depressive symptoms and/or personality disorders, thymectomy did not correct these symptoms.

More recently, an animal model of depression, the olfactory bulbectomized rat, has been used to study the relationship between the thymus and depression. After removal of olfactory bulbs, rats subsequently develop a series of changes in behaviour, neurotransmitter, endocrine and immune aspects which are similar to those occurring in depressed patients. A significantly decreased thymus weight has also been found, which is associated with increased weight of adrenal glands and other physical changes linked to depression. Thymopeptide treatment markedly reverses most of the changes caused by bulbectomy. IL-2, a major cytokine produced by T cells, can also attenuate these changes in olfactory bulbectomized rats.

In another animal model of depression, multiple stressors (footshock, swimming in cold water and isolation) were found to reduce the weight of the thymus gland. In addition, the reduced weight of the thymus glands in rodents has been linked to reduced serotonergic activity and increased emotional reactivity in social stress. Social stress, as occurs when a rat is subjected to repeated defeat by another rat, increases the midbrain serotonin metabolism and 5-HT2A receptor density, and decreases the density of hippocampal 5-HT1A receptors. Following such social stress, the animals showed an increased anxiety in the elevated-plus maze and a reduced thymus weight.

The effects of several factors that are causally related to depression and involve changes in thymus function have also been investigated in animals. As mentioned previously, elevated IL-1 concentrations has been found in both brain and blood of patients with depression and with Alzheimer's disease. As has been discussed elsewhere, the inflammatory responses and abnormalities in glucocorticoid secretion observed in such conditions may result from IL-1 hypersecretion. Central administration of IL-1 for several days causes many depressive symptoms, such as an increase in anxious behaviour, reduction of food intake, loss of body weight, negative balance of nitrogen, and reduction of lymphocyte proliferation. An IL-1-induced reduction in thymus weight is negatively correlated with an increase in adrenal weight and rise in plasma corticosterone concentrations. Sub-chronic CRF administration also causes a similar effect on thymus weight and suppresses lymphocyte functions; an elevation in CRF has been reported to occur in both depressed and schizophrenic patients and there is evidence that IL-1 directly stimulates CRF release in the hypothalamus. Conversely, during stress exposure (such as a conflict test), pretreatment with the thymic hormones thymopentin or T5 can normalize both the gamma-aminobutyric acid (GABA) reduction and corticosterone elevation that occur in rats. The stress-induced anxiety in the elevated-plus maze is also prevented by thymic hormone pretreatment. It is of interest that the effects of these thymic hormones on the stress-induced changes are similar to the effects of antidepressant treatment. This study suggests that thymus hormones may be precursors of new psychoneuromodulatory peptides that could be of value in the treatment of depression.

In elderly men it has been shown that psychosocial factors may be related to an abnormal T-α_1 response to stress. Individuals who are suffering depressive illness or stressful life events have higher concentrations of T-α_1 following physical stress (glucose challenge) when compared to their age- and sex-matched controls, but there is no correlation between psychosocial factors and T-α_1 concentration in the baseline condition. During stressor challenge, interpersonal sensitivity and psychotism are also positively correlated with the blood concentration of T-α_1.

EFFECTS OF ANTIDEPRESSANT AND ANTI-PSYCHOTIC DRUGS ON THYMUS FUNCTIONS

Fluoxetine, a serotonin reuptake inhibitor, is normally used for treatment of depression. In rats, fluoxetine has no effect on thymus functions, but in an activity-based anorexia model of rats, it significantly reduces oxytocin concentrations in the thymus gland. This is due to an abnormal increase in sympathetic activity by fluoxetine that reduces thymus weight.

In olfactory bulbectomized rats, it has been reported that the antidepressants clorgyline and desipramine do not reverse the decrease in thymus weight, but do reverse reduced spleen weight. A higher dose of desipramine has been found to reduce thymus weight in both sham operated and bulbectomized rats, which may result from its toxic effects. Administration of 6-hydroxydopamine (6-OHDA) in mice reduces the weight of thymus and number of T cells, such as CD4+ and CD8+, and causes thymus atrophy or apoptosis. Pretreatment of desipramine can block the effect of 6-OHDA on thymus functions.

Experimental studies have shown that lithium salt also induces thymus involution in both cortex and medulla in mice and rats.

Neuroleptic drugs such as haloperidol incubated *in vitro* with thymocytes largely suppresses this cell proliferation, while there are no available data to show *in vivo* effect on thymus function.

There are very few studies to show the possible role of benzodiazepine drugs in modulation of the thymus gland in psychiatric disorders. One study has reported that clonazepam treatment in mice could reverse auditory stress-induced changes in thymus cellularity, such as T-cell function and subpopulation.

From these data, it can be seen that most studies have only examined thymus weight, a marker that may not completely reflect the functional changes in the thymus gland during psychiatric diseases or stress. Different drug treatments involve different mechanisms which may exert different influences on thymus functions. The interaction between the brain, endocrine system and thymus during treatment is not yet known. Further investigation on changes in thymus structure, thymic hormone production and thymocyte functions needs to be undertaken.

BIBLIOGRAPHY

Dardenne, M. and Savino, W. (1994) Control of thymus physiology by peptidic hormones and neuropeptides. *Immunology Today* **15**: 518–523.

Fabris, N. (1992) Biomarkers of aging in the neuroendocrine-immune domain. *Annals of the New York Academy of Sciences* **663**: 335–348.

Fabris, N., Mocchegiani, E., Muzzioli, M. and Provinciali, M. (1988) Neuroendocrine-thymus interactions: perspectives for intervention in aging. *Annals of the New York Academy of Sciences* **521**: 72–81.

Hill, A. G., Jacobson, L., Gonzalez, J., Rounds, J., Majzoub, J. A., et al. (1996) Chronic central nervous system exposure to IL-1β causes catabolism in the rats. *American Journal of Physiology* **271**: R1142–1148.

Magni, G., Micaglio, G. F., Lalli. R., Bejato, L., Candeago, M. R. et al. (1988) Psychiatric disturbances associated with myasthenia gravis. *Acta Psychiatrica Scandinavica* **77**: 443–445.

Song, C., Earley, B. and Leonard, B. E. (1997) Effect of chronic treatment with piracetam and tacrine on some changes caused by thymectomy in the rat brain. *Pharmacology, Biochemistry and Behavior* **56**: 697–704.

Steinmann, G. G. (1986) Changes in the human thymus during aging. *Current Topics in Pathology* **75**: 43–88.

Wick, G. and Grubeck-Loebenstein, B. (1997) Primary and secondary alterations of immune reactivity in the elderly: impact of dietary factors and disease. *Immunological Reviews* **160**: 171–184.

Zatz, M. M. and Gldstein, A. L. (1995) Thymosine, lymphokines, and the immunology of aging. *Gerontology* **31**: 263–277.

Zhang, Y., Saito, H. and Nishiyama, N. (1994) Thymectomy-induced deterioration of learning and memory in mice. *Brain Research* **658**: 127–134.

12 Animal Models of Stress and Psychiatric Disease and their Potential Application to Psychoimmunology

INTRODUCTION

Animal models are widely used to investigate or illustrate aspects of human psychopathology. The extent to which it is possible to extrapolate from animals to humans, and consequently the value of the information that may be derived from an animal model, depends on the validity of the model.

The two main uses of animal models are as screening tests for the development of new drugs to treat psychiatric illness and as simulations of the behavioural and/or neurochemical changes that are believed to be causally associated with specific psychiatric diseases. The principal reason for using animal models of psychiatric disease in the field of psychoimmunology has been to understand the nature of the changes in the immune system which may relate to the behavioural changes seen in patients. As at this stage of its development, psychoimmunology has only limited application in the development of novel therapeutic strategies, the contents of this chapter will emphasize the importance of those animal models that simulate aspects of the major psychiatric diseases. By its very nature, this implies that an animal model is of value in testing a hypothesis which must ultimately be studied in the patient for its validation.

There are three criteria which should be applied for the validation of an animal model.

1. The *predictive* validity of the model means that the performance of the animal in a specific test situation is essentially similar to the psychiatric state being modelled.
2. The *face* validity implies that there are major similarities between the behaviour of the animal and the clinical condition being modelled.
3. The *construct* validity implies that the model has a sound theoretical basis.

These criteria will now be considered in more detail so that they may be applied to the models that are of potential use in psychoimmunological research.

PREDICTIVE VALIDITY

This usually implies that drugs, or treatments, that are known to influence the clinical state should have a similar effect in the animal model. Thus situations that precipitate or exacerbate the disorder should have a similar effect on the model whereas, conversely, those conditions relieving the condition should normalize the behaviour in the animal model. The assessment of predictive validity is primarily based on considerations of sensitivity and specificity to drugs of actual, or potential, therapeutic use. Thus, drugs known to be effective should be active in the animal model at doses that approximate to those used therapeutically to produce tissue concentrations that are clinically relevant. In most cases, it is essential that the pharmacological effects in the model should only become optimal after chronic administration of the drug, as there are few major psychiatric conditions in which drug treatment produces an immediate therapeutic effect.

FACE VALIDITY

To be valid, an animal model of a psychiatric condition should resemble the disease state in terms of its aetiology, symptomatology, treatment and pathophysiological basis. In practice, this is almost impossible to achieve as, for example, there is no evidence that any species apart from humans suffers from such major psychiatric conditions as depression, schizophrenia, mania, panic disorder or obsessive compulsive disorder. With regard to the pathophysiological basis of these disorders, little is currently known, which makes it largely impossible to fulfil this criterion when developing animal models. For this reason, most models are based on the symptoms that have logical similarities with the disease state in humans.

CONSTRUCT VALIDITY

There is ample evidence to show that the behavioural components of a physiological function or pathological condition differ between species. Furthermore, there is no evidence that species, other than humans, suffer from any of the major psychiatric illnesses. This makes the establishment of construct validity difficult in an animal model. For this reason, the construct validity is the most difficult criterion to establish.

It must be emphasized that, at present, few animal models perform well in terms of the predictive, face and construct validity. However, it is important to remember that an animal model is still useful if it is well suited to address a specific problem. Models are used to expand an understanding of a psychatric disorder and the results obtained from the experimental studies are used to determine whether such changes also occur in the clinical situation.

This may help to refine the animal model. Ultimately, this could lead to a situation whereby the animal model is fully validated.

ANIMAL MODELS OF SCHIZOPHRENIA

Schizophrenia is generally regarded as being a uniquely human disorder and while primates, cats, dogs and rats may exhibit psychotic symptoms under certain experimental conditions, the existence of the full range of symptoms of schizophrenia is, so far, impossible to model in animals. Part of the difficulty in modelling schizophrenia comes from the limitations of the clinical nomenclature. For example, the Diagnostic and Statistical Manual of Mental Disorders (DSM) emphasizes the classical symptoms of schizophrenia such as thought disorder, delusions, hallucinations and inappropriate effect. This definition does not take into account increased response switching followed by perseveration and stereotypy, symptoms which occur in schizophrenic patients and in animals that have been exposed to dopaminomimetic drugs.

In addition to a difficulty that may arise as a consequence of differences in nomenclature, it is also necessary to allow for the changes in the nature of the illness with time. For example, the acute phase of the disease differs from the symptoms seen in the chronic phase. In addition, the proportion of the "positive" and "negative" symptoms varies from the acute to the chronic phases of the illness, the "positive" symptoms referring to the active , overtly recognizable symptoms while the negative symptoms refer to symptoms of neglect or omission (for example, poverty of speech, lack of personal hygiene and "flat" affect).

The clinical symptoms of schizophrenia and the symptoms that can be provoked in animals following various treatments indicate how a detailed assessment of social behaviours can be of practical value in developing animal models. Such models can be somewhat arbitrarily divided into four groups: (1) pharmacologically based models; (2) brain lesion models; (3) genetic and foetal development models and (4) behaviourally based models.

PHARMACOLOCICALLY BASED MODELS

Most of these are based on the use of domaminergic hyperactivity in which stimulants such as amphetamine or metamphetamine are used to induce hyperactivity and stereotyped behaviour in rodents. Other methods, using primates or cats, involve the chronic intoxication of the animals with amphetamine or cocaine. Neuroleptic drugs attenuate these symptoms. Localized injections of dopamine agonists into the nucleus accumbens of primates have been shown to produce many of the positive symptoms of acute schizophrenia listed above.

The discovery that the *N*-methyl-D-aspartate (NMDA) glutamate receptor antagonist phencyclidine may produce many of the symptoms of paranoid schizophrenia in humans has led to the use of this drug as a psychotomimetic agent in animals.

BRAIN LESION MODELS

There is behavioural evidence that the hippocampus, besides being involved in spatial and working memory, is also the source of highly perseverative thought and fixed delusions. There is experimental evidence to show that discrete electrolytic lesions of the hippocampus in rats result in excessive stereotyped behaviour similar to that seen following amphetamine administration.

Lesions of the ventral tegmental area (VTA), a dopamine-rich area of the mesolimbic system, has been shown in rats to cause cognitive learning deficits, while direct stimulation of the nucleus accumbens, another important component of the mesolimbic system, leads to excessive excitability and hypersensitivity to sensory stimulation in the rat.

The discovery that enlargement of the lateral and third ventricles occurs in schizophrenic patients prompted the development of animal models in which the size of the ventricles was experimentally increased. It has been shown that acute ventricular demyelination caused by lysophosphatidylcholine causes profound neurological and behavioural changes that make it a potentially valuable model if schizophrenia.

GENETIC AND FOETAL DEVELOPMENT MODELS

It is known that disturbances resulting from viral infection, radiation exposure and emotional stress during the second trimester of pregnancy are probably critical to the foetal brain changes that may lead to schizophrenia. Such changes are thought to be closely related to periventricular structures such as the basal ganglia, hippocampus and the mesocortical system. Clearly this is an area that requires further research as brain damage, caused by both pre- and perinatal disturbances, are thought to be factors that act together with a genetic predisposition to result in schizophrenia in later life.

BEHAVIOURALLY BASED MODELS

Isolation stress in rodents is associated with a persistent lack of response to other animals of the same species. The isolation of rats immediately after weaning results in hypersensitivity of the dopaminergic system. Social isolation in primates has also been shown to cause symptoms that are similar to those seen in chronic schizophrenia.

SUMMARY

It would appear that some valuable animal models of schizophrenia are already available. Clearly there is a need to increase the models based on abnormalities in foetal development. Most of the animal models in current use are based on changes in behaviour following a disturbance in the dopaminergic system. It would appear that models based on changes in other neurotransmitters (such as endogenous opioids or serotonin) have not been shown broadly to mimic the symptoms of schizophrenia.

ANIMAL MODELS OF ANXIETY

Whereas there is no universal agreement regarding the validity of the animal models of depression and schizophrenia, it is generally agreed that many of the animal models of anxiety fulfil the criteria of face validity (in that they are fear inducing) and predictive validity (they are relatively selective for responding to clinically effective anxiolytics). The models can be broadly divided into:

1. Those using spontaneous unconditional behaviour.
2. Those involving simple or complex classical and/or operant conditioning procedures.
3. Those that concentrate on drug-induced discriminative status.
4. Those involving brain stimulation paradigms.

UNCONDITIONAL BEHAVIOUR TESTS

Many of these tests involve studying the exploratory activity of an animal (usually a rodent) in a novel environment. Exploratory activity appears to be a function of general activity, impulsivity (the need to become familiar with a novel environment) and anxiety (the need to escape from an unpredictable environment).

One of the most widely used unconditional behavioural tests is the "open field" test, whereby the animal is placed in the centre of a brightly illuminated arena from which it cannot escape. The locomotion, sniffing and rearing (indices of exploration), defecation, urination, freezing and grooming (indices of fearfulness) are then measured over a fixed time interval, usually 3–5 min. Drugs that reduce the degree of anxiety tend to increase the locomotor activity and reduce the symptoms of fearfulness. Despite its practicability, the "open field" test is limited by its lack of specificity as stimulants and anticholinergic drugs that lack anxiolytic properties increase locomotor activity. The behaviour of rodents in the hole board apparatus, in which the animal is allowed to explore a square board containing 16 holes, is a less stressful version of the "open field". The apparatus allows the general activity of the animal to be assessed as well as the degree of fearfulness as determined by the number of times it explores the holes in the apparatus. Another unconditional test that has some validity is the light–dark box in which the number of times a rodent emerges from a dark box to explore the brightly lit compartment gives an index of the lack of fearfulness. Many anxiolytics increase the number of times the animal explores the brightly lit area.

Perhaps the best known and widely used test of anxiety is the elevated plus maze. This apparatus consists of four arms arranged in the form of a cross situated 50 cm above the ground. Two of the arms are open and the other two closed. The number of times the animal explores the open arms gives a measure of the lack of fearfulness; this behaviour is increased by most clinically effective anxiolytics.

Whereas the "open field", "hole board", light–dark box and elevated plus maze tests involve observing the behaviour of single animals, the social interaction test is perhaps a more realistic representation of the natural environment. In this test, the amount of social intervention between unfamiliar male rats (sniffing, grooming, wrestling, etc.) is decreased by anxiety and largely antagonized by anxiolytics.

CONDITIONED AVOIDANCE BEHAVIOURS

The presumed advantage of conditioning and operant procedures rests with the increased degree of control which the experimenter has over the behaviour of the animal and also the isolation of any confounding variables by suitable experimental design. Most of the experimental procedures involve aversive stimulus such as mild footshock.

Passive and active avoidance tests are particularly popular for assessing the potential anxiolytic activity of novel compounds. In the passive avoidance tests the animal (usually a rodent) is punished for making a response. Usually this occurs when the animal steps off a platform to explore its surroundings. When the animal is placed in the apparatus 24 hours later, this escape response is inhibited. Many anxiolytics disinhibit the passive avoidance response.

In contrast to the passive avoidance test, in the active avoidance test, the animal is shocked in one area of the apparatus but not the other. These areas are then reversed and in order to avoid the footshock the animal must learn to move from one side of the apparatus to the other to avoid the shock. A sound or light is usually used as the conditioning stimulus. Anxiolytics are generally effective in facilitating performance in the two-way active avoidance task.

The Geller–Seifter conflict test has been widely used to study anxiety in rodents and for the detection of anxiolytics. This paradigm usually consists of several operant components used by different light signals. A period of positive reinforcement (e.g. food reward), usually on a variable interval schedule, is followed by a short period when the responses are neither reinforced nor punished and then by a conflict component in which all responses are simultaneously rewarded with food and punished with a mild footshock. The suppression of responding in the conflict component is attenuated by anxiolytics, relatively specifically and with a potency proportional to their clinical potency.

DRUG DISCRIMINATION MODELS

Anxiolytic and anxiogenic drugs induce internal states that are sufficiently intense for a human being to describe accurately. Thus states of fear can be induced by convulsants such as leptazol (pentylenetetraol), yohimbine (the alpha-2 adrenoceptor antagonist) or beta carboline (an inverse benzoiazepine receptor agonist). Such reactions have also been observed in primates as well as rats. Experimentally it has been shown that rats that are trained to push a lever for a food reward under the influence of leptazol will push the same lever when injected with a different type of anxiogenic drug but not if the drug lacks those properties. Anxiolytics were shown to block the preference of the rats for the leptazol-associated lever.

BRAIN STIMULATION MODELS

Stimulation of different regions of the brain can produce the behavioural symptoms of fear in animals. These brain regions include the amygdala, locus coeruleus, medial raphe nucleus and the dorsal periaqueductal grey area of the midbrain. So far, the brain stimulation paradigms have not been extensively used in psychopharmacological studies, largely because interactions between fear responses produced by brain stimulation have not so far produced a particularly coherent body of data. However, the medial septal hippocampus theta rhythm paradigm has achieved considerable attention in recent years. In this paradigm, the theta rhythm is recorded from electrodes placed in the hippocampus that are stimulated by electrodes placed in the medial septum where the pacemaker cells are thought to be located. The threshold current required to drive the thera rhythm shows a characteristic curve which in the male rat falls to a minimum of 7.7 Hz. Anxiolytics selectively increase the threshold current necessary to drive the theta rhythm. From such studies, it has been argued that the 7.7 Hz theta rhythm is specifically related to the processing of novelty, non-reward and punishment, the effect being to switch on the behavioural inhibition system.

SUMMARY

It is not unreasonable to conclude that experimentally induced conditioned or unconditioned fear responses are not only central to clinical anxiety but can also be stimulated in animals. Thus fear-induced behaviour in animals would appear to represent meaningfully both the aetiology and symptoms of human anxiety and can therefore claim to have predictive, face and construct validity. The drug-induced discriminative states and brain stimulation models are pharmacologically or electrophysiologically elicited rather than being dependent on situational cues which are thought to be important in human anxiety. As such, these models lack construct validity.

ANIMAL MODELS OF DEPRESSION

Hitherto, most animal models that have been used for the selection of putative antidepressants have been based on the monoamine deficiency theory, which postulates that depression arises as a result of a deficiency in biogenic amine neurotransmitters in the synaptic cleft. A valid animal model of depression should fulfil the following criteria:

1. It should show behavioural changes that simulate those occurring in the depressed patient, for example, memory loss, motor retardation, deficits in cognition, irritability, anorexia, loss of libido.
2. It should show a normalization of these symptoms when the antidepressant drugs are administered.
3. As the effective control of depression only occurs following chronic drug treatment, the animal model should only respond optimally to antidepressants that are chronically administered.

Whereas it has been possible to develop rodent models of depression that satisfy the predictive validity, and to some extent the face validity, it has not been possible to develop reliable models of construct validity. This is because of the paucity of data relating to the biochemical changes that are causally related to depression even though there is some evidence that changes in the function of the biogenic amine neurotransmitters may play a crucial role.

Many of the animal models of depression are based on the effect of stress, the changes resulting from the exposure of animals (usually rodents) to stress being reversed by antidepressant treatments. The stressors used vary from mild to severe stress as exemplified by footshock, restraint stress and immersion in water. Chronic mild unavoidable stress has also been used to produce a model of depression which has the advantage over many of the stress models in that the behavioural deficits can be corrected by chronic, but not acute, antidepressant treatment. Other models are based on ethological methods whereby the effects of social defeat are monitored. Most of these procedures are associated with a decrease in motor activity and/or reward behaviour (for example, sucrose consumption) which may be reversed by acute and/or chronic antidepressant treatment depending on the model studied.

A second group of models is based on the effects of social isolation. Such studies have been mainly made on non-human primates but more recently behavioural changes following the social isolation of rats have been shown to be useful. The first and second group of models were largely developed 15–20 years ago and have undergone little change since their introduction.

The third group of models involve the reversal of changes that follow discrete lesions of the limbic system. Thus lesions of the amygdala, septum and the olfactory bulbs produce behavioural changes that can be reversed by the chronic administration of antidepressants.

There is experimental evidence to suggest that social isolation is associated with a reduction in brain serotonin turnover. When rodents are socially isolated for prolonged periods, they exhibit hyperactivity and aggression towards intruders, such behaviour being reversed by antidepressant treatment. Thus social isolation causes symptoms that resemble those caused by destruction of serotonergic pathways in the forebrain which may reflect the aggressiveness and impulsive behaviour reported to occur in a subgroup of depressed patients who have a low cerebrospinal fluid concentration of 5-hydroxyindole-acetic acid (5-HIAA). Such changes in serotonergic function that follow prolonged social isolation are long-lasting, and differ from the rapid returns of the serotonergic system to normal following exposure to acute stress.

While social isolation as such has not been implicated in the aetiology of depression in animals, social isolation may model the failure of social function that can result from adverse events occurring in childhood (such as family discord, loss of a parent) and which may predispose to depression. Low cerebrospinal fluid 5-HIAA concentrations are associated with low scores on socialization scales. The concept that isolation-induced serotonin depletion may serve as an animal model for some aspects of depression is supported by the studies of social co-operation in rats. In these studies, it was found that co-operative behaviour could be disrupted by destruction of forebrain serotonergic pathways but could be restored by the administration of the serotonin agonist fluperazine. It seems possible that one of the main functions of serotonin is to enhance the sensitivity of the animal to social cues. It has been postulated that the activity of forebrain serotonin is controlled by social reinforcement.

LEARNED HELPLESSNESS MODELS

Seligman in 1975 developed a model of learned helplessness which mimics some of the main features of depression, particularly those that are precipitated by unfavourable environmental events. Dogs exposed to an unavoidable electrical shock were subsequently found to be unable to learn to avoid an aversive stimulus and remained motionless and helpless in such a situation.

Even though the relevance of the "learned helplessness" model of depression may be questioned, short-term immobility to stress may provide a useful model for the detection of antidepressant drugs. The method developed by Porsolt involves placing rodents individually into a water-filled glass cylinder at 25°C from which they cannot escape (Porsolt et al., 1978). After a few minutes of vigorous swimming and attempted escape, the animals remain quiet, only making movements sufficient to keep their head above the water. Exposure to the same environment 24 hours later shows that the animals have "learned" not to try to escape from the container and therefore they remain immobile. This model has been widely used as a test for antidepressants. Both "standard" tricyclic antidepressants, such as amitriptyline and imipramine, and atypical antidepressants, such as mianserin and irpindole, increase the time in which the animal struggles to escape from the container on being placed in it on the second occasion. Clearly, drugs that cause marked sedation, reduce the muscle tone, will produce "false positives" in such a test situation, as will anticholinergic or antihistamine drugs. Despite the widespread use of the Porsolt "learned immobility" test as a screening method for antidepressants, a critical evaluation of the test suggests that it suffers from the same fundamental problems as the original Seligman model.

It appears that the immobility may reflect either an adaptive response to the particular situation, physical fatigue or a combination of these factors. Such criticism, together with the observation that such psychotropic drugs as caffeine, antihistamines and pentobarbitone also reverse the "behavioural despair" behaviour, suggests that such a model is an inadequate representation of depression and of limited value in the detection of antidepressant drugs.

CHANGES IN BEHAVIOUR FOLLOWING OLFACTORY BULBECTOMY

The North American psychologist, Watson, in 1907 was probably the first investigator to comment on the behavioural effects of bilateral bulbectomy in rats. Most experimenters have reported an increased irritability and aggressiveness in rats following bulbectomy. More recent evidence suggests that hyperemotionality and aggressiveness do not appear in rats handled frequently before, and during, the postoperative period and are not primarily effects of the lesions per se.

An increased incidence of muricidal (mouse-killing) behaviour has also been reported to occur following bilateral bulbectomy. While such behaviour is relatively uncommon in most strains of intact rats, the frequency of such behaviour is reported to increase dramatically following bulbectomy. However, the pattern of the mouse-killing behaviour is quite different to that seen in spontaneously muricidal strains. This behaviour of the bulbectomized rat has been termed "irritable aggression".

In rodents, bulbectomy is followed by an increase in locomotor activity in a novel environment such as the "open field" apparatus. These changes in locomotor activity and in other types of behaviour are not likely to be due to anosmia, because the reversible inhibition of the functioning of the olfactory nerve in the nasal cavity by zinc sulphate solution does not result in such behavioural changes. The hyperactivity shown by bulbectomized animals in the "open field" must be considered as a failure of adaptation and risk assessment and this "deficit" can be attenuated by the chronic administration of all classes of antidepressants. It should be noted that drugs lacking antidepressant activity do not attenuate this behaviour and neither will antidepressants following their acute administration.

Differences have been found between the active and passive avoidance performance of the bulbectomized rat. Thus, bulbectomized rats have been shown to be deficient in the acquisition of a passive avoidance task, but superior to controls in the acquisition of a two-way active avoidance task (shuttle box). However, other investigators have shown that one-way active avoidance learning is deficient after bulbectomy. Deficits in runway behaviour for a food reward and in conditioned taste aversion also occur in the bulbectomized rat. Changes in social (e.g. increased aggression and irritability), sexual (e.g. maternal and mating behaviour), and non-social behaviours such as exploratory activity of a novel environment have been shown to occur following bulbectomy. In addition, when placed on a holeboard apparatus, the ambulations score, head dipping (a measure of the exploratory activity indicated by the animal investigating a hole), and grooming were significantly reduced in bulbectomized rats when compared with their sham operated controls. Furthermore in a novel test for neophobia, bulbectomy caused a total elimination of the neophobia response when compared with sham operated controls.

IMMUNE CHANGES FOLLOWING OLFACTORY BULBECTOMY

Immunological changes occurring following olfactory bulbectomy (OB) have been the subject of a recent review (Song and Leonard, 1995b) and will only be summarized here (Table 12.1).

The earlier reported change in the immune system associated with OB was a reduction in neutrophil phagocytic response, similar to that found in depression. More recently, a reduction in neutrophil catalase and glutathione peroxidase and an increase in superoxidase dismutase have been found. The altered gluthathione peroxidase was attenuated by chronic desipramine treatment. A reduction in mitogen-stimulated lymphocyte proliferation occurred which has also been reported with depressed patients. In contrast, increased monocyte proliferative as well as mononuclear phagocytic responses, are observed in the OB rat; the latter effect is also found in depressed patients. An increase in positive acute phase proteins and a

Table 12.1   Immune changes following olfactory bulbectomy

Reduced neutrophil phagocytosis
Increased mononuclear cell phagocytosis
Reduced lymphocyte proliferation
Increased monocyte proliferation
Increased positive acute phase proteins
Reduced negative acute phase proteins
Increased neutrophils number
Reduced lymphocytes number
Increased leucocyte adhesiveness/aggregation
Reduced thymus weight
Reduced spleen weight
Increased alpha-1-acid glycoprotein levels

reduction in negative acute phase proteins also occur in OB rats, which are similar to the acute phase protein changes that are observed in depression. Of the acute phase proteins, alpha-1-acid glycoprotein levels are increased in both the OB rats and depressed patients. It is known that alpha-1-acid glycoprotein will suppress immune function and that levels can be increased by monocyte activation as well as by glucocorticoids. The alpha-1-acid glyprotein concentration is not increased significantly until five weeks after surgery.

The differential white blood cell profile is also altered following olfactory bulbectomy, and there is an increase in the percentage of neutrophil and reduction in lymphocytes. Lymphocyte aggregation is a marker of stress and has been shown to be increased following olfactory bulbectomy. A reduction in plaque-forming cells has been observed in OB mice while a reduction in the relative weights of the immune-related organs, thymus gland and spleen, has also been observed. Some of the behavioural changes seen following olfactory bulbectomy can be simulated by the intracerebroventricular administration of proinflammatory cytokines such as interleukin-1.

CHRONIC MILD STRESS MODEL OF DEPRESSION

This model was developed by Willner in an attempt to use relatively realistic but stressful conditions that may act as trigger factors for human depression. In this model, rats or mice are exposed in a sequential manner to a variety of mild stressors (such as continuous illumination, wet bedding, background noise, changes of cage mates, cage tilted) which change every few hours and last for several weeks. This procedure has been found to decrease the sensitivity to reward as indicated by a reduction in the consumption of a weak sucrose selection. Normal sucrose consumption is restored when the rodent is treated chronically with an antidepressant. Most classes of antidepressants which have been tested in the chronic mild stress model have been found to be effective, as has electroconvulsive shock, lithium and the

5-hydroxytryptamine 1A (5-HTIA) partial agonist buspirone. Stimulants, neuropeltics, anxiolytics and opiates are ineffective in reversing the anhedonia (reduced sucrose consumption). Willner has reasoned that the chronic mild stress model has reasonable construct, fact and predictive validity. However, there is an increasing number of reports that the behavioural changes and the effects of antidepressants are difficult to replicate.

SUMMARY

The animal models of depression which have been considered in this short review have contributed to the development of new antidepressants have suggested possible mechanisms of their action and have helped to expand our knowledge of the psychobiology of depression. However, major problems underlying the validity of animal models of any psychiatric condition lie in the uncertainty of the nature of the disease process which they are designed to simulate. Only more research on the biological basis of mental illness will improve this situation. Nevertheless, animal models have the practical advantage of allowing hypotheses that have been developed on the basis of clinical observation to be tested in animals. If the hypothesis is not refuted in the animal model then clinical studies could be devised to assess the validity of the hypothesis in patients. Thus despite the widely recognized limitation in the animal models currently available, they will continue to have a major impact on the development of novel antidepressants and indirectly help in the understanding of the aetiology of mental illness.

ANIMAL MODELS OF ALZHEIMER'S DISEASE

It is generally accepted that the more accurately an animal model mimics the aetiology and symptomatology of human ageing, the greater will be its validity and predictive value. The following criteria have been applied to the development of animal models of dementia:

1. The behaviour being assessed should display natural age-related deficits in the animals being studied.
2. The behaviour should have conceptual and operational similarities to the symptoms seen in humans.
3. The species being studied should show age-related neurochemical changes similar to those seen in humans.
4. Any changes induced experimentally in young animals should produce changes in brain function similar to those occurring in the aged subject.
5. Drugs shown to be effective clinically should also produce positive effects in the animal model.

While the aged animal provides the most valid animal model of human ageing, its validity as a model of dementia is related to the extent to which Alzheimer's disease represents an exacerbation of normal ageing rather than a distinct neuropathological disease. However, while aged models may be of some value in exploring the relationship between specific behavioural deficits and pathological changes associated with the accumulation of amyloid plaques and neuronal loss, they are of limited value as simulations of the disease state. It is well known that while most patients with Alzheimer's disease are over 65 years of age, and that the frequency of the disease is age-related, the majority of aged individuals do not suffer from the disease. The recent finding of a genetically linked factor (apolipoprotein E4) in the late-onset form of Alzheimer's disease is further evidence that Alzheimer's disease is not a consequence of normal ageing. With regard to the neuropathological changes that are causally related to the symptoms of the disease, there continues to be a debate regarding the relative importance of the classical neuropathological changes (amyloid plaques and neurofibrillary tangles) and specific neurotransmitter deficits (such as those occurring in the cholinergic system). Clinical and experimental evidence suggests that memory impairments may be correlated with both the neuropathological changes and the cholinergic deficit but as these indices covary with one another it is difficult to conclude which is of primary importance as the causative factor. An additional problem, which is not applicable to any of the major psychiatric diseases, relates to the absence of effective therapeutic agents. While there is much interest in the recently introduced, centrally acting anticholinesterases in the relatively short-term treatment of the symptoms in the early phase of the disease, there is no evidence that drug treatments prevent the development of the disease. Such factors make Alzheimer's disease difficult to model, particularly in rodents that form the basis of most experimental studies. All animals age and show memory deficits in the later stage of life, yet it is only humans that unequivocally develop Alzheimer's disease. To date, transgenic mice in which the human form of β-amyloid is expressed within the brain have not provided the experimental breakthrough which would have been anticipated from the neuropathological findings in humans. For this reason, three types of models will be considered: (a) behavioural models in aged animals; (b) pharmacological models in which drugs (particularly scopolamine) are used to produce memory deficits; and (c) neurotoxic and electrolytic lesion models.

BEHAVIOURAL MODELS

Motor deficits occur in aged animals in most species. Thus an age-related reduction in motor activity, explanation, habituation and motor co-ordination commonly occurs. Sensory deficits also commonly occur in all species of aged animals. Aged rats, for example, show delayed reaction times to footshock and auditory startle and decreased startle responses to a suprathreshold stimulus. A decline in visual and auditory sensitivity with ageing is well recognized and largely attributable to a decline in peripheral sensory organs.

Apart from these well-established age-related changes, specific tasks based on memory and learning have been widely used. Maze learning tasks have been widely used for the past 70 years. A renewed interest in maze learning in rodents has occurred recently with the focus on the spatial learning abilities of the animals. This emphasis has been aided by the realization that the hippocampus and its central cholinergic innervation is important as a neuronal substrate for spatial mapping strategies used by rats and other mammals. Such deficits can be shown by exposing the rats to the Morris water maze. In this apparatus, the animal must learn to orientate itself in a tank of warm water so that it can escape onto a slightly submerged (invisible) platform.

Such studies show that aged rodents have a specific spatial impairment which can be reversed by centrally acting anticholinesterases that enhance hippocampal cholinergic activity.

Passive avoidance acquisition and retention is also frequently used to assess memory deficits in aged animals (see section on animal models of anxiety, earlier in the chapter). Numerous studies have shown that aged animals manifest deficiencies in passive avoidance retention but it is difficult to conclude whether such deficits are due to an age-related decline in memory as opposed to increasing difficulties in detecting the conditioning stimuli or engaging in the motor response.

The eight-arm radial maze, which consists of a central platform from which eight arms of equal length radiate, is used to assess changes in working memory, particularly in rats. Animals with a good working memory soon learn to go to each arm of the maze in turn to consume the food placed at the end of the arm. Young rats learn to visit each arm in turn only once whereas old rats take longer to learn the task and make more errors. This memory task is particularly sensitive to hippocampal damage. Whether the deficits shown in aged rats are specifically due to a defect in working memory is now uncertain and it may be that a decline in visual sensitivity to the spatial clues necessary for guiding the animal to the food is a contributing factor.

While most memory-related tests have been carried out on rodents, primates have been used to assess delayed response performance. In these tasks, the monkey can see a flashing light but is prevented from obtaining a food reward by an observation window; after a variable delay (0–30 seconds) the window opens and the animal is reinforced. Aged animals show greater impairments than younger animals the longer the delay. Centrally acting anticholinesterases were found to improve the performance of the aged animals.

It may be concluded from these studies that aged animals may provide a good model of natural ageing in humans but the specific pathology of

Alzheimer's disease is minimal in the aged animal. Thus these animal models poorly represent the symptoms and neuropathological basis of Alzheimer's disease.

PHARMACOLOGICAL MODELS

A major advantage of drug-induced changes in behaviour is that they enable specific neurotransmitters to be identified which may be causally linked to specific changes in behaviour. This approach has been widely used to investigate the potential role of the cholinergic system in memory performance and the age-related cognitive decline seen in Alzheimer's disease. The cholinergic muscarinic antagonist scopolamine has been widely used in both human and animal studies to produce memory and cognitive deficits.

In primates, scopolamine has been shown to cause deficits in delayed colour-matching tasks, delayed spatial response tasks and the removal of object discrimination tasks. In the young monkey, these changes are essentially similar to the deficits seen in the aged monkey. Thus the scopolamine-treated young monkey may be regarded as an animal model to study age-related decline in cognitive function and some of the deficits associated with Alzheimer's disease.

The amnesic effects of scopolamine have been extensively studied in rodents. In these animals, scopolamine has been consistently found to impair performance in classical conditioning tasks, passive avoidance, sensory discrimination tasks, spatial working memory tasks and spatial delayed response tasks. In contrast, reference memory tasks do not appear to be adversely affected by scopolamine. Experimental evidence suggests that the effects of scopolamine are primarily on the encoding of new information but the drug has little effect on long-term memory processes. Thus scopolamine-induced amnesia may be of value in modelling the decline in short-term memory that characterizes Alzheimer's disease.

NEUROTOXIC AND ELECTROLYTIC LESION MODELS

Degenerative changes in animal brains have been induced by metallic neurotoxins (such as aluminium and trimethyltin) and by viruses such as the scrapie virus. Thus neurofibrillary tangles have been induced by aluminium, the expression of β-amyloid by trimethyltin and by the scrapie virus. These treatments induce an encephalopathy that can be fatal, but early in the course of treatment it is possible to develop models that resemble the psychopathology of Alzheimer's disease.

The neurotoxic effects of aluminium salts have been observed following the intracerebral administration of the metal to rabbits and cats, when most of the behavioural changes reported following scopolamine administration occur. Rats appear to be more resistant to the effects of aluminium. Less consistent results have been obtained when aluminium salts are given orally. Furthermore, it is now apparent that the structure of the neurofibrillary tangles induced in animals by aluminium salts differs from those occurring in patients with Alzheimer's disease.

Trimethyltin, following a single intraperitoneal dose, induces profound damage to the hippocampus which is associated with deficits in the acquisition of learning. There is evidence of an increased expression of β-amyloid in the brains of the rats. This model would appear to be worthy of further study.

Scrapie virus infections have long been known to occur in sheep and goats leading to motor incoordination and eventually neurodegenerative changes and death. More recently bovine spongiform encephalopathy (BSE) has been shown to cause similar changes in cattle. These spongiform encephalopathies are similar to human Creutzfeld–Jakob disease.

Some strains of the scrapie virus have been shown to induce neuritic and amyloid plaque formation in the brains of infected mice. This appears to be the most convenient experimental model of neuritic plaque formation found in Alzheimer's disease.

Lesions of specific brain nuclei by the use of locally injected neurotoxins have been useful for determining the role of specific neurotransmitters in some of the behavioural changes that occur in Alzheimer's disease. Of these lesions, destruction of the nucleus basalis magnocellularis, the main cholinergic cell body in the rat brain, has been the most widely studied. Such lesions lead to the disruption of learning in both active and passive avoidance tasks. Electrolytic lesions of the nucleus basalis produced similar memory and learning deficits to those produced by neurotoxins such as kainic acid and ibotenic acid.

SUMMARY

Of the three major groups of models that have been described, the advantage of the behavioural models lies in their face validity in that they manifest similar neuropathological and behavioural changes in those seen in humans. However, such models are limited because the major changes that appear to be causally related to Alzheimer's disease are poorly expressed in aged animals. They therefore fail to exhibit construct validity.

In the pharmacological models, in which memory deficits are induced by anticholinergic drugs, some of the symptoms of Alzheimer's disease can be simulated, but most of the central pathological changes seen in the disease are absent. Furthermore, the drugs affect the peripheral as well as the central cholinergic system and are therefore likely to have confounding effects.

The encephalopathic models (aluminium, tin neurotoxicity and scrapie virus infections) have the advantage of modelling the plaques and tangles seen in Alzheimer's disease. However, the nature of these pathological changes differs from those in the human disease. The subcortical lesioning models, involving the electrolytic or chemical destruction of the main cholinergic cell body region, lead to changes in memory and learning without producing any of the other neuropathological changes seen in Alzheimer's disease.

In conclusion, none of the available animal models meet all the conditions necessary for an adequate model of Alzheimer's disease.

ANIMAL MODELS OF DRUG ABUSE AND DEPENDENCE

It is unrealistic to expect that any animal model will account for all the complex interacting processes that are involved in the clinical syndromes of drug abuse and dependence. Thus no model will fulfil all the validation criteria that are desirable (i.e. predictive, face and construct validity).

The notion of predictive validity in an animal model depends on the ability of the model to discriminate accurately between those drugs that are abused by humans and those that are not. Ideally the animal model should enable the ranking of the drugs in terms of their abuse potential. However, it is sometimes difficult to determine the abuse/dependence potential of such drugs in humans in order to assess whether the ranking of such drugs in the animal model is similar to that in humans. Regarding face validity of animal models of drug abuse and dependence, little is known about the aetiology and biochemical basis of these phenomena in humans and therefore it is difficult to see how this criterion can be fully met.

Construct validity presupposes that the animal model has a sound theoretical basis. Again this is difficult to achieve in an animal model. In animals, chronic drug intake is rarely motivated by fear of the withdrawal effects but usually results from the action of drugs as positive reinforcers of behaviour. In humans, and in some animal models, the positive and negative (i.e. fear of the withdrawal effects) interact as determinants of drug self-administration. The uncertainty regarding the relative importance of these two processes in the human situation makes it difficult to develop animal models that have construct validity. Nevertheless, despite these obvious difficulties, models have been developed to assess the abuse and dependence liability of drugs.

MODELS OF ABUSE LIABILITY

These are mainly based on drug self-administration procedures and rely on the principles of operant conditioning which assumes that if the administration of a drug is contingent on a particular behaviour (for example, pressing a lever for the drug to be administered) that leads to an increase in that behaviour, then the drug can be categorized as a positively reinforcing stimulus. This approach has been used for over 30 years to show that a wide range of drugs are self-administered by animals by either the intragastric or intravenous routes. Drugs of abuse may therefore be viewed as positive reinforcers. However, just because a drug is self-administered by an animal does not necessarily mean that it has euphoriant or other subjectively pleasing properties. Numerous different methods have been developed in which the schedules of reinforcement in drug self-administration are varied according to the nature of the drug of abuse. Some of these methods are described in detail in the references supplied at the end of this chapter.

Methods have been developed to assess the efficacy of drugs as reinforcers. Of the methods used, the discrete trial choice procedure enables an animal to show a preference for one drug infusion over another when required to make one or two mutually exclusive responses. In such studies in monkeys, it can be shown that the animals prefer higher doses of cocaine to lower doses and, if given a choice between cocaine or a less potent stimulant such as diethylpropion, prefer the former drug. Similar studies have been conducted in human subjects in which preferences for caffeinated drinks over non-caffeinated drinks were compared. Thus it would appear that there are close links between animal and human studies of drugs and reinforcers and these studies show that drugs which are potent reinforcers (e.g. cocaine) are frequently prone to abuse, whereas those that are less prone to abuse (e.g. the antihistamine chlorphentermine) are poor reinforcers in animal models. Therefore, despite their limitations, the self-administration models are of considerable value for studying the fundamental process in drug abuse.

Drug abuse is generally considered to be a compulsive form of behaviour and this may be simulated in animals by the method of schedule-induced polydipsia. This method is based on the observation that rats trained to press a lever for a small quantity of food (e.g. a single pellet) ingest a small quantity of water prior to the resumption of lever pressing. Even though rats were not deprived of water, it was found that they drank three times the normal quantity of fluid.

The exposure of rodents to an intermittent schedule of food results in the intake of a substantial quantity of fluid for which there is no physiological need. Furthermore, the more food deprived the animals, the greater the degree of polydipsia. Using this method, rats can be induced to self-administer large quantities of drugs including ethanol, benzodiazepines, opiates, phencyclidine, barbiturates, amphetamines and nicotine. A sufficient quantity of these drugs can be consumed over a period of time to lead to dependence. This experimental approach can be modified to enable the animal to self-administer a drug of abuse by injection (for example, opiates, ethanol and nicotine). The main advantage of the schedule-induced drug self-injection is that it prevents the methodological problems associated with the oral administration of drugs such as those that may arise from aversive tastes of the drug solutions and from the delay inherent in drug absorption from the gastrointestinal tract.

With regard to the validity of the schedule-induced polydipsia and drug self-administration, it would appear that they have a low predictive validity since the animals can be induced to consume almost any drug that is in the solution. Regarding the face validity, the mechanism of self-administration relies heavily on the compulsive nature of drug abuse which may not apply to human drug abuse. It is also unclear whether the schedule-induced behaviours of drug abuse have construct validity. Nevertheless, these models of drug abuse offer many advantages over the schedule reinforcement methods.

THE CONDITIONED PLACE-PREFERENCE/AVERSION PARADIGM

The procedure consists of placing the animal in two or more different environments that may be distinguished in terms of the drug or vehicle treatments. Thus rats, for example, are given a drug of abuse in one environment and saline (or the vehicle) in the second environment. Following the training session, the animals are then tested (when drug free) for their preference or aversion for the environment in which they had previously received the drug or saline. Drugs that induce place preference include the stimulants, opiates, barbiturates and the benzodiazepines, while those drugs inducing place aversion include lithium, naloxone, kappa opiate agonists and picrotoxin.

ASSESSMENT OF DRUG DEPENDENCE

This can be determined by noting the extent to which the abrupt cessation of treatment leads to spontaneous withdrawal effects. Alternatively the animals may be made dependent on a drug of abuse and then the extent to which a test drug alleviates the withdrawal effects of a known drug of abuse is determined. Another method involves the use of specific antagonists (for example, flumazenil in the case of the benzodiazepines or naloxone for the opiates). This is an example of precipitated drug withdrawal and has the advantage of being less time-consuming than the spontaneous withdrawal methods.

GENETIC MODELS OF NEUROLOGICAL AND PSYCHIATRIC DISEASE

The use of genetically specified animals (usually rodents) to address fundamental questions in different areas of neuroscience has become a major area of research in recent years. Some 40 years ago, studies showed that inbred mouse strains differed in their preference for 10% ethanol solutions. Such studies were important in laying the basis to *pharmacogenetics*. At the simplest level, a single gene may be considered to influence a drug response (Figure 12.1).

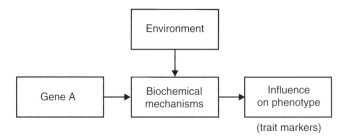

Figure 12.1   Single gene influence on a drug response.

Figure 12.1 shows that the gene A activity, through a number of biochemical mechanisms, leads to a specific response. However, the environment also influences these biochemical mechanisms (for example, by affecting the availability of a substrate) and thereby modulates the effect of the gene expression on the behaviour.

In most cases, multiple genes acting through a number of intermediate biochemical processes influence the response to a drug. Such polygenic mechanisms may be mediated through convergence on a common pharmacological mechanism, or a divergence (Figure 12.2).

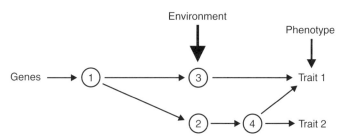

Figure 12.2   Multiple gene influence on a drug response.

Clearly attempts to trace a path from a single gene to a single drug response phenotype is extremely complex, not only because of the numerous mechanisms that may be influenced by a single gene but also because the environment may amplify or diminish the impact of the genetically determined biochemical changes on the phenotype.

Genetic selection for desired traits has been applied in recent years to produce mice that exhibit specific behavioural traits. For example, as a result of such genetic selection, it has been shown that the sensitivity of mice to the benzodiazepine inverse agonists (the beta carboline DMCM) is determined by a single gene, whereas different genes determined the sensitivity of mice to caffeine. Mouse lines that have been produced for experimental studies include:

1. HA/LA mice (high and low alcohol dependence related to the severity of withdrawal seizures following chronic alcohol consumption).
2. FAST/SLOW mice (increase and decrease in motor activity following acute alcohol injection).
3. DS/DR mice (diazepam sensitive and resistant mice as assessed by roto rod ataxia following administration of diazepam).
4. HAR/LAR mice (high and low analgesia response to an acute injection of levorphanol).
5. HAD/LAD mice (high and low voluntary consumption of alcohol).
6. A/ANA mice (alcohol avoiding and non-avoiding as assessed by voluntary alcohol consumption).

In addition to the several strains of mice that show differences in sensitivity to ethanol, several strains have been reported to display differences in sensitivity to central depressants. For example, C57 BL mice have been reported to show a greater susceptibility to the effects of the environment (so-called phenotypic buffering) than DBA mice and are the most susceptible to the effects of phenobarbitone administration. The C57 BL mice also have a shorter barbiturate-induced sleeping time than the DBA strain. These differences may be partly due to the ability of the C59 BL mice to metabolize the barbiturate faster than the DBA mice, as shown by the latter strain having a lower sensitivity to the sedative effects of the barbiturate than the C57 BL strain. It has also been reported that Ethanol Withdrawal Seizure Prone (WSP) and Withdrawal Seizure Resistant (WSR) mice, which were bred to demonstrate severe or minimal handling-induced convulsions after three days of exposure to ethanol, show similar differences in behaviour when a barbiturate is substituted for the ethanol. Thus ethanol and barbiturates may exert their differential effects by acting on similar genetically linked biochemical mechanisms.

ANIMAL MODELS OF NEUROLOGICAL DISEASES: MULTIPLE SCLEROSIS AND AMYTROPHIC LATERAL SCLEROSIS

The aetiology of *multiple sclerosis* is still unknown and pathogenesis of myelin degeneration is still the subject of debate. There is circumstantial evidence that a viral infection may play a role in the initiation of the disease process in patients with the appropriate genetic background. It is hypothesized that a viral infection in the first two decades of the patient's life may initiate an immune process which will eventually result in the destruction of myelin. There is still controversy regarding the role of T-cell activation against encephalitogenic epitopes of the myelin protein components. With regard to other possible immunological mechanisms, a delayed-type hypersensitivity response against viral antigens in the central nervous system (CNS) is a possibility. A mouse model of this type of lesion is provided by Theiler's encephalomyelitis virus infection. This virus is a piconavirus which produces a gastrointestinal infection that may be complicated by an infection of the CNS.

Following intracerebral administration of the virus, a mild neuronal infection occurs which is noticeable in the anterior horn of the spinal cord. This phase is transient and decreases spontaneously within two to three weeks. However, the animals soon begin to develop lesions of the white matter of the spinal cord which then persist for the lifetime of the animal.

Behaviourally, this is manifested by hind limb spastic paralysis and finally incontinence. The pathological changes are manifested by lymphocytic infiltrations of the meninges and perivascular spaces of the white matter of the spinal cord. Lymphoid cells eventually invade the surrounding parenchyma which is associated with demyelination. It appears that the myelination is directly related to the presence of the inflammatory cells, which suggests that the lesion is immune mediated rather than a reflection of the pathological changes caused by the viral infection. This is confirmed by the ultrastructural changes. These changes are similar to those identified in another model of multiple sclerosis, the *experimental autoimmune encephalomyelitis* (EAE) model, whereby the destruction of the myelin laminae by the infiltration of macrophages, and the vesicular degeneration of myelin due to activated mononuclear cells, is a common feature of both Teiler's infection and EAE. These changes have been interpreted as examples of receptor-mediated phagocytosis and/or structural repression of a stage in antigen processing.

The mechanism whereby macrophages cause the destruction of myelin in these animal models appears to be due to the secretion of proinflammatory cytokines, free radicals and proteases, which are known to have a major inflammatory effect on brain tissue. In the EAE and Theiler's infection it is known that the macrophages and microglia are the active participants in the pathological processes that lead to the tissue damage; this would appear also to occur in multiple sclerosis. With regard to the genetic susceptibility of different strains of mice to the virus infection, it is now well established that there is a wide variation between the most sensitive strains (such as the DBA/1 and DBA/2) and the most resistant (as exemplified by the BALB/C and C57 BL/6) with strains such as the CBA being intermediate in their sensitivity.

Unlike the animal models of psychiatric illness, for which the face and construct validities to the human condition are, at best, marginal, the virus infection models of multiple sclerosis appear to have good face, construct and predictive validity. In the human disease, however, a specific virus that causes the condition has not been identified, though several have been implicated. Indeed a specific virus may not necessarily be the causative agent because the virus acts primarily to initiate the immune changes that reflect the underlying genetic vulnerability of the patient.

The neurodegenerative diseases that include motor neuron disease are a heterogeneous group of diseases in which neurons of the motor system undergo programmed atrophy and degeneration without an apparent cause. Amyotrophic lateral sclerosis (ALS), and its variants, are the most important members of this group. ALS has received considerable attention in recent years because it has recently been discovered that there is a gene mutation which is closely linked to about 20% of familial cases of the disease.

A mouse model of human mutant Cu, Zn SOD (superoxide dismutase) has been developed as a model of ALS. While there have been several animal models (including those induced by viruses, genetic manipulation and by toxic chemicals), the novel mutant mouse model carries the human transgene corresponding to the defective gene that has been characterized in one of the families that has the familial form of ALS. Several lines of mutant mice have been developed, some of which (the G1 line) are characterized by a high expression of ALS, while a second line (the G20 line) has a lower expression of the transgene. The high expressers of the gene develop evidence of the pathological changes at about 60 days and the initial clinical signs at 80 days of age. These animals do not survive longer than 187 days of age whereas the low expression line live for about one year, at which time they are paralysed. The pathological changes seen in the high expresser line involve fine vacuolation of the axoplasm in the motor neurons of the lumbar and cervical areas of the spinal cord; this later spreads to the brain stem. Changes also involve the vascular degeneration of the mitochondria and the Golgi apparatus. Similar subcellular changes have been reported to occur in patients with ALS.

The link between the mutant gene for ALS and the pathological changes involves the expression of Cu, Zn, SOD, an enzyme that leads to the scaveging of free radical oxygen; SOD converts the superoxide anion into the hydrogen peroxide and oxygen. Thus a mutant form of this enzyme appears to be defective in ALS, thereby leading to an accumulation of the neurotoxic superoxide anion. The mutant SOD transgenic mouse is one of the first models that expresses the mutant human gene and therefore has major importance as a relevant model of the human disease. It therefore is likely to have predictive, face and construct validity.

KNOCKOUT AND TRANSGENIC MICE AS MODELS OF HUMAN NEUROLOGICAL AND PSYCHIATRIC DISEASE

There is evidence that most major psychiatric diseases have many causes, both genetic and environmental, and it is unlikely that a single mutant gene is primarily responsible for the pathological state. It is therefore unlikely that genetic manipulation of rodents to produce animals that either over- or under-express a gene (*transgenic animals*) or in which a specific gene for a receptor or key enzyme is deleted (*knockout animals*) can be produced to mimic the psychiatric disorder accurately. However, it might be possible to consider the disease in terms of its major behavioural elements (for example, cognitive and attentional deficits, negative symptoms, psychotic symptoms) and develop a mouse model that models subsets of those symptoms.

One aspect of schizophrenia that can be developed in this way is the loss of auditory gating. In normal individuals, two tones presented close together will not evoke a response to the second tone; schizophrenics respond to both tones. In rodents, a soft tone that will not startle the animal when presented immediately before a louder tone will significantly reduce the startle response to the louder tone. This behaviour is called pre-pulse inhibition. Knockout mice, which lack the 5-HT1B receptor, behave more like schizophrenics in terms of their behaviour when a soft tone is paired with a loud tone in that they respond equally to both tones.

To date, depression models of learned helplessness behaviour have not been applied to transgenic or knockout mice, but with the development of mouse lines that differ in their response to unavoidable stress it is anticipated that appropriate models of this aspect of human behaviour will be developed in the near future.

Two neurological diseases that have been extensively studied using knockout and transgenic mice include ALS, mentioned previously, and Alzheimer's disease. Thus transgenic mice have been produced that develop amyloid plaques and show behavioural consequences that are linked to the mutant expression of amyloid precursor protein (APP) and severe cognitive impairment.

In these mice, the concentration of highly fibrillogenic β-amyloid protein was increased more than 14-fold over the normal endogenous levels; learning and memory deficits preceded the histological changes. However, unlike the human condition, no neuronal loss is apparent in these transgenic models, which suggests that β-amyloid alone is not acutely toxic or solely responsible for the behavioural deficits seen in Alzheimer's disease. Mouse models have begun to identify the possible causes that may underline the pathology associated with Alzheimer's disease which could lead to the elucidation of the relationship between the protein linked to the disease and the nature of the intervention that can reverse or impede the neurodegenerative changes associated with the disorder.

Despite the rapid growth in research in which knockout or transgenic mice have been used to study diseases of the nervous system, the field is still in its infancy. However, even with improved technology, one knockout or transgenic mouse will not be identical to another. Technically, copy number and insertion sites are likely to influence the pattern of expression even when a large number of promoter fragments are used in transgenesis. In addition, strain differences will be an ongoing source of variability. Nevertheless, the use of different background strains to examine knockout or transgenic phenotypes could lead to the identification of interacting genes that modify the function of the gene under investigation.

CYTOKINE ABNORMALITIES IN THE CEREBELLAR MUTANT MICE

Interleukin-1 (IL-1) and tumour necrosis factor (TNF), in addition to their proinflammatory actions, are well known as immunomodulatory factors. Thus IL-1 has been shown to be a growth factor for astrocytes *in vitro* while TNF has a growth-promoting effect on human astrocytoma and glioma cell lines. In addition, TNF enhances class II antigen expression of interferon gamma (IFN-γ) stimulated astrocytes *in vitro*. There is evidence that, in addition to their physiological roles, proinflammatory cytokines can promote gliosis. IL-1 has been shown to induce the excessive expression of the β-amyloid precursor gene and alpha-1 chymotrypsin, the two major components of the extracellular accumulation of amyloid deposits in Down's syndrome and Alzheimer's disease (see Chapter 9).

Such observations have led to the search for strains of mice that exhibit neurodegenerative disorders which may also show abnormalities in the expression of proinflammatory cytokines. So far, more than 20 point mutations have been described in mice that affect the development of the cerebellum. Some of these mutants result in neuropathological changes that resemble the hereditary ataxia seen in Friedreich's ataxia or olivopontocerebellar atrophies. Four strains of mice have been identified that show various forms of ataxia, namely the staggers, Purkinje cell degeneration, lurcher and nervous mouse. In these mutant strains, the Purkinje cells are partially or totally absent, which leads to an indirect degeneration of other cerebellar and precerebellar neurons, mainly the granule cells and inferior olivary neurons. In the homozygous stagger mouse, atrophy of the spleen, thymus and an abnormal immunological response are also apparent. More specifically, macrophages from these mice were found to hyperexpress IL-1β RNA; in addition, following a lipopolysaccharide (LPS) challenge, the macrophages from the homozygous stagger mice released a higher concentration of the cytokine than macrophages from the wild-type strain.

The mRNA expression of TNF-α and IL-6 was also greater following LPS stimulation. Regarding the other cerebellar mutant strains of mice, it has been shown that the lurcher and Purkinje cell degeneration, and nervous strains also show an elevated expression of IL-1 mRNA. Not all mutant strains show such immunological abnormalities, however. Thus the spinal mutant strains (such as the Wobbler and motor neuron degeneration strains) and the neurological mutants (jimpy and motor end-plate disease) show only a slight increase or no changes in IL-1 mRNA expression.

From such studies, it would appear that the cytokine hyperexpression is an indirect consequence of the mutation that affects cerebellar function. One possibility is that the degenerating Purkinje cells produce a factor or factors that increase IL-1 expression by the peripheral macrophages. The nature of this signal remains obscure, but could act on the second messenger system leading to increased IL-1 expression. Another possibility is that the macrophage membrane is modified in the mutant mouse strains; this is indicated by the increased release of IL-1 from the macrophages by long-term potentiation (LTP).

The consequence of the hypersecretion of proinflammatory cytokines by macrophages, particularly those occurring in the brain, would be the destruction of central neurons. It is of interest to note that there is a correlation between the hyperexpression of IL-1 in the cerebellar mutant mice strains and gliosis; a proliferation of astroglial cells has been shown to occur in the stagger, lurcher and Purkinje cell degeneration strains, but not the weaver mutant strain. The advantage of such genetic models is that they illustrate how a genetically linked increase in proinflammatory cytokines could be involved in neurodegenerative diseases in which amyloidogenesis and astrogliosis form the pathological basis.

ANIMAL MODELS OF STRESS AND IMMUNITY

Hans Selye, who devoted his life to the study of the effects of stress on behaviour and the endocrine system, defined stress as the response of the organism to the demands made upon it by the internal and external environment. Selye's definition of stress helped to emphasize its subjective nature by indicating that what is stressful for one individual is not necessarily so for another. Similarly, the response of an individual to a stressful stimulus often varies with time. Selye proposed that the basic physiological response to stress was non-specific in that all stressors tended to produce similar physiological response regardless of the nature of the stressor. This led to the concept of stress resulting from an activation of the hypothalamic–pituitary–adrenal axis and the sympathoadrenomedullary system. These responses to most types of stressor are summarized in Figure 12.3.

Despite the pioneering research of Selye and his collaborators over 40 years ago, it is only within the past three decades that the relationship between stress, the immune system and mental illness has been explored. This has led to the following conclusion, which will form the basis of the present section on animal models of stress and its relationship to immunity:

1. Alterations in immune responses can be conditioned.
2. Electrical stimulation or surgical lesions of specific brain regions, alter immune functions.
3. Stress can change the immune responses and growth of tumours and infections.

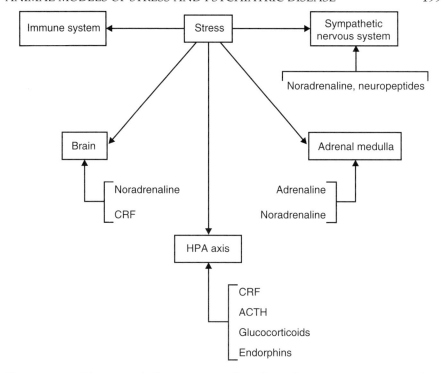

Figure 12.3 Diagram of the primary physiological response to stress. CRF, corticotrophin-releasing factor; ACTH, adrenocorticotrophic hormone.

A wide variety of stressors have been used in experimental studies to investigate the effects of the environment on immunological function. These stressors range from a physical stimulus such as loud noise, rotation, cold, restraint or immobilization stress and electric footshocks, to stressors which are of a psychological nature such as aversive conditioning. Those stressors which may be more relevant to the human condition include social models using crowding, isolation or aggression. There have also been studies conducted on the effects of "natural" stressors on animals in the wild. Although it is customary to distinguish physical (e.g. cold) and psychological (e.g. restraint) stressors, this type of classification is of limited value since there is evidence that most stressors have strong emotional elements which account for their activating effects on the immune–endocrine–neurotransmitter axes.

RESTRAINT MODELS

Physical immobilization of an animal (usually a rodent) is widely used as a stressor and involves both physical and emotional components. This is achieved by confining the animal to a restriction cage, usually a narrow tube, that does not allow the animal to move. Other procedures involve restraining the rodent on a board by means of adhesive tape. Such procedures allow an extensive manipulation of the frequency and the duration of the stressor. As a consequence of this type of stress, a suppression of both cellular and humoral immunity generally occurs. For example, it has been frequently reported that a marked reduction in the *in vitro* proliferation of lymphocytes occurs in response to stimulation by mitogen, together with a reduction in natural killer (NK) cell activity. Severe restraint stress of several hours duration has been reported to reduce the expression of MHC class II glycoproteins on peritoneal macrophages. Although such findings serve to differentiate the effects of prolonged and severe stress on different aspects of the immune system, the ethical basis for conducting such experiments is surely questionable.

In addition to the changes in cellular and humoral immunity that occur following restraint stress, there is also evidence from such studies that the susceptibility of the animal to infection is increased. For example, it has been shown that restraint stress modulates the pathogenesis of an acute toxoplasmosis infection in mice. However, the susceptibility to infection appears to depend on the virulence of the viral strain. Nevertheless, not all stressors adversely affect the immune system. For example, in an animal model of diabetes mellitus, an autoimmune disease, it has been shown that chronic restraint stress administered once weekly protects the rodents against the disease, presumably due to the enhanced glucocorticoid secretion exerting an immunosuppressive effect.

ELECTRIC SHOCK MODELS

The immunosuppressive effects of electric shocks to the tail or feet of rodents has been widely used to investigate the effects of stress on the immune system. The results of such studies indicate that electric shocks decrease the *in vitro* proliferation of lymphocytes to mitogens, decrease NK cell activity and suppress the *in vivo* IgG antibody production to an antigenic challenge.

Several of these experimental studies have focused on the importance of psychological factors in the activation of the immune system and the pathological changes that follow moderate to severe stress. For example, it has been shown that when rats could form a behavioural response to avoid or terminate the aversive shocks, the severity of stomach ulcers was reduced compared to those rats that could not terminate the shocks. Similarly, it has been shown that whereas uncontrollable electric shock to the tails of rats reduced the lymphocyte proliferative response, rats exposed to a similar stressor from which they could escape failed to exhibit the immunosuppressive response.

DIFFICULTIES IN REPLICATING THE EFFECTS OF ELECTRIC SHOCKS ON THE IMMUNE SYSTEM

Several investigators have repeated such experiments with variable results, largely due to the lack of standardization of the *in vitro* tests and stress procedures used. Researchers often overlook the fact that mitogen proliferation is highly variable so that detection of the effect of the stressor may be compromised when superimposed on the larger individual differences that exist with regard to the mitogen proliferation. Another problem that is frequently ignored concerns the sampling bias associated with the collection of cells from a single site such as the peripheral blood or spleen. It is well known that the lymphocyte population found in the blood or any other site represents only a small portion of the total pool available. Stressors are known to affect the dynamic interchange of lymphocytes between the blood, bone marrow, lymph nodes, thymus and spleen. Thus different subsets of cells may be sampled in different studies which could lead to difficulties in replicating the results. Moreover, stress can cause changes in the circadian pattern of corticosterone secretion and as a consequence shift the circadian pattern of lymphocyte subsets at the sampling site. Thus, because of the integrated nature of the immune system, *in vitro* measures do not always exactly mirror the activity of the intact immune system. Despite these pitfalls, it is generally agreed that the psychological aspect of stressor controllability is an important factor in the relationship between stress and immunity.

EFFECT OF LEARNING AND MEMORY ON THE IMMUNE RESPONSE TO A STRESSOR

It is not unreasonable to conclude that the previous experience of an animal to an inescapable electric shock will affect the immune response. The acute stressor will activate learning and memory processes within the brain which will result in a conditioned stress response upon re-exposure to the same stressor. Conditioned stress had been reported to reduce the *in vitro* proliferative responses of splenocytes to mitogen stimulation and also lead to the antigenic challenge. Similarly, it has been shown that a conditioned aversive stimulus can suppress the development of adjuvant arthritis. However, not all conditioned stress situations lead to immunosuppression. For example, in a passive shock avoidance paradigm, immune activation has been found to occur which was presumably mediated by an activation of the sympathetic innervation of the spleen. Such activation of the immune system by an aversive stimulus does not appear to be restricted to electric shock stress. For example, a combination of saccharin in the drinking water and a lithium chloride injection with the odour of camphor on the conditioning stimulus has been shown to augment NK cell activity. This conditioned increase in NK cell activity would not appear to be due to a change in interferon release but could be associated with the conditioned release of enkephalins/endorphins or the release of a neuromodulator from the sympathetic system at local sites near the effector cells of the spleen.

The previous experience of a stressor may also have a major impact on the immune response of an animal. For example, it has been shown that footshock stress delivered to rats 24 hours after a mild antigen priming will suppress immunological memory formation and hence the secondary humoral immune response. In addition to the effects of learning and memory of a stressor on the immune response, it is also evident that following exposure to a chronic stress (e.g., repeated footshocks), the stress response can produce desensitization of the response (a decrease from session to session), sensitization (an increase from session to session) or no change. Thus when mice are injected with tumour cells and exposed to acute inescapable footshocks, subsequent exposure to the stressor led to an attenuation of the tumour-enhancing effects of the stress. Similarly, repeated exposure to electric shocks resulted in an attenuation of the enhanced mitogenic responsiveness of splenic T lymphocytes which had been enhanced in the mice exposed to acute footshock. Repeated exposure to restraint stress was also found to be necessary to induce a decrease in the number of helper and suppressor T cells.

The results of these experimental studies emphasize the difficulties that may arise when trying to interpret the results of the effects of acute or chronic electric shock on immune changes in rodents. Nevertheless, providing the numerous variables (such as the effect of the circadian rhythm at the site from which the immune cells are derived, standardization of the assay methods used etc.) are carefully controlled, experiments using the electric shock paradigm allow the relative contribution of psychological factors such as stressor controllability and predictability (learning and memory processes) to be evaluated for their effects on the immune system.

SOCIAL STRESS MODELS

Despite the obvious utility of the restraint and electric shock induced stress, such studies are limited because they do not mimic any real life situations of animals. However, all mammals may experience socially induced stress and the few studies that have been carried out in the field on wild animals (usually rodents) indicate that social stress has a major impact on the immune system. These social stress models are particularly relevant when studying the influence of environment on immune function. Such models may be separated into three major groups, namely social group models, dyadic interactions (resident–intruders) models and social isolation models.

Social group models may be illustrated by the effect of daily grouping for a few hours of male mice that were otherwise isolated. It was shown that such a situation results in significantly lower antibody responses to bovine serum albumin in contrast to the permanently group housed mice where the dominant male has the highest antibody titres. Similarly, it has been shown that the crowding of rats results in a diminished response to an antigen challenge. In general, it would appear that social stress due to high density housing in animals increases disease vulnerability and decreases the survival of the animals.

Other studies have analysed the relationship between the position of the animal within the social structure and to the endocrine and immune status of the animal. Thus several studies have reported that the dominant male in a colony has a higher *in vitro* proliferation response of splenocytes than subordinate males, whereas the subordinate animals in particular show signs of immunosuppression. Differences have also been found in the distribution of T-cell subsets in dominant and subdominant males, dominant males having the opposite ratios of T-cell subsets to subdominant males, who were characterized by the lowest T-helper : T-suppressor ratios.

Dyadic interactions between male rodents is also a useful model for the study of the impact of social stress on the immune system. The basis of this model is the capability of male rodents to establish a territory and to defend it against any intruder. This method enables the effects of offensive and defensive behaviour on the immune system to be studied. Of the few studies that have been conducted so far, it is clear that social defeat reduces the antibody response in both rats and mice. In a more detailed study of the behaviour of aggressive and non-aggressive rats, non-aggressive rats were found to have consistently smaller thymus glands, and reduced *in vitro* proliferative responses of lymphocytes to plant mitogens, than aggressive rats. In addition, in a model of territorial intrusion, intruder rats showed a decrease of IgG antibody titre as long as three weeks after immunization with a protein antigen.

Changes also occur in the central neurotransmitter systems in response to aggression and submission. Thus in mice conditioned to show aggressive or submissive behaviour, the formation of aggressive behaviour was accompanied by an activation of the dopaminergic system, whereas the development of submissive behaviour was characterized by an increase in the activity of the serotonergic system. As the biogenic amine neurotransmitters are known to be actively involved in the modulation of the immune system, it is possible that the changes in the immune responsiveness of the rodents that are subjected to dyadic interaction stress could be a consequence of the changes in these neurotransmitters.

Social isolation models may be used to study the effects of isolation in those animals that normally live in social groups. However, the results obtained from such models are not always consistent, with some investigators reporting lower antibody titres in isolated male mice as compared to group housed controls whereas others have reported that isolated male mice had a higher antibody response to sheep erythrocytes and a better macrophage-mediated host defence than group housed mice.

A number of studies have shown that maternal deprivation and/or early weaning suppresses adult immunocompetence. In non-human primates, the separation of infants that had been raised together for a period of 11 days resulted in reduced lymphocyte function which rapidly normalized following the regrouping of the infants. Despite the relevance of social stress models for investigating the effects of environmental stress on the immune system, the conflicting results regarding changes in immune function may arise as a consequence of the degree to which the animals can cope with the stressor. It seems that the ability of an animal to cope depends not only on the nature of the stress but also on the genetic and/or phenotypic characteristics of the animal. These variations in coping, in addition to the numerous factors already discussed above regarding a source of variation in the immune response, help to compound the problem. With regard to the difference in coping strategies, aggressive male rodents usually adopt an aggressive coping strategy whereas non-aggressive males generally adopt a passive coping style. These strategies are reflected in the activity of the sympathoadrenal system, with the aggressive males having a more highly reactive sympathetic system, while the non-aggressive males had a more reactive pituitary–adrenal axis. Such factors could play an important part in the differences in the immune response of these animals. Other studies on Roman-high and Roman-low avoidance rats selected on the basis of their active avoidance behaviour have shown that the low avoidance male animals have a lower NK cell activity and splenocyte proliferative response than the high avoidance males.

EFFECTS OF DIFFERENT TYPES OF STRESSOR ON THE IMMUNE RESPONSE

In addition to the various animal models in which a specific stressor is investigated for its effect on various parameters of cellular and non-cellular immunity, studies have also been undertaken to determine whether different types of stress influence the immune function in a similar manner. For example, rats of the Lewis strain when subject to a single electric shock had a marked reduction in the response of the spleen and blood lymphocytes to the plant mitogen concanavalin A; this effect was attenuated following exposure to an increased frequency of electric shocks. Thus the magnitude of the effect of the stressor on the immune response depends on the compartment of the immune system assayed as well as the frequency with which the stressor is presented. By contrast, the chemical stressor 2-deoxyglucose, an antimetabolite that produces an acute intracellular deprivation of glucose, causes changes in behaviour that are markedly different from the effects of electric shocks; electric shocks increase the locomotor activity of the rats whereas 2-deoxyglucose decreases it. Furthermore, the reactivity of blood and spleen lymphocytes was decreased following electric shocks, an effect that was attenuated by chronic treatment with 2-deoxyglucose. However, examination of the lymph from the mesenteric lymph nodes and the thymus of the rats treated with 2-deoxyglucose showed that no changes occurred in the mitogenic responses of lymphocytes in the lymph nodes. Conversely, the immune responsiveness of the lymphocytes from the thymus gland differed from changes seen in the spleen; a single injection of 2-deoxy-glucose had no immunosuppressive effect, whereas several injections of the metabolite reduced the mitogenic responsiveness of the lymphocytes. These studies demonstrate that different types of stressor may have similar effects on some aspects of cellular immunity, but there are subtle differences in the responsiveness to the different stressors of lymphocytes from compartments of the immune system. These immune changes were not correlated with the effects of the stressors on behaviour.

Sickness Behaviour Precipitated by LPS: an Animal Model to Study the Actions of Endogenous Cytokines

LPS is an integral component of the outer membrane of Gram-negative bacteria which, by stimulating myeloid cells to synthesize cytokines such as IL-I, IL-6 and TNF-α, causes marked changes in the behaviour of rodents and in the metabolic and endocrine systems. These cytokine-mediated agents are part of the general homeostatic reaction which form the first line of defence against infection.

Stimulation of the HPA axis with the resultant increase in plasma glucocorticoids is one of the first and most dramatic effects of LPS. The cascade of cytokine release that is initiated by LPS has been postulated to be part of the important inhibitory feedback mechanism that mediates the immunological responses. Behaviourally, LPS causes a change in the sleep–wake cycle, anorexia, anhedonia, loss of libido as well as fever. For these reasons LPS may be considered to induce depression-like symptoms and be a useful model for investigating the effects of proinflammatory cytokines on the immune, endocrine and neurotransmitter systems. For example, there is evidence from *in vivo* microdialysis studies in rats that the LPS challenge results in an increase in the release of noradrenaline and serotonin in the hippocampus and in noradrenaline and dopamine release in the hypothalamus and prefrontal cortex. Presumably such changes in central neurotransmitter function impact on the immune and endocrine systems as well as causing some of the behavioural changes. It is also evident that the prostaglandins play a crucial role in modulating the central effects of the cytokines that are released by LPS. Thus the LPS-induced behavioural and neurotransmitter changes are largely attenuated by pretreatment with the cyclo-oxygenase inhibitor indomethacin. There is also experimental evidence to show that corticosterone modulates the behavioural and metabolic effects of LPS, which may account for the rapid reduction in the biological activity of LPS when it is administered to rats for several days.

The Importance of Strain Differences in the Effects of Stress on Immune Function

There is ample experimental evidence to show that the effects of stress on immunity are dependent on the strain of animals used. For example, it has been shown that when different strains of mice are exposed to acute inescapable footshock, only CD+1 and C57B/6J strains exhibit a decrease in NK cell activity, whereas the C3H/HEJ strain were unaffected. Similarly mice of the HLA-SW/ICR, C57 B/6N and C3H/HEJ strains showed an enhanced mitogenic response of the splenocytes, whereas the C3H/HEN strain were unaffected. In addition to the differences in immune response to stress shown by different mouse strains, large differences in lymphocyte reactivity have also been found in rodents that differ in their behavioural reactivity, which suggests that some immune responses can covary with behavioural traits.

Such findings emphasize not only the importance of assessing the interaction between genetic factors and the immune responses to stress but also how subtle changes in behaviour and physiology that are influenced by the genetic substrate can modulate the way in which the immune system responds to external and internal stressors.

SUMMARY

Various animal models (mainly rodent models) that have been developed to investigate the effects of various internal and external stressors in the immune system have been described. These may be divided into three main types, namely those based on restraint or electric shock induced stress, social stress models and brain lesion models. In addition, sickness behaviour induced by the administration of cytokines or lipopolysaccharide have been used to elucidate the effects of the immune system on behavioural, central neurotransmitters and the immune system. Of these various models, the social stress models are perhaps the most valid in that the type of stressor has biological relevance to the animal. Nevertheless, the restraint and electric shock models are of practical value in that they enable the severity and duration of the stressor to be accurately determined. Other factors that may compound the interpretation of the results, and their difficulty in replication, include the differences in responsiveness of the strains of rodents used, the variability in the reproducibility of some of the methods used to assess immune function, the lack of suitable controls, particularly when electric shock is used as the stressor, and failure to take into account the coping skills which animals adopt when repeatedly subjected to a stressor. An overview of some of the changes reported to occur when these different animal models are used is shown in Table 12.2.

Table 12.2 Effects of different types of stressor on the immune system of rodents

Restraint models	Reduced lymphocyte proliferation Reduced NK cell activity Increased susceptibility to infection
Electric shock models	Reduced lymphocyte proliferation Reduced NK cell activity Reduced IgG antibody formation
Social group models	Short-term isolation of grouped male mice leads to reduced antibody response to an antigen Dominant male mice have higher antibody titres than submissive mice Crowding of rats causes reduced antigen response Dominant male rodents have higher proliferative splenocyte response than submissive males Subordinate male rodents have lower T-helper: T-suppressor ratios than dominant males
Dyadic interactions	Offensive and defensive behaviour causes differences in immune responses: social defeat reduces the antibody response Non-aggressive rats have smaller thymus glands and reduced proliferative responses of lymphocytes to mitogens than aggressive rats. These rats also show decreased IgG antibody titres
Social isolation models	Isolated rodents, changes in antibody titres have been reported but the results are equivocal Maternal deprivation in non-human primates results in reduced lymphocyte function
Sickness behaviour (induced by LPS or proinflammatory cytokines)	Behavioural changes in rodents that simulate many of the symptoms of depression Immune, endocrine and behavioural changes largely reversed by chronic antidepressants or by cyclo-oxygenase inhibitors
Brain lesion models	The olfactory bulbectomized rat model has been the most extensively studied Behavioural, endocrine, immune and neurotransmitter changes reversed chronic antidepressants IL-1 exacerbates the deficits whereas IL-2 largely attenuates the deficits

CONCLUSION

This chapter has presented an overview of some of the animal models that have been developed to mimic some of the major psychiatric and neurological diseases. It is self-evident that the conventional models at best express some of the symptoms of the human disease, which is to be expected as the pathological basis of the severe psychiatric diseases is largely unknown and their genetic basis (if present) is unlikely to be due to a single gene mutation. Of all the models described, the mouse model of amytrophic lateral sclerosis is unique in that it simulates both the behaviour and neuropathological changes seen in the human disease. The success of this model is largely due to the identification of the gene mutation and the production of transgenic mice that express the function of this mutant gene. Hopefully, the further development of knockout and transgenic mice will enable animals to be developed that over-express or under-express cytokines and their receptors. Such models should be invaluable in elucidating the functional relationship between cytokines and disorders of the central nervous system.

BIBLIOGRAPHY

Monographs

Boulton, A. A., Baker, G. B. and Martin-Iverson, M. T. (Eds) (1991) *Neuromethods*, Vol. 18. *Animal Models in Psychiatry* Humana Press, Clifton, NJ.
Boulton, A. A., Baker, G. B. and Martin-Iverson, M. T. (Eds) (1991) *Neuromethods*, Vol. 19. *Animal Models in Psychiatry II* Humana Press, Clifton, NJ.
Boulton, A. A., Baker, G. B. and Butterworth, R. F. (Eds) (1992) *Neuromethods*, Vol. 21. *Animal Models of Neurological Disease I.* Humana Press, Totowa, NJ.
Boulton, A. A., Baker, G. B. and Butterworth, R. F. (Eds) (1992) *Neuromethods*, Vol. 22 *Animal Models of Neurological Disease II.* Humana Press, Totowa, NJ.
Boulton, A. A., Baker, G. B. and Wu, P. H. (Eds) (1992) *Neuromethods*, Vol. 24. *Animal Models of Drug Addiction.* Humana Press, Totowa, NJ.
Iannaccone, P. M., and Scarpelli, D. G., (Eds) (1997) *Biological Aspects of Disease— Contribution from Animal Models.* Harwood Academic Publishers, Amsterdam.
Vogel, H. G. and Vogel, W. H. (Eds) (1997) *Drug Discovery and Evaluation— Pharmacological Assays.* Springer Verlag, Berlin.
Willner, P. (Ed) (1991). *Behavioural Models in Psychopharmacology—Theoretical, Industrial and Clinical Perspectives.* Cambridge University Press, Cambridge.

Review Articles

Crawley, J. N. and Paylor R. (1997). A proposed test battery and constellations of specific behavioural paradigms to investigate behavioural 1 phenotypes of transgenic and knockout mice. *Hormones and Behaviour* **31**: 197–211.
Kelly, J. P., Wrynn, A. S. and Leonard, B. E. (1997) The olfactory bulbectomized rat as a model of depression: An update. *Pharmacology and Therapeutics* **74**: 299–316.
Picciotto, M. R. and Wickman, K. (1998) Using knockout and transgenic mice to study neurophysiology and behaviour. *Phsyiological Reviews* **78**: 1131–1163.
Woolman, E. E., Kopmels, B., Bakalian A. et al. (1992) Cytokines and neuronal degeneration. In Rothwell, N. and Dantzer, R. (Eds) *Interleukin-1 in the Brain.* Pergamon Press, Oxford.

Selected Publications on Specific Animal Models

Bohus, B. (1989) Psychosocial environment and the immune system. In: Schonpflug, W. (Ed.), *Bericht über den 3b Kongress den Deutchen Gesellschaft für Psychologie in Berlin*, Vol. 2, pp. 81–93. Verlag für Psychologie-Hogrefs. Göttingen.

Connor, T. J. and Leonard, B. E. (1998) Mini review—Depression, stress and immunological activation: the role of cytokines in depressive disorders. *Life Sciences* **62**: 583–606.

Connor, T. J., Song, C., Leonard, B. E., Merali, Z., and Anisman, H. (1998) An assessment of the effects of central IL-1 beta, IL-2, IL-6 and TNF alpha administration on some behavioural, neurochemistry, endocrine and immune parameters in the rat. *Neuroscience* **84**: 923–933.

Dantzer, R. (1993) *The Psychosomatic Delusion*. Free Press, New York.

Esterling, B. and Rabin, B. S. (1987) Stress-induced alterations of T-lymphocyte subsets and humoral immunity in mice. *Behavioural Neuroscience* **101**: 115–119.

Felten, D. L., Felten, S. Y., Bellinger, D. L. et al. (1989) Noradrenergic sympathetic neural interactions with the immune system: structure and function. *Immunology Reviews* **100**: 705–713.

Kelley, K. W. (1989) Growth hormone, lymphocytes and macrophages. *Biochemical Pharmacology* **38**: 705–713.

Koolhaas, J. M. and Bohus, B. (1991) Animal models of human aggression. In: Boulton, A. A., Baker, G. B. and Martin-Iverson, M. T. (eds). *Neuromethods 19, Animal Models in Psychiatry II*, pp. 249–271. Humana Press, Clifton NJ.

Laudenslager, M. L., Flesher, M., Hofstadter, P. et al. (1988) Suppression of specific antibody production by inescapable shock: stability under varying conditions. *Brain, Behaviour and Immunity* **2**: 92–101.

Maier, S. F. and Landenstager, M. L. (1988) Inescapable shock, shock controllability and mitogen stimulated lymphocyte proliferation. *Brain, Behaviour, and Immunity* **2**: 87–91.

Porsolt, R. D., Anton, G., Blavet, N. and Jaffre, M. (1978) Behavioural despair in rats. *European Journal of Pharmacology* **47**: 379–399.

Seligman, M. E. P. (1975) *Helplessness: On Depression, Development and Death*. Freeman, San Francisco.

Selye, H. (1955) Stress and disease. *Science* **122**: 625–631.

Song, C. and Leonard, B. E. (1994) SSRI's reverse the impairments in behaviour, neurotransmitter and immune functions in the olfactory bulbectomized rat. *Human Psychopharmacology* **9**: 135–146.

Song, C. and Leonard, B. E. (1995a) Interleukin 2 induced changes in behavioural, neurotransmitter and immunological parameters in the olfactory bulbectomized rat. *Neuroimmunomodulation* **2**: 263–272.

Song, C. and Leonard, B. E. (1995b) The effect of olfactory bulbectomy in the rat, alone and in combination with antidepressants and endogenous factors, on immune functions. *Human Psychopharmacology* **10**: 7–18.

Weisse, C. S. (1992) Depression and immunocompetence: a review of the literature. *Psychological Bulletin* **111**: 475–479.

Willner, P. (1985) Antidepressants and serotonergic neurotransmission: an integrated review. *Psychopharmacology* **85**: 387–404.

13 Psychoneuroimmunology of HIV Infection and Chronic Fatigue Syndrome

INTRODUCTION

Immune deficiency disorders can be divided into those disorders with a deficiency or malfunction in one or more aspects of the immune response. These may be classified as (a) a B-cell- or antibody-mediated immunity, as exemplified by recurrent bacterial infections; (b) T-cell-mediated immunity, as shown by an increased susceptibility to viral, fungal or protozoal infections; (c) both B- and T-cell-mediated immunity, leading to acute and chronic infections; (d) immunity mediated by the action of non-antigen-specific cells such as phagocytic cell or natural killer (NK) cell deficiency; (e) immunity associated with the activation of serum complement leading to autoimmunity.

Anyone with such immunodeficiencies generally suffers from recurrent infections. The various disorders can be diagnosed by specific laboratory tests and are indicated by the types of infection suffered by the patient. Furthermore, immune deficiency disorders are frequently divided into *primary disorders*, which may be hereditary or acquired and in which the immune deficiency is the cause of the disease, and *secondary disorders*, in which the immune deficiency is the result of other diseases. A detailed discussion of the different types of primary and secondary immune deficiency diseases is outside the scope of this volume and readers who are interested in more details should consult the standard texts mentioned in the bibliography.

ACQUIRED IMMUNE DEFICIENCY SYNDROME (AIDS)

AIDS has become the focus of global concern largely as a result of the epidemic proportions it has reached in many developing countries. Currently there are over half a million cases of AIDS in the USA, and over 90% of the diagnosed cases may result in premature death. The World Health Organization estimates that there are at least 14 million people infected with HIV worldwide. This is a conservative estimate and other estimates range from 40 to 120 million infected individuals. Thus it is clear that HIV infection constitutes a serious threat to a significant proportion of the world population. Despite the extensive research that has been undertaken into the nature of the virus causing the disease, prevention of the disease by means of specific vaccines has so far proved impossible.

For many years it has been known that the human immune deficiency virus (HIV) is the cause of AIDS. Two to four weeks following infection, some individuals experience fever, a sore throat and general malaise which usually rapidly disappear. This is followed by an asymptomatic period which usually lasts for years and is followed by the overt disease, AIDS. AIDS patients exhibit various manifestations of the syndrome typified by severe immune deficiency accompanied by opportunistic infections that eventually overwhelm the patient; infection with *Pneumocystis carinii* is frequently the cause of death. However, common opportunistic pathogens include bacteria, viruses, fungi and protozoa. In addition, AIDS patients often exhibit a pronounced susceptibility to Kaposi's sarcoma, a rare skin cancer previously confined to the elderly or those receiving immunosuppressive therapy. A rare type of non-Hodgkin's lymphoma may also frequently occur in these patients. About 35% of AIDS patients also show profound changes in both the central and peripheral nervous systems which brings their disease to the attention of psychoimmunologists. When one takes into account the projected numbers that will be infected with HIV, and who will develop AIDS as a consequence, by the year 2000 some 28 million people will probably show severe psychiatric and neurological complications.

PATHOLOGY OF HIV INFECTION

HIV is a retrovirus and like other viruses it requires the nuclear processes of other cells to replicate. However, unlike other viruses, HIV utilizes the conversion of genetic information of the host cell from RNA to DNA, a reversal of the usual mechanism of action of viruses. HIV is attached to the target cell through a specific glycoprotein (gp 120) on the CD4 protein located on the T cells. After attachment, the viral envelope fuses with the cell membrane and the viral core, containing two strands of RNA together with structural protein enzymes, enters the host cell. Information is then passed from the viral RNA to the host cell DNA by RNA dependent DNA and the resulting DNA is used as a template to form double-stranded DNA. The double-stranded DNA then migrates into the nucleus of the host cell and is inserted, by the viral enzyme integrase, into the host cell genome. Completion of the reverse transcription of the viral RNA is dependent on the activation of the host cell, a process that is essential for the biosynthesis of new viral particles that can infect new cells. It now appears that the virus can remain in a fairly dormant state for several years, which accounts for the long and variable period called the *latent* or *asymptomatic phase*.

The precise origin of HIV is still uncertain, but recent evidence suggests that it originated in the Congo. Two strains have been clearly identified, HIV-I and HIV-II, the latter mainly confined to Africa. The HIV-II virus appears to be less pathogenic than the HIV-I form. HIV is known to be related to other retroviruses and it appears to be similar to simian immune deficiency virus (SIV), which causes symptoms of AIDS in monkeys that are similar to AIDS. Recent research suggests that a mutant form of SIV may have given rise to HIV as a result of individuals in the Congo having eaten infected monkeys. SIV-infected monkeys have provided a valuable model of HIV and for the development of drugs to treat the infection.

The decline in the proportion of CD4+ cells infected with HIV increases dramatically with the progression of the disease. This suggests that the destruction of the CD4+ cells during HIV infection is the direct result of the virus infection. In addition, even in cells that are not damaged by HIV, there is a major impairment in their immune function. This is apparent even in the early asymptomatic phase of the infection and may be due to the impairment of antigen-specific CD4+ function which arises from a block in the interaction of CD4+ cells with MHC class I molecules on the surface of the antigen-presenting cells. Such an interaction is essential for the activation of CD4+ cells by an antigen.

A consequence of reduced activation of the CD4+ cells is the reduction in the release of interleukin-2 (IL-2), a cytokine which is essential for the activation of many T-cell subtypes. In addition, it is now known that HIV can infect monocytes and macrophages that phagocytose the virus; this implies that monocytes may act as a reservoir for HIV, transporting the virus throughout the body which includes the brain. There is now evidence that various microorganisms that can infect the patient during the asymptomatic phase of the disease could lead to the activation of CD4+ infected cells thereby increasing the transcription of HIV, destruction of CD4+ cells and the development of AIDS. Thus the vital role played by CD4+ lymphocytes, not only in cell-mediated immunity but also in T-cell dependent antibody production and immune regulation, explains the generalized immune deficiency of AIDS patients who are then prone to various opportunistic infections and malignancies.

Although there has been a major emphasis on the detrimental effect of HIV on CD4+ cells, it has recently been observed that stimulation of CD8+ T cells, through the T-cell receptor complex, leads to *de novo* expression of the CD4 antigens on the cell surface; this results in the susceptibility of CD8+ T cells to HIV infection. In addition, activation of monocytes in HIV infected individuals results in the appearance of double positive CD4+/CD8+ T cells which become infected by endogenous HIV. This could provide another mechanism whereby HIV could attack the immune system and also help to explain why CD8+ T-cell defects, as well as CD4+ defects, occur in patients with AIDS.

While failure of T-cell homeostasis is an important feature of HIV-I infection, there is substantial evidence that T-cell homeostasis is independent of CD4+ and CD8+ subsets. Failure of T-cell homeostasis appears to precede the development of clinically defined AIDS by approximately 1.5 to 2 years and this could be an important feature of the progression of HIV-I infection. It has been hypothesized that T-cell turnover and depletion of memory cells in patients with HIV-I infection can be viewed as the reverse of the process whereby immune reconstruction occurs after stem cell transplantation, and that changes in the functional activity of T-cell memory may be critical to both processes.

The eventual loss of CD4+ lymphocytes contributes substantially to the development of AIDS in those infected with the HIV-I virus. There is evidence that in HIV-I infection, there is a shift in the CD4+ lymphocytes from Th1 cells (which produce cytokines that favour cell-mediated immune responses) to Th2 cells (which favour humoral immunity). This observation has concentrated the attention of researchers on IL-12, a cytokine which is produced by antigen-presenting cells. IL-12 plays a central role in the development of Th1-type immune responses and, *in vitro*, has been shown to inhibit HIV-1 replication. Whether this will have useful therapeutic application is uncertain. Similarly, IL-2 has been shown to decrease the expression of CD4, the primary HIV receptor and CC-chemokine receptor 5 (a co-receptor used by macrophagotrophic viruses), suggesting that IL-2 may be of benefit in the restoration of immune function in AIDS patients and possibly prevent the infection of healthy macrophages by decreasing the expression of HIV-I receptors. Finally, IL-6 has been shown to be elevated in patients with HIV infection, and may contribute to the pathogenesis of the infection. It has been shown that a subunit of the IL-6 receptor (CD126) is over-expressed on monocytes, B cells and CD4+ T cells in HIV-infected individuals. It would therefore appear that the increased expression of the IL-6 receptor (CD126) may directly or indirectly contribute to immune dysfunction and to AIDS pathogenesis in HIV-infected patients.

In addition to the cytokines IL-2, IL-6 and IL-12, which appear to play different roles in the pathogenesis of AIDS, there are a number of chemokines present which act as chemotactic factors for leucocytes and thereby play a role in leucocyte recruitment and trafficking. Some chemokines have been shown to suppress HIV-I infection. In addition, chemokine receptors serve, along with CD4+, as obligate co-receptors for HIV-I entry. The identification of these chemokine co-receptors could be important in the development of drugs that act as receptor antagonists, thereby enabling the pathogenesis of AIDS to be better understood. It is already apparent that the production of some chemokines in response to immune cell activation is initially enhanced by the immune suppressive proteins interferon alpha

(IFN-α) and TAT but then inhibited in parallel with the induction of immunosuppression. This accounts for the clinical observation that uninfected T cells are suppressed and the decline in C-C chemokine release found in the advanced stages of HIV-I infection parallels the rise in IFN-α and extracellular TAT. These could form future targets for drug development.

AIDS DEMENTIA

HIV infection is frequently associated with the development of a broad spectrum of central nervous system (CNS) and neuropsychological deficits now termed HIV-associated dementia. Motor slowing may begin early in HIV infection whether the patient is asymptomatic or not and resembles the changes seen in basal ganglia related disorders such as *Huntington's disease*. Once AIDS has developed, symptoms increase rapidly, assisted by an increased permeability of the blood–brain barrier, and can become an incapacitating dementia. These symptoms appear to be unrelated to any opportunistic infection. Postmortem studies have shown the presence of multinucleated giant cells, microglial nodules, perivascular monocyte infiltrates, astrogliosis, white matter pallor and neurodegeneration or neuronal injury. Vacuolar neuropathy occurs in about 20% of patients, particularly those with dementia.

The search for the mechanism responsible for the neuropsychological deficits has focused on the lesions within the brain. HIV appears to be localized in the macrophage infiltrates and microglia rather than in the neurons and astrocytes. This suggests that the neurological deficits are mediated indirectly by either virus or endotoxins that produce the neurological symptoms by killing or damaging the neurons, disrupting neuronal electrolyte transport and impairing neurotransmission. Attention has been particularly directed at the macrophages because of their close association with HIV.

While the precise mechanism whereby HIV exerts its neurotoxic effects is still unclear, there is evidence that glycoprotein 160 (gp 160), a component of the HIV envelope, is neurotoxic to hippocampal cells in very low concentrations. It has been found that gp 120, which is also a component of the HIV envelope, causes a similar excitotoxic response in neurons as excitatory transmitters such as glutamate, kainate and quinolinate. The precise mechanism whereby gp 120 interacts with the glutamate and N-methyl-D-aspartate (NMDA) receptors is uncertain. Experimentally, it has been shown that gp 120 stimulates nitric oxide synthesis in a human astrocyte cell line. Nitric oxide has been implicated in NMDA receptor mediated neurotoxicity. There is experimental evidence that the neurotoxic effects of gp 120 can be blocked by NMDA receptor antagonist, which is further evidence that at the cellular level, HIV neurotoxicity may therefore be associated with an excessive activation of the glutamatergic system.

When gp 120 was injected intracerebroventricularly into rats, there was a significant decrease in spatial learning. This could be blocked by vasoactive intestinal polypeptide (VIP), which shows a certain analogous sequence with gp 120 for some HIV strains. Administration of low doses of gp 120 for 28 days to newborn rats was found to result in morphological damage of pyramidal neurons in the cortex. Many other developmental changes were also delayed in these animals.

Within the CNS, some cytokines are well known to be toxic to neurons and oligodendrocytes, to stimulate astrocytic proliferation and act as mediators of fever. Although selective increases in cytokine expression in the brain have been shown to occur in HIV-infected patients, there is a minimal correlation with the severity of the encephalitis. The most consistent response is an increase in tumour necrosis factor alpha (TNF-α) co-cultures of astrocytes and HIV-infected monocytes have been shown to produce neurotoxic factors that include TNF-α and IL-1β; in addition, arachidonic acid metabolites have been implicated in the synthesis of these agents together with platelet-activating factor, leucotrienes B4 and D4 and tipoxin A4. Of these, platelet-activating factor when added to cultures of unaffected monocytes and astrocytes was shown to be neurotoxic. These results suggest that arachidonate metabolites, cytokines and neurodegenerative responses are linked and that an interaction between monocytes and astrocytes is required for HIV-induced neurotoxicity.

In addition to the various immunotoxic agents that have been implicated in HIV-associated dementia, there is also evidence that specific neurotoxins such as quinolinic acid play a significant role in the neurotoxicity. Thus the concentration of this neurotoxin has been shown to rise in the cerebrospinal fluid of patients in association with the development of the motor deficits. The concentration of quinolinic acid is highest in those patients with neurological deficits and inflammatory lesions. In addition, the cerebrospinal fluid concentration is correlated with measures of immune activation (for example, neopterin and beta-2 microglobulin). It is now apparent that macrophages rather than astrocytes are the important source of quinolinic acid, while cytokines released from activated lymphocytes, macrophages and microglia are an important link between immune activation and the synthesis of quinolinic acid.

However, it should be noted that more than a decade after the detection of DNA for HIV in the brain, the pathophysiology of HIV infection remains an enigma. Nevertheless, there are a number of key observations, which may be summarized as follows:

1. HIV dementia is caused by the virus itself as no other pathogen has been consistently found in the brains of patients with HIV.
2. In comparison with other virally induced encephalopathies, there is a discordance between the viral content of the brain and the degree of neurodegeneration.

3. The cell types in the brain which are responsible for the viral synthesis are the resident macrophages and microglial cells.
4. The astrocytes are also probably infected with HIV, but such infection is highly restricted in terms of viral synthesis.
5. At least one neurotoxic component of HIV infection is derived from the infected microglia.

It would appear that the cognitive dysfunction that develops as a result of HIV-I infection is at least partly mediated by excitotoxins and free radicals. These HIV-infected macrophages and microglia, or immune-activated macrophages and astrocytes (activated by the shed HIV-I envelope protein gp 120 or other viral proteins and cytokines), secrete arachidonic acid, platelet-activating factor, free radicals such as nitric oxide, glutamate, quinolinate, etc. Such a pathway also leads to neurodegeneration in the case of stroke and other neurodegenerative diseases and operates via the NMDA-glutamate receptor. The use of NMDA antagonists may therefore be of value in reducing the neurodegenerative impact of HIV-I in the future. The modulatory influence of the growth factor NF kappa B on normal T-cell responses including IL-2, IL-6, IL-8 and several T-cell surface receptors is also an important component of both the central and peripheral actions of HIV. A reduction in the activity of NF kappa B has been found in T cells from aged individuals and also in HIV-I infection. The ability of hydrogen peroxide, or other reactive oxygen species, to induce T-cell signals and functional responses could also help to account for the neurodegenerative changes that occur following HIV infection.

Stress has been postulated to play an important role in the progression of HIV-I infection to AIDS. HIV-I-infected patients frequently experience severe psychiatric complications and major depression is a common presenting symptom of the disease. It is therefore not unreasonable to assume that various neuropeptides and neurohormones (such as the enkephalins, endorphins, vasoactive intestinal peptide, ACTH) could affect the function of macrophages and monocytes, thereby contributing to the development of the HIV infection. Specific receptors for these neuropeptides and neurohormones occur on these types of immune cell. However, so far little attention has been paid to the determination of the blood concentrations of such substances in stressed, HIV-I-infected patients.

DRUGS OF ABUSE AND AIDS

Intravenous drug abuse is frequently associated with HIV infection and the drug of abuse could play a significant role in the pathogenesis of the infection. Opiates, such as morphine, have been postulated to promote the progression of HIV infection and the consequent development of secondary opportunistic infections. Opioids are known to have a diversity of effects on the immune system. These effects may be mediated indirectly via the brain or via the opioid receptors situated on the immunocytes. Indeed it has been argued that the opiates (and the endogenous opiates, the enkephalins and endorphins) can operate as cytokines. Evidence from *in vitro* studies suggests that the immunomodulatory actions of opioids are mediated by ultra high affinity receptors on monocytes and glial cells, which could explain the immunosuppressive actions of the opiates. However, the effect of opiates such as morphine on immune cells would appear to depend on the concentration. It has been shown, for example, that the secretion of IL-6 by activated macrophages is stimulated by low concentrations of morphine (nanomolar range) but inhibited by high concentrations (micromolar concentrations) of the drug. Furthermore, the expression of the genes for such cytokines is dependent on the activation of the trancription factor NF kappa beta. However, as morphine differentially affects NF kappa beta dose dependently, it seems unlikely that these immune changes are clinically relevant when opioids are abused in high doses.

Other drugs of abuse may also act as immune suppressants. Cannabinoids have long been known to impair various aspects of cellular immunity and thereby contribute to the pathogenesis of HIV infection while recently attention has been directed towards the effect of both intravenous and smoked ("crack") cocaine. While sometimes contradictory, both human and animal studies show that cocaine can suppress the function of NK cells, T cells, neutrophils and macrophages and can suppress the ability of these cells to secrete immunoregulatory cytokines. *In vitro* studies have also shown that cocaine can enhance the infectivity and/or replication of HIV in human cell lives.

Nitric oxide type inhalants are widely used by male homosexuals and epidemiological studies now indicate that inhalant abuse is a cofactor in HIV infection and in Kaposi's sarcoma. Inhalation of nitrites is associated with non-specific cytotoxicity that affects both humoral and cell-mediated immunity. In addition, there is evidence that nitrites increase macrophage synthesis of TNF-α which can directly stimulate HIV replication and the growth of Kaposi's sarcoma cells. Nitrite abuse could therefore be an important trigger factor in the progression of HIV to AIDS.

SUMMARY

Neurotoxicity associated with HIV-I infection may be related to the presence of the virus and agents that are derived from it. The toxicity may be exacerbated by toxins released from the host (e.g. quinolinic acid) in response to the presence of the virus and/or due to immune activation. The clinical signs of HIV-associated neurological disease may be a consequence of the combined or separate effects of these neurotoxins but it would appear from experimental studies that the NMDA receptors may play a key role in neurotoxicity.

CHRONIC FATIGUE SYNDROME (CFS)

CFS is a disabling illness characterized by persistent and overwhelming fatigue. Fatigue can be defined as a profound sense of tiredness, lack of energy and a feeling of exhaustion. It is distinguished from depression which includes symptoms of lack of self-esteem, despair and feelings of hopelessness. Patients with CFS experience most profound tiredness and become exhausted after minimal physical exertion. The fatigue can appear suddenly or gradually and persist throughout the period of illness. Patients are forced to function to a level of activity which is substantially lower than their usual capacity. Other symptoms of CFS include fibromyalgia (generalized muscle aches and pains), weakness, sleep disorder, impaired memory and poor concentration; infections are also a common feature of the condition. These symptoms may persist for months or even years. Significant fatigue without any obvious cause must be present for at least six months in order to fulfil the diagnostic criteria of CFS. Although the symptoms of CFS were described about 150 years ago (Charles Darwin and Florence Nightingale probably being sufferers) CFS was only finally accepted as a neurological disease by the World Health Organization in 1993.

The *neuropsychiatric symptoms* have been estimated to occur in about 80% of patients. The most consistent finding is mild depression, often accompanied by anxiety, intense introspection and hypochondriasis. Cognitive deficits are common. Many patients are forced to abandon intellectual pursuits. However, CFS patients usually do not suffer from the anhedonic or suicidal symptoms which typify depression. Emotionality and a tendency to tearfulness are common; the emotional changes usually fluctuate with the severity of the fatigue symptoms.

Patients with CFS often complain of symptoms that suggest CNS involvement including difficulty with concentration, attention, memory, photophobia and a paraesthesias. Such symptoms may be related to the neurological abnormalities which have been detected by magnetic resonance imaging (MRI), suggesting that an abnormality in the structure of the white matter occurs in subcortical areas of the brain. Such changes are distinct from those seen in multiple sclerosis.

Single photon computerized tomography (SPECT) abnormalities have also been detected in the brains of CFS patients that more closely resemble those seen in patients with AIDS encephalopathy than in patients with major depression, a condition which may coexist with CFS. These SPECT changes may be a consequence of reduced blood flow through the small cerebral vessels and/or a dysfunction of neuronal or glial cells.

Unlike depression, where there is ample evidence of pituitary–adrenal hyperactivity, in CFS there is evidence that corticotrophin-releasing factor (CRF) secretion is reduced. In addition, disruption of both the serotonergic and noradrenergic pathways occurs in CFS with changes in

5-hydroxyindole-acetic acid (5-HIAA), vasopressin and prolactin that are the opposite of those found in major depression.

Impairment of cognition is one of the most common and disabling symptoms of CFS and while cognitive functioning is usually confined to the normal range, there is evidence that these patients often have detectable abnormalities of memory and/or attention during timed psychological tasks. One study to date has reported that the immunological and cognitive abnormalities are correlated but are unrelated to coexisting depression.

IMMUNITY AND THE PATHOPHYSIOLOGY OF CFS

The pathophysiology of CFS remains unknown but circumstantial evidence suggests that the condition may result from a disordered immune response to a precipitating infection or antigenic challenge. Thus CFS is frequently reported to occur following an acute virus infection, although in only a minority of cases has the initiating infectious agent been documented during the acute phase of the illness. In those cases where the infective agent has been documented, a range of common viral infections were implicated and these include varicella, Epstein–Barr virus, rubella, mumps and enterovirus. Non-viral infections that have been implicated include toxoplasmosis and brucellosis. Thus it may be questioned whether the host response to these antigens may be disturbed, resulting in the chronic symptoms, or whether some undocumented infection may initiate CFS.

One of the major problems resulting from attempts to implicate a disordered immune system in patients with CFS results from the probable heterogeneity of the patients being studied and the difficulties that have arisen in the standardization of the assays used.

A defective humoral immune response to infections thought to precipitate CFS may allow antigens to evade the immune system crucial to the effective clearance of the infection. Serum concentrations of total immunoglobulins G, A and M have been shown to be within the normal range. When the subclasses of IgG were determined, there was some evidence of a partial reduction in IgG1, 2 and 3. Such changes are not typical of patients with significant humoral immune deficiency, but rather suggest a mild abnormality in the synthesis of immunoglobulins. These reduced immunoglobulin concentrations occur transiently in acute viral infections and are likely to be due to alteration in T-cell control; both IFN-α and IFN-γ, as well as IL-4, are known to modulate immunoglobulin synthesis. Further studies have shown that the intrinsic capacity of T and B cells to initiate immunoglobulin synthesis is not defective.

Studies of the humoral immune response to specific agents thought to initiate CFS have focused on herpes virus and enterovirus. Although the pattern of development and persistence of IgG antibodies to these viral infections has been proposed as a laboratory marker of CFS, recent evidence suggests that the presence of these antibodies has little diagnostic value. However, an apparent association exists between atopy and CFS. A history of atopy (allergies to food, drugs or inhaled antigens) and skin test reactivity to food and inhaled antigens occurs in the majority of patients with CFS when compared to the appropriate controls. Such studies revealed that patients with CFS had higher serum IgE concentrations and increased lymphocyte responsiveness to specific antigens. It thus seems possible that atopy is a manifestation of a disorder of cell-mediated immunity which can predispose the individual to an aberrant response to viral or intracellular infection, possibly due to an altered production of cytokines.

Aspects of cellular immunity have also been the topic of attention. There is some evidence of reduced NK cell function in CFS but the results have been variable and no attempt has been made to control for the effects of medication, alcohol in gestation, smoking or for the possible impact of anxiety or mood disorders.

Variable results have also been obtained from CFS patients in which the T-cell subsets have been determined. There is some evidence that CD8, but not CD4, T-cell subset numbers are reduced when compared with healthy controls and patients with major depression, but so far none of the studies has assessed the consistency of T-cell subsets with time, or demonstrated any correlation with the course or the severity of the disorder.

The ability of T cells to proliferate in response to a mitogen has also been investigated in comparison to a group of control subjects and depressed patients. The T-cell response to the mitogen phytohaemaglutinin (PHA) was found to be significantly reduced in CFS patients in comparison to controls; the T-cell response in the depressed patients was also reduced but not so markedly as in the CFS patients. The ability of CFS patients to respond to an intradermally administered challenge (a delayed hypersensitivity test) indicates that these patients tend to be allergic.

The regulation of a cell-mediated immune response to an antigen is dependent on the activity of cytokines. These immune transmitters are not only important for effective immunity but may also directly produce psychiatric symptoms. Of the wide variety of cytokines determined in patients with CFS, only the serum concentration of transforming growth factor beta has been shown to be elevated. However, the synthesis of cytokines for monocytes *in vitro* in response to lipopolysaccharide has been shown to result in an elevation in IL-1β, TNF-α and IL-6; IL-1α does not apparently change. In the cerebrospinal fluid, a slight increase in IFN-α, but not other cytokines, has been reported. It should be emphasized that numerous factors may contribute to the difficulties in detecting the cytokines in patients with CFS. Thus there is a need to control for the assay methods used, to assess changes throughout the course of the disease (rather than at one time point only) and to determine concurrently the presence in the serum of the cytokine inhibitors which could interfere with the detection of the cytokines.

The absence of inflammatory symptoms in patients with CFS (for example, fever and leucocytosis; elevated acute phase proteins) further suggests that the concentrations of the cytokines in the serum will be minimal.

Whether the abnormalities in the immune system of patients with CFS have any relationship to the symptoms of the disease is presently unclear. In the only study that attempted to examine this question, clinical improvement in CFS was not associated with changes in lymphocyte subsets or the degree of immune activation. Thus while it may be postulated that the state of immune activation could lead to the synthesis of cytokines that disrupt neurotransmitter function, thereby causing the symptoms of the disease, definitive evidence in favour of this hypothesis is still lacking.

SUMMARY

There is evidence of a disordered immune system in patients with CFS and several studies have led to the conclusion that there is an association between CFS and immune dysfunction, the pattern of changes being similar to that seen in patients with an acute viral infection. Nevertheless the prevalence of a magnitude of changes in cell-mediated immunity cannot be explained by the concurrence of depression in CFS patients. Thus there remains the need to assess changes in humoral and cellular immunity in CFS patients over time. Some of the possible immune changes that occur in CFS patients are shown in Table 13.1.

Table 13.1 Immune changes reported to occur in patients with CFS

1. Immunoglobulins—total IgG decreased, as are IgG1, 2, 3 subsets

2. History of atopy to various allergens increased

3. Cellular immunity
   reduced NK cell cytotoxicity (? due to depression)
   evidence of increased CD8+ subset of T cells in some studies
   impaired T-cell proliferative response to PHA mitogen
   reduced response to intradermally injected antigen

4. Cytokines
   monocytes challenged with LPS *in vitro* show increased IL-1β, TNF-α, 1 IL-6
   in cerebrospinal fluid, increased IFN-α detected

BIBLIOGRAPHY

Bock, G. R. and Whelan, J. (Eds), (1993) *Chronic Fatigue Syndrome*, Ciba Foundation Symposium **173**. John Wiley and Sons, Chichester.
Buchwald, D. and Komaroff A. L. (1991) Review of laboratory findings of patients with CFS. *Review of Infectious Diseases* **13** (Suppl. 1): S12–S18.

Epstein, L. G. and Gendelman, H. E. (1993) Human immunodeficiency virus type 1 infection of the nervous system: pathogenic mechanism. *Annals of Neurology* **33**: 429–436.

Fukuda, K., Straus, S. E. Hickie, I. et al. (1994) The chronic fatigue syndrome, a comprehensive approach to its definition and study. *Annals of Internal Medicine* **121**: 959–963.

Genis, P., Jett, M. et al. (1993) Cytokines and arachidonic acid metabolites produced during human immunodeficiency virus infected macrophage–astrocyte interactions: implications for the neuropathogenesis of HIV disease. *Journal of Experimental Medicine* **176**: 1703–1718.

Gow, J. W. and Behan, P. O. (1996) Viruses and CFS. *Journal of Chronic Fatigue Syndrome* **21**: 67–83.

Greene, W. C. (1993) Aids and the immune system. *Scientific American* **269**: 99–105.

Harbuz, M. S. and Lightman, S. L. (1992) Stress and hypothalamo-pituitary-adrenal axis: acute and chronic immunological activation. *Journal of Endocrinology* **134**: 327–329.

Linde, A., Anderson B. et al. (1992) Serum levels of lymphokines and soluble cellular receptors in primary Epstein–Barr virus infection in patients with CFS. *Journal of Infectious Diseases* **165**: 994–1000.

Lloyd, A., Hickie, I., Hickie, C. et al. (1992) Cell mediated immunity in patients with CFS, healthy controls and patients with major depression. *Clinical and Experimental Immunology* **87**: 76–79.

Spencer, D. C. and Price, R. W. (1993) Human immunodeficiency virus and the central nervous system. *Annual Review of Microbiology* **46**: 655–693.

Studd, J. and Panay, N. (1996) Chronic fatigue syndrome. *Lancet* **348**: 1384.

Tyor, W. R., Glass, J. D., Griffin, J. W. (1992) Cytokine expression in the brain during AIDS. *Annals of Neurology* **31**: 349–360.

14 The Effects of Drugs of Abuse on the Immune System

INTRODUCTION

The adverse effects of drugs of abuse on health are a major source of concern for health authorities throughout the world. As an illustration of the extent of the problems that result from drug abuse, it has been estimated that over 54 million individuals smoke tobacco in the United States alone, the extent of the problem being far greater in non-industrialized countries, probably because of the lack of government-sponsored health measures to control the problem in these countries. Alcoholism, and heavy social drinking of alcohol, accounts for 10–15 million in the United States. Proportionally there is an even greater degree of alcohol abuse in many northern European countries. In Ireland, for example, a small country of 3.5 million, it has been estimated that 75 000 people are alcohol dependent, while alcohol-related brain damage is now the most important cause for first admissions to psychiatric hospitals.

Cocaine has become a popular drug of abuse among more educated, professional individuals in many industrialized countries. In the United States, over 23 million have used cocaine on an occasional basis while 600 000 to 1 million are regular users and are psychologically dependent on its stimulant effects. The opiates, particularly heroin and morphine, have been used for medicinal purposes and as drugs of abuse for well over a century in industrialized countries, while the impure form of the drug has been widely used as a drug of abuse in Asian societies since antiquity. Approximately, 2.7 million individuals in the United States have used heroin on an occasional basis and of these, over 1 million are now estimated to be dependent on heroin and other opiates. Proportionally, the extent of opiate abuse is probably similar in many other industrialized countries.

With regard to the so-called "soft drugs" of abuse (cannabis, the amphetamine-like stimulants and the hallucinogens), the abuse of cannabis has been the most widely recognized and the adverse effects of its abuse in general health clearly identified. In most industrialized countries, a substantial minority of young persons have experimented with cannabis on an occasional basis, a small proportion becoming regular abusers of the drug.

Most of the evidence linking chronic cannabis use to adverse effects on general health has come from developing countries in which the social use of cannabis is the accepted alternative to alcohol abuse.

It must be emphasized that the poor health of those individuals abusing drugs may not be directly related to the drug itself but due to a complex interaction between the unhealthy lifestyle of the abuser that is often necessitated in order to maintain the drug dependence leading to infection and the immunosuppressive effect of the drug of abuse. This has led to debate regarding the need to legalize the use of some drugs of dependence so that adopting an antisocial and unhealthy lifestyle to maintain the habit is reduced. However, it must be emphasized that there is sufficient clinical and experimental evidence already available to suggest that all drugs of abuse, including alcohol, can adversely affect the general health of the individual, which cautions against changing the law in the mistaken belief that the so-called "soft drugs" are relatively harmless. In this chapter, a general overview will be presented of the effects of alcohol, the "soft drugs" of dependence (nicotine, the amphetamines, cannabis and the hallucinogens), cocaine and the opioids in the immune system.

THE EFFECTS OF ALCOHOL ON THE IMMUNE SYSTEM

Anecdotal reports have appeared in the clinical literature from several centuries indicating that chronic alcohol abuse leads to poor health, changes that would now be recognized as being due to impaired immune function. It has long been known, for example, that alcoholics are prone to infections by pathogens and have a decreased ability to fight infection and an increased risk of developing cancer of the head, neck and upper gastrointestinal tract. While alcohol-induced malnutrition, particularly vitamin deficiencies and advanced liver cirrhosis, is likely to contribute to the immune deficiency, alcohol itself is also known to be a potent immunomodulator. The mechanisms whereby alcohol can modulate immune function will now be considered.

EFFECT OF ALCOHOL ON THE INFLAMMATORY RESPONSE

During an inflammatory response, chemotactic agents, such as the activated components of the complement system, the leucotrienes and the cytokines which are released from activated macrophages and monocytes, induce phagocytes to migrate to the site of inflammation. The neutrophils and monocytes adhere to, and migrate through, the cells lining the blood vessels at the site of infection and destroy the pathogens by engulfing them; intracellular free radicals and enzymes are responsible for this toxicity.

Alcohol had been shown to affect the sequence of events that lead to death of the invading microorganisms in several ways. It has been shown in experimental studies, for example, that alcohol can increase the expression of CD8 molecules on the neutrophil surface; these molecules are required for cellular adhesion. In addition, IL-8 secretion by liver macrophages (the Kupffer cells) is increased by alcohol, which enhances the influx of neutrophils into the liver. This can result in liver damage and forms the basis of alcoholic hepatitis. In clinical studies, it is well established that the blood interleukin-8 (IL-8) concentration is higher in alcoholics and is associated with the accumulation of neutrophils in the liver. Chronic, and even acute, alcohol consumption also reduces the ability of phagocytes to ingest and destroy pathogens. Thus abnormal neutrophil adherence and chemotaxis and reduced functional activity of the macrophages may contribute to the impaired defence against pathogenic microorganisms, thereby reducing the resistance to infection.

Contact between a macrophage and an invading micro-organism induces the release of numerous proinflammatory cytokines such as IL-1, IL-6 and tumour necrosis factor alpha (TNF-α) which play a pivotal role in initiating and maintaining the inflammatory response. In addition, neutrophils, lymphocytes and other white blood cells can release cytokines as part of a major inflammatory process. Should the release of cytokines become excessive, tissue damage will occur. Chronic alcohol abuse, particularly in combination with liver damage, is associated with elevated blood concentrations of TNF-α, IL-1 and IL-6. These cytokines probably contribute to the symptoms associated with alcoholic hepatitis (for example, fever, weight loss, raised liver enzymes in the blood). In contrast to the chronic effects of alcohol, acute moderate quantities of alcohol tend to reduce the release of the proinflammatory cytokines. This could result in the immune system becoming compromised, even if only for a short period.

Under normal conditions, the release of the proinflammatory cytokines decreases during the later phases of an infection due to the release of the immunoregulatory cytokines, the most widely studied being IL-10 and transforming growth factor beta (TGF-β). IL-10 inhibits cell-mediated immunity and promotes humoral immunity by reducing the release of proinflammatory cytokines and T-cell proliferation. Acute alcohol exposure increases the synthesis of IL-10, at least in cultured human monocytes. TGF-β is also increased by pharmacologically relevant concentrations of alcohol in cell culture. Some of the functions of TGF-β are shown in Table 14.1.

Table 14.1 Effects of TGF-β *in vivo*

Inhibition of proinflammatory cytokine synthesis from monocytes and macrophages
Inhibition of T-cell proliferation
Augmentation of humoral immune response
Increased collagen synthesis which can accumulate in the liver

Thus alcohol elevates the concentration of TGF-β which, together with its effects on IL-10, interferes with the body's defence against invading microorganisms by reducing the synthesis and release of proinflammatory cytokines and by inhibiting T-cell proliferation.

Experimental studies have shown that both acute and chronic alcohol administration reduces the production of free radicals by macrophages. These free radicals (for example, O^{2-}, OH^-, hydrogen peroxide and nitric oxide (NO)) are crucially involved in the destruction of microorganisms that have been engulfed by activated macrophages. These changes are particularly apparent in the macrophages produced by the lungs, which may account for the high incidence of tuberculosis found in chronic alcoholics. In the liver, however, oxygen free radicals are over-produced following chronic alcohol abuse, which may contribute to the alcohol-related liver damage.

In addition to the adverse effects of alcohol in cytokine and free radical production, both clinical and experimental studies have shown that alcoholics have a reduced number of T cells in the blood, thymus and spleen. The precise mechanism is unknown but it has been speculated that alcohol induces programmed cell death, or apoptosis, in immature T cells in the thymus and possibly also in mature lymphocytes and monocytes in the blood. T-cell proliferation is also inhibited by alcohol, possibly due to an alcohol-related reduction in IL-2 and to the increased synthesis of IL-10 and TGF-β. Thus the overall effects of alcohol exposure result in a weakened cell-mediated immune response.

Another characteristic change in the immune system that occurs in alcoholics is an elevation of antibodies in the blood, indicating that alcohol alters the number or function of B cells. It is suggested that alcohol may interfere with antibody synthesis indirectly by inhibiting T-cell-derived cytokines that are essential for B-cell function. A reduction in antibody synthesis may also be a consequence of a disordered protein synthesis caused by the alcohol-induced increase in acute phase proteins in the liver.

Natural killer (NK) cells are critically involved in the destruction of virus-infected and cancerous cells and therefore play a crucial role in preventing tumour development. The effect of alcohol on NK cell function is far from clear but chronic alcohol consumption is frequently associated with an increased incidence of cancer which might imply impaired NK cell activity.

There is also evidence that alcohol can directly affect the synthesis of the interferons (IFN-α, IFN-γ) and IL-2; these lymphokines are reduced in the blood of alcoholics. The reduction in the blood concentration of IFN-γ may be particularly important because this cytokine, together with the macrophage-derived cytokine IL-12, is crucial for the induction of the cell-mediated immune response. This could contribute to a greater susceptibility to infections that usually involve the T-cell response.

Clinical studies support the role of a disordered cytokine network in producing the signs and symptoms of alcholic liver disease. Thus such patients show high blood concentrations of IL-1, IL-6 and IL-8 as well as tumour necrosis factor alpha (TNF-α) and monocyte chemoattractant protein-1 (MCP-1). Elevated plasma TNF concentrations are generally correlated with a poor prognosis; the increased concentration of IL-6 and acute phase proteins that occur during the active phase of alcohol liver disease subside as the liver function improves on treatment.

IL-8 may promote neutrophilia as well as neutrophil infiltration of liver tissue; MCP-1 similarly promotes monocyte infiltration. Conversely, the synthesis of IL-10 by monocytes is decreased in alcoholic patients. This cytokine usually acts as an anti-inflammatory factor so that a reduction in the synthesis of IL-10 probably contributes to the increase in the synthesis of proinflammatory cytokines.

These changes that have been observed in alcoholic patients have also been found in rats that have been chronically treated with alcohol. Indeed, many of the experimentally observed defects of proinflammatory cytokines are similar to the symptoms seen in alcoholic patients with alcoholic liver disease. In addition, collagen, which is an important component of scar tissue and aids wound healing, is abnormal in such patients and is associated with excessive deposition in the liver (i.e. fibrosis). The following changes occur both clinically and experimentally after the administration of proinflammatory cytokines and in alcoholics who have cirrhosis: fever, anorexia, neutrophilia, disturbed protein synthesis leading to reduced antibody synthesis, decreased tissue glutathione, decreased serum zinc, increased collagen deposition, increased endothelial permeability, increased metabolic rate and disordered intellectual function (associated with depression and anxiety). Such changes strongly suggest that proinflammatory cytokines play a pathogenic role in alcoholism, producing changes not only in the liver and other peripheral organs but also directly in the brain. Such changes in brain function may vary from an increased incidence of anxiety states and depression (see Chapter 5 on the role of proinflammatory cytokines in the affective disorders) to alcohol-induced dementia as a consequence of increased neuronal death.

CONSEQUENCES OF IMPAIRED IMMUNITY CAUSED BY ALCOHOL

Alcoholics may be considered to be immunocompromised because of the incidence and severity of infections that are increased in these individuals. These infections include increases in pneumoncoccal pneumonia, tuberculosis and AIDS. It is self-evident that an increased risk of AIDS and other sexually transmitted diseases could result from impairment of socially responsible behaviour which the drug brings about. In addition to an increased incidence of severe infections that may occur in the alcoholic, there is also evidence that the healing of traumatic injuries (for example, following a car crash or severe burns) is slower, possibly due to impaired cell-mediated immunity and increased humoral immunity. Additional problems can arise due to the chronic effects of alcohol abuse on neuronal structure and function. Of the regions of the brain which are susceptible to alcohol-induced damage, the hippocampus is particularly vulnerable. As this region is concerned with short-term memory, it is understandable why memory defects are a common feature of alcoholism.

SUMMARY

Both clinical and experimental studies have shown that both acute and chronic alcohol administration can compromise the ability of the individual to resist infection. Following acute alcohol administration, the immuno-compromised state is likely to be transient. The possible mechanisms whereby alcohol produces these effects on the immune system are sum-marized diagramatically in Figure 14.1.

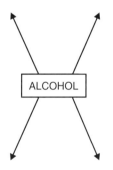

T cell and B cell function

- Reduced T cell numbers

- Elevated antibodies in blood

- NK cells may be functionally impaired in alcoholics

- Decreased IFN-α, IFN-γ and IL-2 reduced cell-mediated immunity

Immunotoxic activity

(Free radical synthesis)

- In lung tissue, alcohol reduces free radical synthesis by macrophages

- In liver, alcohol increases free radical synthesis, increasing liver damage

Liver

- Increased neutrophil infiltration leading to liver damage

Phagocytosis

- Reduced macrophage activity

- Increased TNF-α, IL-1, IL-6, fever, weight loss, increased liver enzymes in blood in those alcoholics with liver damage

- Increased immunoregulatory cytokines (IL-10 and TGF-β) leading to reduced proinflammatory cytokine synthesis, T cell proliferation and antigen-presenting capacity of monocytes

ALCOHOL

Figure 14.1 Changes in the immune system directly or indirectly caused by alcohol. *Consequences of impaired immune system caused by alcohol*: (a) increased susceptibility to infection, particularly lung infections and cancer; (b) reduced healing of traumatic injuries, e.g. burns; (c) increased susceptibility to sexually transmitted diseases (e.g. AIDS) due to risk-taking behaviour and impaired immunity.

THE EFFECTS OF COCAINE ON THE IMMUNE SYSTEM

The euphoria and sense of well-being engendered by cocaine is undoubtedly responsible for its widespread use as a recreational drug. However, in recent years, there has been increasing concern over its acute cardiotoxicity and its long-term effects on the immune system. The adverse effects of cocaine on the immune system are reflected in the rise in the incidence of infectious diseases among cocaine abusers. Such observations have stimulated research into the possible mechanism whereby cocaine may affect immune function. Most of the studies to date have been on rodents, in which it has been shown that both acute and chronic cocaine administration can cause a disturbance in both cellular and humoral immunity and a reduced resistance to bacterial and viral infections. *In vitro*, studies have also shown that cocaine may have a direct effect on the functioning of immune cells. For example, when cocaine is added to mouse or human lymphocytic cultures, the proliferation of T cells is suppressed at relatively high drug concentrations. However, at low *in vitro* concentrations the replication of HIV added to the culture is increased. Such findings could help to explain the increased susceptibility of chronic cocaine abusers to both bacterial and viral infections.

The precise mechanism whereby cocaine can cause immunomodulation is unclear. Cocaine has long been known to have a major pharmacological action on the sympathetic system, the hypothalamic–pituitary–adrenal (HPA) axis and on sodium channels whereby it acts as a potent local anaesthetic. The sympathomimetic effects are a consequence of cocaine blocking the neuronal transporter for noradrenaline and dopamine, thereby enhancing both the central and peripheral function of these amines. The euphoria produced by cocaine has largely been ascribed to the increase in dopaminergic activity in the prefrontal cortex, the peripheral symptoms being a reflection of the increased peripheral sympathetic activity. In addition to the effects on the sympathetic system, cocaine also activates the pituitary–adrenal axis, causing an increased release of both cortisol and the catecholamines. These changes may be crucially important to the immunomodulatory action of the drug.

The local anaesthetic effect of cocaine is related to the ability of cocaine to block fast sodium channels and to displace calcium from cell membranes. There is *in vitro* experimental evidence to suggest that the effect of cocaine on viral replication could be due to its ability to modulate the intracellular calcium concentration. In addition, there is experimental evidence to show that cocaine can cause apoptosis of thymocytes and increase the percentage of thymocytes that go into the S-phase of the cell cycle. These effects of cocaine appear to be due to a direct action of the drug, as qualitatively similar changes were found when the drug was added to a culture of thymocytes. The precise mechanism whereby this occurs is uncertain.

Immune cells, especially lymphocytes, are known to contain both adrenergic and steroid receptors and are therefore readily influenced by both the adrenergic system and circulating glucocorticoids. Experimental evidence has shown that acute cocaine exposure induces a transient inhibition of alloantigen-stimulated T-cell replication. This effect does not appear to be due to an inhibition of calcium uptake by the T cell but could be related to the decrease in IL-2 release, an effect that has been reported to occur in some experimental studies. However, a more likely explanation for the effect of cocaine on the immune system relates to its sympathomimetic effects that result from inhibition of the catecholamine transporters and stimulation of the adrenal medulla. It is known that catecholamines inhibit mitogen-stimulated T-cell proliferation by activating the beta-2 adrenoceptor, which results in a rise in the intracellular concentration of cAMP. The spleen is a rich source of noradrenergic fibres, the distribution of which closely follows those of the macrophages and T cells. Thus it may be hypothesized that the increase in the release of noradrenaline that follows the administration of cocaine causes an activation of the beta receptors on the T-cell membrane with a consequent inhibition of T-cell replication. In addition, the rise in the plasma glucocorticoid concentration following cocaine administration may contribute to the immunosuppressive effect of the drug.

SUMMARY

There is experimental evidence to indicate that cocaine can adversely affect the immune system after acute and chronic administration. Whether these effects occur indirectly, by modulating the HPA axis or the peripheral sympathetic system, or directly, by interacting with specific binding sites on lymphocyte membranes, is unclear. Nevertheless, the results of such studies indicate that the increased susceptibility of cocaine abusers to bacterial and viral infections may be due, at least in part, to an alteration of immune function. These various possibilities may be summarized as shown in Figure 14.2.

CANNABIS AS AN IMMUNOMODULATOR

There are three main components of the cannabis plant. *Cannabis sativa*, which are used for their psychotropic properties, namely the flowering tops of the plant (herbal cannabis or marijuana), cannabis resin (obtained from the excretions of the stem and leaves) and cannabis oil (obtained by distillation of cannabis resin). Apart from alcohol and nicotine, cannabis is undoubtedly the most widely abused drug throughout the industrialized world and also in many developing countries, particularly those Muslim countries where alcohol is illegal. It has been estimated that 78% of illegal

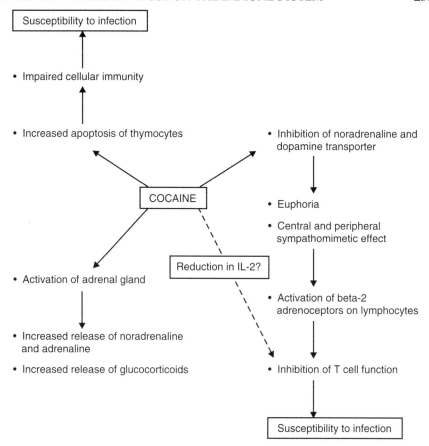

Figure 14.2 Summary of immunotoxic action of cocaine. IL-2, interleukin-2.

drug users abuse cannabis in the United States, the number of current cannabis users in that country exceeding 8.9 million. The extensive use of cannabis as a recreational drug has caused concern regarding the detrimental long-term effects, particularly as there is evidence that long-term users are more liable to infections and cancer.

The cannabis plant contains more than 60 cannabinoids, many of which are pharmacologically active. The major psychoactive component is delta-9-tetrahydrocannabinol (THC), which comprises 1–6% of the weight of the flowering heads, up to 15% of the resin and 40% of the semi-purified cannabis oil. Despite its use in medicine since antiquity (the Chinese used it as a soporific over 2000 years ago), and the more recent evidence of its potent antiemetic and antispasmodic action in the treatment of multiple sclerosis, the potent psychoactive properties and its potentially toxic effects on the brain, lungs and reproductive system have largely limited its use in medicine. Following its acute administration, cannabis has been shown to cause tachycardia, carboxyhaemoglobin and a rise in diastolic blood pressure shortly after the peak drug concentration is reached. In addition, tars from the cannabis smoke are known to be carcinogenic.

THC is metabolized in the liver via the cytochrome P450 oxidase system into 11-hydroxy THC, which is also pharmacologically active; the inactive metabolite is 11-nor-9-carboxyl tetra 9THC. Most of the parent compound and its metabolites, are excreted via the liver and intestines by a process of enterohepatic recirculation.

Over 20 years ago it was reported that smoking cannabis contributed to an increased occurrence of lesions due to the herpes simplex virus. This observation was followed by numerous studies in which the cannabinoids were shown to enhance the susceptibility of rodents and guinea pigs to viral and bacterial infections. There is also anecdotal evidence showing that heavy chronic smokers of cannabis have an increased incidence of neck cancers but it is unclear whether these changes are primarily due to the inhibition of immune function by THC, or due to the carcinogenic content of the smoke or a combination of these processes.

Circumstantial evidence has shown that decreased cellular immunity and reduced immunoglobulin G (IgG) concentrations occur in cannabis smokers. Experimental evidence has shown that THC is able to inhibit both human and rodent NK cell activity, lymphocyte proliferation in response to mitogens and neutrophil activity. In addition, the suppression of splenocyte antibody formation, delay and hypersensitivity responses and interferon synthesis by splenocytes has also been reported following the administration of THC to rodents. However, the precise mechanism whereby these changes occur is unclear. Furthermore, some of the effects of THC on aspects of cellular immunity appear to be restricted to *in vitro* observations and could not be convincingly replicated in *in vivo* studies. One possible reason for the differences between *in vivo* and *in vitro* effects of THC lies in the observation that different serum proteins (alpha, beta, gamma globulins) bind to THC and thereby prevent it reaching toxic levels.

There is more convincing evidence that THC adversely affects the synthesis of immunoglobulins in cannabis users. It is now known that cannabinoid receptors occur in the immune system and are particularly dense in B-lymphocyte enriched areas (for example, the marginal zone of the spleen, cortex of the lymph nodes and the nodular corona of Peyer's patches). This implies that the suppression of B-cell function may be a specific cannabinoid receptor mediated process.

The adverse effect of THC on the activity of macrophages has been known since the early 1970s, when differences in alveolar macrophages were observed between cannabis smokers and non-smokers. *In vitro* studies also demonstrated that alveolar macrophages showed decreased bactericidal activity and reduced superoxide release after THC. Similar changes had been noted *in vitro* regarding the ability of monocytes to phagocytose particles and invading microorganisms. Such observations suggest that THC may alter the functional competence of macrophages by suppressing the expression of macrophage effector molecules. IL-1 and TNF-α secretion is increased following the activation of macrophages and there is evidence that THC can inhibit IL-1 and TNF synthesis by activated macrophages. Experimental evidence suggests that THC reduces TNF production at the translocational step before the TNF precursor is inserted into the cell membrane.

The activation of T cells involves complex signal transduction pathways. THC has been shown to suppress intracellular cAMP accumulation in both human and rodent mononuclear cells and mouse splenic cells. One possibility is that the effect of THC is mediated via an inhibitory G protein. As lymphocytes are known to carry cannabinoid receptors, functional changes caused by THC may be either receptor mediated or receptor independent. To date, it is not known how the cannabinoid receptors are distributed on T, B and other immune cells or how the natural ligand for the cannabinoid receptor, anandamide, may modulate the actions of THC.

In vitro studies have also demonstrated that THC can influence immune function by decreasing the intracellular mobilization of calcium ions from its stores. This may subsequently influence phospholipase A activity and ultimately cellular activation.

While there is considerable evidence supporting the immunosuppressive effects of THC and other pharmacologically active ingredients of cannabis smoke, there is also evidence that in some circumstances THC can stimulate immune cells *in vitro* to release cytokines, arachidonic acid and leucotrienies. These are important components in the initiation and regulation of immune responses. For example, experimental studies *in vitro* have also shown that THC increased the blood concentrations of TNF-α and IL-6 in *Legionella pneumophila* infection.

Another possible mechanism whereby the cannabinoids may enhance immune function under some conditions is provided by the observation that arachidonic acid release is enhanced by THC in a variety of non-lymphoid cells; the lipoxygenase pathway products 12-hydroxyeicosatetraenoic acid (12-HETE) and leucotriene B4 (LTB4) are increased, suggesting that the lipoxygenase rather than the prostaglandin pathway is primarily altered by the drug. This could account for the immune enhancing effect of THC, at least under some conditions and concentrations. These changes in arachidonic acid mobilization may reflect an increase in intracellular calcium originating from intracellular stores. In addition, there is experimental evidence that a low concentration of THC *in vitro* increases tyrosine phosphorylation of intrinsic cellular proteins in macrophages following its immediate addition to the medium but decreases the phosphorylation after prolonged incubation. If this also occurs *in vivo*, it might help to explain the enhancement of immune function that has been reported to occur at low concentrations of THC.

SUMMARY

There is both clinical and experimental evidence to suggest that the cannabinoids, particularly the main pharmacologically active principle THC, are immunosuppressive. Experimental studies also show that, at low concentrations, THC may stimulate some immune cells and enhance cytokine release; high concentrations of THC *in vitro* are immunosuppressive. *In vivo*, the high lipophilicity of THC and related cannabinoids, and the binding of the cannabinoids to serum proteins, complicate the possible adverse effects of these drugs on the immune system. There is evidence that cannabinoid receptors occur in brain and on B cells and macrophages, which could account for the direct immunomodulatory effects of the cannabinoids. A summary of the possible effects of the cannabinoids on the immune system is shown in Figure 14.3.

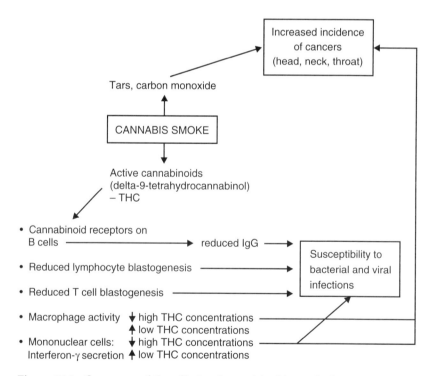

Figure 14.3 Summary of the effects of cannabinoids on the immune system.

THE EFFECTS OF OPIOIDS ON THE IMMUNE SYSTEM

Intravenous drug abusers have long been known to be susceptible to infection, particularly hepatitis B, C, tuberculosis and in recent years AIDS. The extent of the AIDS problem may be illustrated by studies conducted in New York, where it was found that the HIV virus entered the population of opiate addicts as early as 1978 and then increased rapidly, eventually reaching a plateau in 1983–1984 with 50% or more of all untreated heroin addicts becoming infected with HIV. Clearly, because intravenous drug abuse is likely to render an individual susceptible to infection once AIDS has become established, the immune system is further compromised.

In addition to the cannabinoids (which produce their pharmacological effects by activating the cannabinoid receptors on immune cells and other tissues), the opiates such as morphine and heroin also produce their pharmacological effects by acting on specific opioid receptors. These receptors are usually activated by endogenous opioids, namely the endorphins, the enkephalins and the dynorphins. Of the three main classes of opioid receptors (mu, delta and kappa), the pharmacological effects of morphine and heroin are mostly due to their agonist action on the mu receptors.

The endogenous opioid system is involved in normal bodily functions that range from the modulation of pain, the stress response, control of immune function and even the control of reproductive biology. With regard to the stress response, corticotrophin-releasing factor (CRF) releases the endogenous opioid precursor pro-opiomelanocortin (POMC) from the anterior pituitary to yield adrenocorticotrophic hormone (ACTH) and beta-endorphin, which activate the pituitary–adrenal axis and the central opioid system. Following the acute administration of morphine or heroin, the release of ACTH and beta-endorphin is suppressed but following withdrawal from these drugs the HPA axis is activated to cause a marked rise in these hormones.

The effects of the opiates on the immune system are complex. One of the major problems that arises when seeking to relate changes in the immune system to the direct effects of the drugs relates to the effects of opiate withdrawal. Heroin, for example, has a half-life of only one to two hours in humans and with its major active metabolite has a duration of action of about four to six hours. Morphine will act for about this length of time also. With such short-acting drugs, withdrawal effects are common and are expressed by a dramatic rise in pituitary–adrenal function. By contrast, methadone (commonly used in opiate recovery programmes) has a long half-life (approximately one day) and therefore the stress effects of withdrawal on the immune system are less likely. Thus the changes in many aspects of cellular immunity that have been reported to occur in opiate abusers (such as a decrease in NK cell activity) are probably a consequence of an indirect effect of opiate withdrawal and reflect a rise in the activity of the HPA axis.

CHANGES IN THE IMMUNE SYSTEM *IN VIVO*: INDIRECT EFFECTS

Anecdotal reports linking the administration of the opioids morphine and heroin with impaired immune function have been known for several decades. However, until recently it was uncertain whether the immune changes seen in opiate abusers were a consequence of an unhealthy lifestyle or due to the direct immunotoxicity of the drugs.

Experimental evidence, however, has clearly shown that the opiates can act as immodulators in their own right. Thus some twenty years ago it was shown that morphine inhibited *in vitro* antibody formation to sheep red blood cells (SRBCs) in mice. It was later shown that morphine inhibited the ability of human peripheral blood containing mononuclear cells to form rosettes with SRBCs, an effect which is mediated by the cell surface marker CD2. Naloxone, the morphine antagonist, was shown to block this effect of morphine, thereby clearly showing that morphine was producing a direct effect upon the mononuclear cells by stimulating opioid receptors. Further studies showed that opiate abusers also lacked an ability to form rosettes when the lymphocytes were challenged *in vitro* with SRBCs, an effect attributed to a reduction in the number of T cells in the peripheral blood due to a failure to express the antigen that binds to SRBCs. This was reversed by the addition of naloxone to the medium.

One of the major problems that arises in attempting to elucidate the immunomodulatory actions of the opiates in dependent individuals arises from the fact that a substantial proportion of these individuals are multiple drug abusers. Cocaine, for example, was shown to reverse the effect of heroin on T-cell function, whereas alcohol, when used with cocaine and heroin, caused an intermediate effect on T-cell function. Nevertheless, there is evidence that NK cell activity is suppressed in opiate abusers, with a reduction in the CD4+/CD8+ ratio. It is interesting to note that former opiate addicts on methadone maintenance have normal NK cell activity and normal CD4+/CD8+ ratios, whereas heroin-dependent individuals have also been found to have elevated IgA, IgM and IgG concentrations compared to individuals on methadone maintenance. This illustrates the problems of interpreting changes in the immune status of opioid addicts, as such changes could be the result of concurrent infections, poor diet, etc.

It is for this reason that much attention has been given to the action of opioids on the immune function of animals where factors such as the nature, dose and duration of drug treatment, effect of diet and environment etc. can be carefully controlled. In summary, these experimental studies show the following:

- Subchronic morphine administration to rodents causes a suppression of NK cell activity; single injections of morphine had negligible effects.

- The administration of the slow release form of morphine to rodents caused splenic and thymic atrophy, while the splenocytes failed to respond to B- or T-cell mitogens. There was some evidence of the rapid development of tolerance to these immunosuppressive effects of morphine, the immunosuppressive effect being dose dependent.
- In rats, morphine administration was shown to depress the delayed hypersensitivity response following 13 days of morphine administration. The effect on the hypersensitivity response was opioid dependent as an opiate antagonist reversed the effects.
- Increases in the CD4+/CD8+ ratio in both the spleen and thymus have been reported in several species of animal, including the monkey, following the administration of slow release morphine pellets. There is also evidence that morphine may indirectly cause apoptosis of immature thymocytes.
- Macrophage and polymophonuclear leucocyte activities in rodents are suppressed by morphine, an effect that is reversed by naxolone administration. These changes are reflected in the reduced cytokines (IL-2, IL-4 and IFN-γ) in peritoneal macrophages and also suggest that exposure to morphine acutely, or for a few days, can suppress cytokine production by lymphocytes.

CHANGES IN THE IMMUNE SYSTEM: DIRECT EFFECTS

The question now arises whether opiates cause their immunosuppressive action indirectly or directly on cells of the immune system. It is known that the opioids can directly activate the HPA axis and therefore as a consequence of the increase in circulating glucocorticoids suppress cellular immunity. Similarly, a well-established effect of the opioids is to enhance indirectly both peripheral and central sympathetic activity. As has been discussed above (see effects of cocaine on the immune system), enhanced sympathetic activity and increased circulating glucocorticoids can account for the immunosuppressive effects of cocaine and possibly other drugs of abuse.

However, there is experimental evidence to show that morphine, and other opioids, have direct effects on cellular immunity *in vitro*, which suggests that, *in vivo*, the opioids may also have a direct immunosuppressive action. The evidence can be summarized thus:

- Central administration of morphine to rats has been shown to suppress NK cell activity, an effect that is reversed by the opiate antagonist naltrexone. Similar effects have been shown by a mu-receptor selective agonist (DAMGO), whereas selective kappa and delta agonists are ineffective. Thus it would appear that stimulation of the mu receptors is important for the immunosuppressive action of the opioids. However, it must be emphasized that there is also experimental evidence to show that activation of the central sympathetic system, and increased glucocorticoid activity, caused by the opioids can also lead to suppression of NK cell activity.

- Mitogen-stimulated T-cell proliferation is inhibited *in vitro* by morphine; similar changes have been noted following the chronic administration of morphine to mice. It has been shown that splenic lymphocyte proliferative responses are inhibited by morphine, possibly as a result of impaired intracellular calcium mobilization; this effect was glucocorticoid mediated in the CD4+ T lymphocytes, but not in the CD4+, CD8+ splenocytes, and is further evidence that opioids may act through both a glucocorticoid and opioid receptor mediated mechanism. Nevertheless, it would appear that the main mechanism whereby the opioids exert their immunosuppressive effect is through centrally mediated opioid receptors. Activation of nitric oxide synthesis, and the sympathetic system, may also contribute to the immunomodulatory effects of morphine and the mu-receptor activating opioids.

SUMMARY

There is convincing evidence that morphine and related opioids are immunosuppressive. These effects may be mediated by a direct activation of mu-opioid receptors on immune cells. In addition to the direct effects of opioids on immune function, there is also evidence that immunosuppression may occur indirectly through increased HPA activity, sympathetic activity not involving the stimulation of nitric oxide synthase activity leading to increased nitric oxide synthesis. Immunosuppression as a consequence of opiate abuse has major implications with regard to resistance of the individual to infection, including AIDS and tuberculosis, diseases that are disproportionally prevalent in intravenous opiate abusers. Figure 14.4 summarizes the immunosuppressive effects of the mu-type opioids on the immune system.

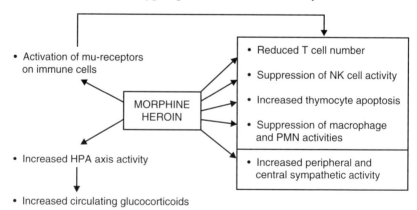

Figure 14.4 Summary of the effect of morphine and related opioids on cellular immunity. (It must be emphasized that most of these changes have been observed in experimental animals. However, circumstantial evidence suggests that these changes are relevant to the action of the opioids in the dependent individual.) NK, natural killer; PMN, polymorphonuclear; HPA, hypothalamic–pituitary–adrenal.

THE EFFECTS OF AMPHETAMINES ON THE IMMUNE SYSTEM

The amphetamines (*d*-amphetamine, methamphetamine) are potent CNS stimulants that also adversely affect the cardiovascular and peripheral nervous system. Their dependence potential is related to the decreased sense of fatigue, mood elevation, euphoria and increase in locomotor activity. Although these stimulant amphetamines were first introduced as anorexians, their abuse potential was soon recognized, which led to them being classified in the USA and most European countries under the Controlled Substance Acts in the 1970s. Their principal clinical use now lies in the control of hyperkinesis in children and in the treatment of narcolepsy. Their pharmacological effects are primarily attributed to an increase in the central release of noradrenaline and dopamine.

In addition to the stimulant amphetamines, this group also contains drugs that primarily release serotonin centrally. Fenfluramine has been used for many years as a non-stimulant anorexiant drug but evidence from rodent studies of its neurotoxicity and occasional cardiotoxicity in clinical studies has resulted in its discontinuation as a therapeutic agent. In addition, two amphetamines that have become widely used as recreational drugs in Europe, methoxydimethylamphetamine (MDMA, "ecstasy") and methoxy-*d*-amphetamine (MDA), have received much attention in recent years because of their potential neurotoxicity following their chronic administration and their acute cardiotoxicity.

Another important drug of abuse that is largely confined to East Africa and the Arab peninsula in countries such as the Yemen and Somalia is khat (or qat). Khat is obtained from the shrub *Catha edulis*, and the active ingredient with stimulant, amphetamine-like properties is the phenylalkylamine cathinone. The leaves are mixed with sodium carbonate or bicarbonate and chewed to extract the active ingredient. Once extracted, cathinone is rapidly converted to cathine and (–) norephedrine, which are much weaker stimulants. The (S)-form of cathinone is the main psychoactive isomer.

Despite the widespread illicit use of the amphetamines for several decades, few studies have been conducted to evaluate the possible adverse effects of these drugs on the immune system. No studies appear to have been conducted on the immunomodulatory effects of khat. The most authoritative text on khat, by Kennedy, suggests that evidence of ill health that is specifically related to long-term use of the drug is very sparse. Of the limited evidence available, an increase in bronchitis and related respiratory illness may be associated with a disturbance of immune function. Clearly, there is a need to survey the effects of all stimulant amphetamine-like drugs for their immunomodulatory effects.

While there is a paucity of data relating to the effects of the stimulant amphetamines on the human immune system, there is experimental evidence from rodent studies that subchronic administration of *d*-amphetamine causes a suppression of T-cell function in the spleen and thymus. Macrophage phagocytosis was also reduced following exposure of mice to *d*-amphetamine. In both these studies, there was a gradual return of the T-cell function to control values by the 20th day of treatment. As has been discussed with respect to cocaine, it is possible that these effects of amphetamine are modulated by an increased peripheral sympathetic activity which returns to control levels due to the development of tolerance when the drug is continually administered.

In vitro studies have also been conducted on the direct effects of the stimulant amphetamines on immune cells. Such studies show that low concentrations (10^{-10}) enhance NK cell activity. Higher concentrations (that could be pharmacologically relevant) of *d*-amphetamine were found to cause a suppression of IL-2 augmented NK cell activity, whereas methamphetamine caused an enhancement of both basal and augmented NK cell activity. Cathinone, *in vitro*, had no effect on either basal or augmented NK cell function. The results of these studies suggest that the stimulant amphetamines probably exert their immunomodulatory effect indirectly by increasing peripheral sympathetic activity.

With regard to the non-stimulant amphetamines such as MDMA, MDA and fenfluramine, there is no clinical data available to indicate whether these drugs have immunomodulatory effects. Preliminary experimental data on MDMA suggests that a high acute dose of the drug does significantly impair T-cell replication. Whether this is due to a direct or indirect effect of the drug is unknown. With the widespread abuse of MDMA and MDA there is clearly a need for extensive clinical and experimental research to evaluate the actions of these drugs on the immune system.

CONCLUSION

It is evident from this brief survey of the actions of the different types of drugs of abuse on the immune system that these effects are complex and vary according to their mode of action at the cellular level. Thus direct immunomodulatory effects on cellular immunity may arise as a result of the drug interacting with specific receptors located on the immune cells (e.g. mu-receptors, cannabinoid receptors), while many of the effects reported are more likely to be due to changes in the activity of the HPA axis and/or the peripheral and central sympathetic systems.

BIBLIOGRAPHY

Carr, D. J. J. and France, C. P. (1993) Immune alterations in morphine treated Rhesus monkeys. *Journal of Pharmacology and Experimental Therapeutics* **267**: 9–21.

Donahoe, R. and Klein, T. W. (1996) Cocaine, alcohol and host defenses. *Journal of Immunology* **69**: 53–62.

Eisenstein, T. K., Hiburger, M. E. and Lawrence, D. M. P. (1996) Immunomodulation by morphine and other opioids. In: Friedman, H., Klein, T. W. and Spector, S. (Eds) *Drug Abuse, Immunity and Infections* pp. 103–120. CRC Press, Boca Raton, FL.

Hall, N. R. S., O'Grady, M. P. and Menzies, R. A. (1991) Neuroimmunopharmacologic effects of drugs of abuse. *Advances in Experimental Medicine and Biology* **288**: 13.

Kennedy, J. G. (1987) *The Flower of Paradise—the Institutionalized Use of the Drug Qat in North Yemen.* D. Reidel, Dordrecht.

Lefkowitz, S. S., Vaz, A. and Kefkowitz, D. L. (1993) Cocaine reduces macrophage killing by inhibition of reactive nitrogen intermediaries. *International Journal of Immunopharmacology* **15**: 717–721.

Pillai, R. M. and Watson, R. R. (1990) *In vitro* immunotoxicology and immunopharmacology: studies of drugs of abuse. *Toxicology Letters* **53**: 269–283.

Szabo, G. (1997) Alcohol's contribution to compromised immunity. *Alcohol Health and Research* **21**: 30–41.

Watson, R. R. (Ed.) (1993) *Alcohol, Drugs of Abuse and Immunomodulation.* Pergamon Press, New York.

Yahya, D. M. and Watson, R. R. (1987) Immunomodulation by morphine and marijuana. *Life Sciences* **41**: 2503–2510.

Zheng, Z-M. and Specter, S. (1996) Marijuana as an immunomodulator. In: Friedman, H., Klein, T. W. and Spector, S. (Eds) *Drugs of Abuse, Immunity and Infections* pp. 59–70. CRC Press, Boca Raton, FL.

15 Sigma Receptors and the Link Between the Immune and Endocrine Axes

INTRODUCTION

Knowledge of the existence of the sigma receptor is closely linked to the unravelling of the complexity of the opiate receptor. Although the therapeutic effects of the natural opiates such as morphine have been known since antiquity, the mechanism whereby morphine produces its pharmacological actions at the cellular level has only been recently discovered. Studies of the actions of various opiate agonists and antagonists greatly assisted in the exploration of the mechanism of action of the opiates. One of the first partial antagonists, nalorphine, was found to combine an analgesic action with marked dysphoric effects, which limited its use as a replacement for morphine. This discovery stimulated the development of more potent analgesics that, hopefully, would not have an abuse potential. Pentazocine resulted from this search but, like nalorphine, was found to cause dose-related dysphoric effects; the dysphoria was associated with hallucinations at high doses.

A major advance in differentiating the hallucinogenic effects of pentazocine and related opioids from their analgesic actions came with the studies of the benzomorphan derivative N-allyl normetazocine (NANM, also known as SKF-10047) in dogs, where it was shown that NANM caused a characteristic delirium that was somewhat similar to the hallucinations seen in humans. Studies on the enantiomers of NANM showed that the (–) form had a high affinity for the mu and kappa opioid receptors whereas the (+) enantiomer had an affinity for the same receptor complex that was occupied by the hallucinogen phencyclidine (PCP). Subsequently it was shown that NANM not only had an affinity for the same receptors as PCP but, additionally, had a high affinity for a unique non-opiate, non-PCP, non-dopamine receptor subsequently called the sigma receptor. However, the use of non-selective ligands to characterize sigma receptors ultimately resulted in over a decade of confusing and conflicting data which impeded progress in understanding its importance.

Recently, progress has been made with the discovery of novel ligands which have a high affinity and selectivity for sigma receptors. As a result, the pharmacological properties of sigma ligands have helped to delineate their function in the dystonias, their neuroprotective mechanisms and possibly importance in depression and psychoses. In addition, the affinities of the selective sigma ligands have enabled the receptors to be differentiated into two main types (sigma 1 and sigma 2) that are differentially distributed in the brain and non-nervous tissues. These receptors have now been cloned.

It would appear that the sigma receptors are unique with respect to the very diverse range of naturally occurring compounds that have affinity for them. These compounds range from neuropeptides such as neuropeptide Y (NPY) and peptide YY (PYY), and steroids such as progesterone, testosterone and corticosterone. In addition, a varied group of drugs also show affinity for the sigma receptors. These include some neuroleptics (for example, haloperidol and remoxipride), cytochrome P450 inhibitors such as lobeline, some antidepressants such as sertraline and clorgyline and some antihistamines. However, direct affinity for the sigma receptors is not a common feature of most of these drugs in the therapeutic group.

With regard to their subcellular distribution, unlike the conventional neurotransmitter receptors the sigma receptors are largely associated with the microsomal fraction of neurons and are particularly enriched in the plasma membranes.

The sigma receptors were originally described in the brain, and further identified in various endocrine organs, the gastrointestinal tract, liver and kidney. More recently, sigma receptors have been detected on mouse lymphocytes, rat splenocytes and human mononuclear cells. The location of these receptors in brain, endocrine and immune cells therefore raises the possibility that the sigma receptors could play a role in the integration of neurotransmitter, endocrine and immune systems. This possibility will now be considered.

EFFECTS OF SIGMA LIGANDS ON CELLULAR AND NON-CELLULAR IMMUNITY

In vitro studies on T lymphocytes and splenocytes from mice show that the sigma ligands (+) pentazocine, haloperidol and di-*o*-tolyguanidine (DTG) all regulate mitogen-induced lymphocyte proliferation. The suppressive effect elicited by most of these drugs on concanavalin A (Con A) stimulated lymphocyte proliferation only at high concentrations (10^{-5} M) which far exceed the relevant pharmacological concentrations of these drugs. In some experiments, however, pharmacologically relevant concentrations of (+) pentazocine (10^{-8} M) were found to suppress lymphocyte proliferation; the (−) isomer of pentazocine, which has a low affinity for sigma receptors, was shown to be inactive. In addition, (+) pentazocine was shown to suppress the release if IL-2 and IL-4 by Con A stimulated lymphocytes at concentrations of 10^{-6} and 10^{-8} M. These results suggest that the suppression of mitogen-stimulated lymphocyte activity by sigma ligands such as haloperidol, phencyclidine and DTG may occur by a receptor independent mechanism. There is evidence that both haloperidol and (–) pentazocine enhance lipopolysaccharide (LPS) induced lymphocyte proliferation in pharmacologically relevant concentrations (10^{-7}–10^{-9} M), which further suggests that these drugs may operate through different receptors to (+) pentazocine. The enantiomers of pentazocine also differ in their effects on interleukin-4 (IL-4) release from LPS-stimulated lymphocytes. Thus (–) pentazocine potentiates IL-4 release while (+) pentazocine was without effect.

Other studies have shown that (+) pentazocine enhances antigen-specific antibody production by splenic lymphocytes to the stimulatory effects of sheep red blood cells and LPS *in vivo*. This suggests that (+) pentazocine may regulate the humoral immune response, a view supported by the observations that (+) and especially (–) pentazocine affects lymphocyte responses to the B-cell mitogens at low concentrations, whereas these enantiomers modulate Con-A-induced lymphocyte responses only at high (10^{-5} M) concentrations. The results of such studies suggest that multiple receptors exist on immune cells that are differentially affected by sigma ligands. These include the sigma 1 and 2, kappa opioid and possibly dopamine receptors.

There is now evidence that both the sigma 1 and 2 receptors on immune cells exhibit a high affinity for haloperidol and DTG whereas (+) pentazocine has a high affinity for the type 1 sigma receptor. Thus LPS induced IgM synthesis, which is enhanced by haloperidol and DTG but not by (+) pentazocine, would appear to involve an activation of sigma 2 receptors. However, the ability of haloperidol, DTG and both (+) and (–) pentazocine to enhance pokaweed mitogen-induced IgM synthesis at different concentrations suggests that both sigma 1 and 2 receptors are active. In addition, dopamine (specifically D2) and kappa opioid receptors (responsive to pentazocine) could also contribute to the effects of these drugs on immunoglobulin synthesis.

A better understanding of the effects of sigma ligands on the immune system has been provided by the synthesis of highly specific compounds which have no direct action on dopamine and *N*-methyl-D-aspartate receptors that often complicate the interpretation of the results obtained from earlier studies with non-selective sigma ligands. The cyclohexylamine derivative SR 31747 has been shown to bind with a high affinity to both sigma 1 and 2 receptors human and rat lymphocytes. *In vitro* studies show that SR 31747 inhibits the proliferative response to mitogens on mouse and human lymphocytes while, *in vivo*, the compound has been shown to prevent delayed-type hypersensitivity granuloma formation.

Studies on the distribution of sigma receptors on immune cells show that SR 31947 specifically binds with a high affinity to macrophages. As these cells produce proinflammatory cytokines following activation, it is not surprising to find that *in vivo* the compound suppresses LPS-induced release of IL-1, IL-6 and tumour necrosis factor alpha (TNF-α) in a dose-dependent manner. These effects were not observed *in vitro*, which suggest that the changes induced by SR 31747 are indirect, possibly involving the elevation of glucocorticoids. This has been substantiated by a study in which the steroid receptor antagonist mifepristane blocked the effects of SR 31747 on cytokine release. Furthermore, adrenalectomy was also found to block the effects of the compound on the immune system. Thus it would appear that the sigma 1 and 2 receptors on macrophages indirectly modulate immune function by elevating glucocorticoid secretion after stimulating ACTH release. This effect could be attributable to the stimulation of sigma receptors in both the hypothalamus and anterior pituitary gland. In addition, steroid receptors have also been located in the adrenal cortex and therefore the immunosuppressive effect of this sigma 1 and 2 receptor ligand is probably due to a direct, and indirect, increased release of glucocorticoids.

An increased synthesis and release of IL-1, IL-6 and TNF-α has been detected in such autoimmune diseases as psoriasis, systemic lupus erythematosus, multiple sclerosis, multiple myeloma and rheumatoid arthritis. These cytokines are believed to act additively or synergistically to induce the persistence of the inflammatory processes. Selective sigma ligands such as SR 31747 may therefore have an important role to play in the treatment of autoimmune diseases and the subsequent inflammatory responses that are involved.

Another mechanism whereby sigma ligands could protect against the harmful effects of proinflammatory cytokines involves an elevation of the anti-inflammatory cytokine IL-10. SR 31747 was shown to protect mice against the toxicity of staphylococcal enterotoxin B infection, an effect which has been ascribed to the enhanced synthesis and release of IL-10 and an inhibition of the release of IL-2, IL-4, IL-6, TNF and granulocyte-macrophage colony-stimulating factor (GM-CSF). In addition, T cells appear to play a role in the action of SR 31743. Thus T-cell activation by *Staphylococcus* requires T-cell receptor and CD28 costimulatory signals delivered by the antigen-presenting cell. Thus the inhibition of T-cell proliferation by the compound may result from an effect on an antigen-presenting cell or indirectly by elevating the release of glucocorticoids.

The anti-inflammatory cytokine IL-10 is synthesized by various immune cells including CD4+ cells, monocytes, B cells and T cells. As SR 31747 raises IL-10 concentrations in nude mice that lack T cells, it would appear that CD4+, monocytes and/or B cells are responsible.

EFFECTS OF SIGMA LIGANDS ON BEHAVIOUR AND ENDOCRINE CHANGES

While there has been considerable interest shown in the action of sigma receptor ligands on the immune system, few studies have been concerned with the concurrent effects of such ligands on the behaviour, immune and endocrine systems in an attempt to elucidate the interrelationship between the changes induced in these systems by sigma ligands. The selective sigma ligand igmesine (JO-1784) has been investigated for its effects on these systems following the observation that it suppresses stress-induced colonic motor disturbances and reverses corticotrophin-releasing factor (CRF)-induced inhibition of gastric acid secretion in the rat. This suggests that igmesine may have an anti-stress property, an effect which was confirmed by the observation that it antagonized the anxiogenic effect of CRF in rats placed on the elevated plus maze or in the brightly lit "open field" apparatus. Despite the anti-stress effects of igmesine as shown by the behavioural antagonism of CRF, it did not attenuate the changes in brain amine transmitters (as shown by a slight increase in the turnover of noradrenaline and a greater increase in the turnover of serotonin and dopamine in the hypothalamus). Also igmesine did not attenuate the increase in corticosterone caused by the intracerebral injection of CRF, even though it did reverse the reduction in mitogen-induced proliferation of lymphocytes caused by CRF. Furthermore, igmesine did not reverse the changes in lymphocyte and neutrophil numbers caused by the peptide. Thus the specific sigma ligand igmesine antagonizes some of the effects of centrally administered CRF on behaviour and the immune system which suggests that it may have anti-stress properties. However, unlike SR 31743, it does not apparently activate the pituitary–adrenal axis or significantly reverse corticosterone-induced elevation by CRF and therefore the reversal of the effects of CRF on mitogen-induced lymphocyte proliferation may be a consequence of the direct action of the drug as the lymphocyte sigma receptors.

It must be emphasized that all the studies so far published on the effects of sigma ligands on the immune and endocrine systems are based on experimental data. So far, none of the specific sigma ligands have been subject to extensive clinical use although several such drugs (such as rimicazole BMY-14803 and remoxipride) were assessed for their antipsychotic activity and igmesine is currently undergoing extensive clinical trials for the treatment of depression. It therefore remains to be seen if the selective sigma ligands will be useful for the treatment of stress-related disorders including autoimmune disease, where the increase in proinflammatory cytokines appears to play a crucial role.

MODULATION OF SIGMA RECEPTORS ON IMMUNE CELLS BY NEUROPEPTIDE Y (NPY) AND STEROIDS

Steroid use is known to cause psychiatric disturbances and immunosuppression. The routine use of high doses (10–100 times the usual clinical dose) of steroids results in depression, paranoia, euphoria, irritability, hyperactivity, and visual and auditory hallucinations. The precise cause of these psychiatric symptoms is largely unknown but the fact that hallucinogenic opioids produce some of the symptoms that simulate those caused by steroids suggests that the sigma receptors may be involved. There is *in vitro* evidence to show that of some 40 steroids tested, only progesterone, testosterone, deoxycorticosterone, 11-beta-hydroxyprogesterone, pregenalone and corticosterone had affinity for brain sigma receptors. In addition, the relative potencies of these steroids for the sigma receptor sites in the spleen were similar to those in the brain. This raises the interesting question whether steroids modulate the immune system at least partly by a direct action on sigma receptors.

This view is supported by experimental studies showing that steroids could displace 3H-NANM from sigma sites on immune cells. It is of interest to note that progesterone, deoxycorticosterone and corticosterone are effective anti-inflammatory agents and prevent granuloma formation, whereas steroids such as the oestrogens, pregnenolone and hydrocortisone were inactive both at sigma receptors and as anti-inflammatory agents. Testosterone would appear to be the exception to this rule because although it is a potent ligand for sigma receptors it does not have an anti-inflammatory action. Nevertheless, such observations may help to explain the complicated changes in the immune, endocrine and neurotransmitter systems caused by anti-inflammatory steroids.

Besides some steroids, other endogenous candidates for the sigma receptors include some peptide-like compounds from brain called sigmaphins, the identity of which is unknown. Of the neuropeptides that have been investigated, NPY and PYY, though lacking in affinity for sigma receptors, do modulate the functional activity of sigma receptors in the gastrointestinal tract and possibly the hippocampus. Zinc has also been shown to competitively displace some selective sigma ligands from hippocampal slices. However, of these putative endogenous ligands, only NPY has been investigated for its affects on endocrine and immune functions. Thus both NPY and igmesine were found to reduce neutrophil phagocytosis and decrease mitogen-stimulated lymphocyte proliferation *in vitro*. However, differences between those agents occurred when they were administered centrally to rats. Thus the selective sigma ligand igmesine significantly reduced neutrophil phagocytosis but enhanced lymphocyte proliferation without affecting the corticosterone concentration, while NPY, although it reduced lymphocyte proliferation, raised the corticosterone concentration. These results suggest that whereas sigma ligands such as igmesine exert their immunomodulatory effects on the immune and endocrine system directly through actions on the pituitary gland and immune organs, NPY may act indirectly on the immune system by activating the sympathetic system which innervates the lymphoid tissue. These differences in the sites of action may be responsible for experimental changes observed and add to the view that it is unlikely that NPY is an endogenous ligand for sigma receptors.

SUMMARY

There is substantial experimental evidence to show that sigma 1 and 2 receptors occur on many types of immune cells and may play an important role in the immunomodulatory action of many psychotropic drugs (Figure 15.1). So far, there are few clinical studies in which the effects of selective sigma ligands on the immune and endocrine systems have been assessed. However, there are a reasonable number of experimental studies showing the immunomodulatory effects of sigma ligands on sigma receptors (for example, mitogen-stimulated lymphocyte proliferation). An increase in IL-10 secretion occurs independently of changes in circulating glucocorticoids, whereas other immune changes (such as the proinflammatory cytokines) probably reflect an increase in glucocorticoid release that may modulate immune function via the steroid receptors. Clearly the role of

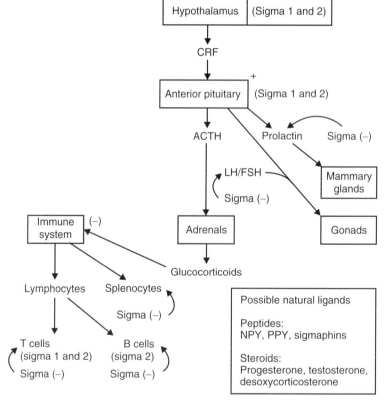

Figure 15.1   Relationship between the HPA axis and sigma receptors. Activation of sigma receptors leads to inhibition (–) of the immune system. CRF, corticotrophin-releasing factor; LH, luteinizing hormone; FSH, follicle-stimulating hormone; NPY, neuropeptide Y; PYY, peptide YY.

sigma receptors in modulating immune changes that occur following exposure to stress, in anxiety or affective disorders requires further attention. In addition, there is an urgent need not only to assess the therapeutic efficacy of some of the recently developed specific sigma ligands, but also to evaluate their effects on immune and endocrine function.

BIBLIOGRAPHY

Carr, D. J. J., Mayo, S., Woolley, T. W. and De Costa, B. R. (1992) Immunoregulatory properties of (–) pentazocine and sigma ligands. *Immunology* **77**: 525–531.

Derocq, J.-M., Bourrie, B., Segui, M., Le Fur, G. and Casellas, P. (1995) In vivo inhibition of endotoxin-induced pro-inflammatory cytokines production by the sigma ligand SR 31747. *Journal of Pharmacology and Experimental Therapeutics* **272**: 224–230.

Gudelsky, G. A. and Nash, J. F. (1992) Neuroendocrinological and neurochemical effects of sigma ligands. *Neuropharmacology* **31**: 157–162.

Junien, J. L., Gue, M. and Bueno, L. (1991) Neuropeptide Y and sigma ligand (JO 1784) act through a Gi protein to block the psychological stress and corticotrophic-releasing factor induced colonic motor activity in rats. *Neuropharmacology* **30**: 101–110.

Leonard, B. E. (1998) The potential contribution of sigma receptors to antidepressant action. In: Skolnick, P. (Ed,) *Antidepressants: New Pharmacological Strategies*, pp. 159–172. Humana Press, Totowa, NJ.

Martin, W. R., Eades, C. G., Thompson, J. A., Huppler, R. E. and Githert, P. E. (1976) The effects of morphine and nalorphine-like drugs in the non-dependent and morphine dependent chronic spinal dog. *Journal of Pharmacology and Experimental Therapeutics* **197**: 517–532.

Roman, F. Pascard, X. Duffy, O., Vanche, D., Martin, B. and Junien, J. L. (1990) JO 1784: a potent and selective ligand for rat and mouse brain sigma sites. *Journal of Pharmacy and Pharmacology* **42**: 439–440.

Song, C. and Leonard, B. E. (1998) Comparison between the effects of the sigma receptor ligand JO 1784 and neuropeptide Y on immune functions. *European Journal of Pharmacology* **345**: 79–87.

Song, C., Earley, B. and Leonard, B. E. (1997) Effect of chronic pre-treatment with the sigma ligand JO 1784 on CRF-induced changes in behaviour, neurotransmitter and immunological function in the rat. *Neuropsychobiology* **35**: 200–204.

Strausbaugh, H. and Irwin, M. (1992) Central corticotrophin releasing hormone reduces cellular immunity. *Brain, Behavior, and Immunity* **6**: 11–17.

Su, T.-P. (1993) Pharmacological characterization of sigma receptors. *NIDA Research Monographs* **133**: 41–53.

Su, T.-P., London, E. D. and Jaffe, J. H. (1988) Steroid binding at sigma receptors suggests a link between endocrine, nervous and immune systems. *Science* **240**: 219–221.

Wolfe, S. A., Kulsakdinum, C., Battaglia, C., Jaffe, J. H. and De Souza, E. B. (1988) Initial identification and characterization of sigma receptors on human peripheral blood leucocytes. *Journal of Pharmacology and Experimental Therapeutics* **247**: 1114–1119.

Appendix 1 Summary of the Characteristics of Cytokines (Monokines) and Lymphokines

	No. of amino acid units	Cell sources	Functions	Associated pathological disorders	Therapeutic uses
IL-1-alpha, beta	159 (α), 153 (β)	Monocytes Lymphocytes Keratinocytes Endothelia Microglia Chrondrocytes	Cytokine induction in many different cell types Haematopoiesis Co-stimulate T cells Activate endothelium Neuroendocrine activation Acute phase protein response Pyrogenic	Inflammation Sepsis Diabetes Autoimmune disease Osteoporosis	None?
IL-2	133	Activated T cells	Stimulates T-cell function, differentiation etc. Stimulates thymocyte proliferation Stimulates B-cell proliferation Stimulates Ig secretion Stimulates growth and proliferations of monocytes and oligodendrocytes	Adult T-cell leukaemia and lymphoma Decline in immune response with age	Treatment of cancers and AIDS Use in bone marrow transplantation Anti IL-2 or IL-2R therapy used for immunosuppression
IL-3	133	Activated T, NK and mast cells Human thymic epithelial cells	Supports proliferation of differentiation of myeloid cells Prevents apoptosis Induces MHC class II and the adhesion molecule LFAI in macrophages	Myelodysplastic syndrome (MPS)	Support of haematopoiesis Patients with bone marrow failure

(Continued over)

	No. of amino acid units	Cell sources	Functions	Associated pathological disorders	Therapeutic uses
IL-4	129	T cells Mast cells Eosinophils Basophils	B-cell proliferation B-cell differentiation T-cell proliferation Activation of monocytes Mast cell proliferation	Asthma Dermatitis Multiple sclerosis Allergy Inflammatory bowel disease	Anti-tumour agents Immune stimulator
IL-5	115	T cells Mast cells Eosinophils	Eosinophil growth and differentiation Eosinophil chemotaxis Eosinophil activation Basophil activation	Eosinophil Asthma Allergy Dermatitis Biliary cirrhosis	? None
IL-6	186	Monocytes/ macrophages Fibroblasts T lymphocytes Endothelial cells Chrondrocytes Astrocytes and microglia Mast cells	Stimulates B-cell antibody production Stimulates T-cell growth Stimulates heamatopoiesis Stimulates liver acute phase proteins	Multiple myeloma Rheumatoid arthritis Systemic lupus erythematosus Trauma Bacterial infection	Potential anti-tumour activity Potential platelet stimulator
IL-7	152	Bone marrow stromal cells Foetal liver cells Thymic stroma Thymic epithelia Keratinocytes	Pre/pro B-cell proliferation Pre/pro B-cell differentiation T-cell proliferation NK cell activity Monocyte cytokine secretion	Juvenile arthritis T-cell lymphoma B-cell leukaemia Hodgkin's disease	Lymphopoiesis post bone marrow transplantation

IL-8	72-77	Monocytes–macrophages Lymphocytes Endothelial cells Epithelial cells Fibroblasts Keratinocytes Synovial cells	Neutrophil chemotaxis/activation T-cell chemotaxis Keratinocyte mitogenesis/chemotoxis Angiogenesis	Rheumatoid arthritis Ulcerative colitis Cystic fibrosis Alcohol hepatitis Psoriasis	? None
IL-9	126	T cells	Erythroid and myeloid growth and differentiation T-cell activation B-cell activation Mast cell and neuron differentiation (in mice!)	Hodgkin's disease Some leukaemias	? None
IL-10	160	Monocytes T cells B cells Epithelial cells Melanoma Tumour cells	Inhibition of proinflammatory cytokines by monocytes, mast cells etc. Inhibition of IL-2 by T cells Inhibition of MHC class II Inhibition of NO synthesis by monoctyes/macrophages Mast cell growth factor	Systemic lupus erythematosus Leishmaniasis Inflammatory bowel disease	Prevention of graft vessel heart disease Anti-inflammatory and immunosuppressant Autoimmune diseases

(Continued over)

	No. of amino acid units	Cell sources	Functions	Associated pathological disorders	Therapeutic uses
IL-11	178	Bone marrow stromal fibroblasts Lung fibroblasts Trophoblasts Osteosarcoma cells Articular chondrocytes Synoviocytes	Synergistic stem and progenitor cell growth factor Acute phase protein inducer Inhibitor of adipocyte differentiation Inducer of neuronal differentiation Stimulates osteoclast development	None known	Treatment of septic shock Accelerates platelet recovery in myelosuppressed patients
IL-12	? (197-306)	Monocytes B lymphocytes	Stimulates proliferation of T and NK cells Enhances lytic activity of NK cells Induces cytotoxic T-lymphocyte responses to tumour cells Increases IFN-γ synthesis by T and NK cells Promotes development of Th1 over Th2 cells Inhibits IgE synthesis Enhances haematopoietic stem cell proliferation Regulates number of cell surface markers	Endotoxin-induced shock Autoimmune encephalomyelitis Insulin-dependent diabetes Rheumatoid arthritis	Treatment of infectious diseases and opportunistic infections Vaccine adjuvant Anti-tumour agent

IL-13	112	Activated T cell Mast cells B cells	B-cell growth and differentiation IgE switch factor Anti-inflammatory activity on monocytes and macrophages Increases ICAM-I on most cells Stimulates chemotoxis	Nephrotic syndrome	Anti-inflammatory agent Anti-tumour activity
IL-14	483	T cells B lymphoma	Proliferation of activated B cells Inhibits immunoglobulin secretion	Non-Hodgkin lymphoma B-cell lymphoma	? None
IL-15	114	PBMCs Monocytes Placental tissue Skeletal tissue	Stimulation of activated T, B, NK cells Induction of differentiation of CD34+ to NK cells Chemoattraction of T cells	? None	Immunotherapy in cancer patients In rheumatoid arthritis as T-cell attractant Anti-tumour therapy
IL-16	? 130	CD8+ T cells Eosinophils Epithelial cells	Chemotaxis CD4+ cells Competence factor for CD4+ T cells Induce eosinophil adhesion	Asthma Sarcoidosis Inflammation	Anti HIV

(Continued over)

	No. of amino acid units	Cell sources	Functions	Associated pathological disorders	Therapeutic uses
IL-17	?	Activated CD4+ memory T cells Activated CD8+ T cells?	Activates on transcription factor FkB Induces IL-6 and IL-8 by fibroblasts Induces secretion of GM-CSF by fibroblasts Induces secretion of PGE2 by fibroblasts Co-stimulates activated T-cell proliferation	? None	? None
IL-18	193	Monocytes Macrophages Epithelial cells	Activates NK cells Enhances IFN-γ, GM-CSF, IL-2 synthesis by activated T cells Inhibits IL-10 synthesis by activated T cells	Possibly inflammatory disorder	Possibly anti-tumour or anti-microbial
GM-CSF	144	T cells Macrophages Endothelial cells Fibroblasts B cells	Inhibits apoptosis Proliferation Differentiation into granulocytic and macrophage lineages	Inflammatory mediator Some eosinophilic states	Mobilization of peripheral blood-stem cells Stimulation of myelopoiesis Use in fungal infections
TNF	233	Macrophages T cells Many other cells	Cytotoxic for tumour cells Antiviral activity etc. Growth stimulation Immune modulation Proinflammatory	Cachexia Cerebral malaria Multiple sclerosis Rheumatoid arthritis Crohn's disease	Cancer

Lymphotoxins	205 (alpha), 244 (beta)	T cells B cells	Lymphoid organogenesis Immune reponse regulation Cytotoxic for tumour cells	? None	? None
IFN-α, β	189	Leucocytes Fibroblasts Epithelial cells Endothelial cells	Anti-viral Anti-tumour NK cell enhanced cytoxicity MHC antigen	Various autoimmune disorders, e.g. SLE AIDS Graft host rejection	Hepatitus B, C MS (IFN-β) Genital warts AIDS-related Kaposi's saracoma Polycythaemia
IFN-γ	166	Monocytes and macrophages Dendritic cells T cells NK cells	MHC class II expression Macrophage activation NK cell and T-cell activation Ig isotype regulation Anti-viral anti-bacterial	Autoimmunity	Infections with *Leishmania* and *Toxoplasma*

Data abridged from *Cytokines* (1998), edited by A. Mire-Sluis and R. Thorpe; Academic Press, New York.

Appendix 2 Glossary

Activation of T cells or B cells: A sequence of events that results when a T or B cell is stimulated by antigen. The cells then proliferate and differentiate into cells that eliminate the stimulating antigen.

Acute phase proteins: These include alpha-l-antichymotrypsin, alpha-l-antitrypsin, haptoglobin, alpha-l-acid glycoprotein, coeruloplasmin, albumin and transferrin. Depressed patients have reduced concentrations of negative acute phase proteins (albumin and transferrin) and elevated positive acute proteins (antichymotrypsin), antitrypsin, acid glycoprotein, heptoglobin and coeruloplasmin).

Agranulocytosis: White blood cell count < 2000 cells/mm^3, a polymorph count < 500 cells/mm^3 and relative lymphopenia. The eythrocyte and platelet counts are usually normal. The two basic catogories of drug-induced agranulocytosis are immunological and toxicological. In the first type (allergic reaction), the drug triggers the development of an antibody against the antigen on the granulocytes or their bone marrow precursors. In the second type, the drug kills the precursor cells, resulting in the depletion of the bone marrow.

Allotype: Genetically determined differences in antigens that are directed by their antigenic properties.

Alpha-l-acid glycoprotein: See Acute phase proteins.

Amyotrophic lateral sclerosis (ALS): Adult onset paralytic disorder caused by the degeneration of large motor neurons of the brain and spinal cord. It causes generalized and progressive wasting and weakness of skeletal muscles and usually results in death from respiratory complications within five years. Autoimmunity has been proposed as a possible cause.

Antibody: A protein that is produced in response to, and interacts with, an antigen. B cells produce antibodies, also known as immunoglobulins (Igs) of different classes designated IgF, IgM, IgA, IgD and IgE.

Antigen: Any substance that is recognized by B or T cells and that stimulates these cells to mount an immune response.

Autoimmune reactions: Immune responses directed against the body's own cells and tissues. These reactions can result in autoimmune diseases such as rheumatoid arthritis and insulin-dependent diabetes mellitus.

Basophil: A white blood cell containing secretory granules. The secretory granules contain local hormones (e.g. histamine) that are released in response to tissue injury and contribute to an inflammatory response.

B cells or B lymphocytes: White blood cells originating in the bone marrow (hence B cells) and distributed throughout the blood and lymphoid organs. B cells produce antibodies when stimulated by antigens.

CD4 cells: T-helper lymphocyte, a subset of lymphocytes identified by their differential functions and specific cell surface markers. A decline in CD4 cells predicts the development of AIDS in HIV seropositive individuals.

Cell-mediated immunity: Immune protection provided by the direct action of immune cells as opposed to protection provided by circulating antibodies which provide humoral immunity.

Chronic fatigue syndrome: A symptom complex of extreme fatigue in combination with signs of impaired immune function (e.g fever and lymphadenopathy). The onset is often associated with the aftermath of an acute viral infection (post-viral fatigue syndrome).

Complement: Group of blood proteins that are activated by antibodies that are bound to antigens or by complex carbohydrate molecules found on the surface of some bacteria. These reactions result in the attraction of phacogytes to an infection site, the release of cytokines that amplify the immune response and the direct lysis of invading bacterial cells.

Cytokines: These complex proteins regulate cellular interactions and functions. Cytokines are produced and secreted by a variety of cell types throughout the body including the brain where microglia and astrocytes form part of the immune system. Cytokines that control functions of the immune system are referred to as interleukins (ILs). The cytokines also activate the hypothalamic–pituitary–adrenal (HPA) axis, which suggests that changes in endocrine function that occur during immune activation may be partly modulated by the interleukins. Cytokines contribute to cell growth and differentiation.

Cytotoxic T cell: See T lymphocyte.

Delayed-type hypersensitivity T cell: See T lymphocyte.

Dendritic cell: A cell with long thread-like projections found in lymph nodes, spleen and the blood. Dendritic cells present antigens in association with major histocompatibility complex (MHC) proteins to T cells.

Differentiation: A developmental process by which cells become increasingly specialized, involving the acquisition of new characteristics and new functions.

Drug allergy: Adverse reactions evoked by drugs or toxins that activate the immune system in undesirable ways. The changes may include skin eruptions, oedema, anaphylactoid reactions, fever and eosinophilia. The major types of hypersensitivity are: type I: IgE mediated allergic reactions including anaphylaxis and urticaria; type II: autoimmune syndromes such as thrombocytopenia and agranulocytosis, type III; serum sickness; and type IV: cell-mediated allergy such as contact dermatitis from topically applied drugs.

Effector cell: A T or B cell that has been stimulated by an antigen and, as a consequence of activation, eliminates the antigen.

Epitope: Portion of a protein molecule that elicits an antibody response. Any protein contains many epitopes. Monoclonal antibodies can be produced that will recognize only a specific epitope on a protein. Thus alterations of an epitope can lead to an altered antigenicity to a monoclonal antibody.

Granulocyte-macrophage colony-stimulating factor (GM-CSF): Glycoprotein that stimulates proliferation of precursor cells in bone marrow. Produced by T lymphocytes, endothelial cells, fibroblasts and keratinocytes. GM-CSF regulates granulopoiesis. Specific receptor located on neutrophils and eosinophils, monocytes and leukaemoblasts. May be used in the treatment of drug-induced agranulocytosis.

Guillain–Barré syndrome: Acute idiopathic polyneuritis characterized by muscle weakness and paraesthesia.

Helper T cell: (See T lymphocyte).

Human granulocyte colony-stimulating factor (G-CSF): Haematopoietic glycoprotein that promotes proliferation of neutrophils. Has been used to treat neutropenia.

Human leucocyte antigens (HLAs): Polypeptide chains on surface of all nucleated cell surfaces whose expression is controlled by the individual's HLA genotype. Each individual has a total of eight alleles at these loci, allowing considerable polymorphism. There are five components of the human major histocompatibility complex (MHC): A, B, C, D and DR. These are potent antigens and act as targets for cytotoxic T cells.

Humoral immunity: Immune protection provided by antibodies that circulate in the blood and lymph as opposed to protection provided by the direct actions of the immune cells (i.e. cellular immunity).

Hypersensitivity: Components of the immune system overreact or respond in an inappropriate manner causing tissue damage. Criteria for determining hypersensitivity reactions include: (a) only occurs in a small proportion of exposed individuals; (b) there is a latent period between exposure and the immune reaction; (c) occurs with small doses of the antigen; (d) is associated with other known hypersensitivity phenomena (e.g. eosinophilia).

Immunoassay: Laboratory test that uses specific antibodies as reagents to interact with antigens (e.g. a drug). These assays are about 100 times more sensitive than thin-layer chromoatography.

Immunoblot: See Western blotting.

Immunocompetence: Property of T and B cells that have acquired the ability to recognize antigens via antigen-specific receptors. Term also used to describe the status of the immune systems (i.e whether functioning normally or not).

Immunodeficiency disease: Disease in which congenital or acquired defects in one or more components of the immune system (e.g. T- or B-cell function) reduce the effectiveness in protecting the organism against pathogens.

Immunoglobulins: Any class of structurally related proteins with antibody activity (IgA, IgM etc.).

Inflammatory responses: Redness, swelling and pain produced in response to tissue injury or infection as a result of increased blood flow and an influx of white blood cells and inflammatory mediators into the affected site.

Interferons: A group of proteins (lymphokines) that increase the resistance of cells to viral infections. They also augment the activity of NK cells, cytotoxic T cells and macrophages.

Interleukins (ILs): Lymphokines, or cytokines, that regulate immune cell growth, maturation and function. Eighteen different types of interleukins have been identified so far (see Appendix 1).

Leucocyte: General term for any type of white blood cell (i.e. lymphocytes, monocytes, neutrophils, basophils).

Lymphocyte: Immune cell genetically programmed to recognize specific antigens that bind to the lymphocyte and stimulate the development of more lymphocytes that react with the antigens. The two main lymphocyte subpopulations are T and B cells.

Lymphocyte mitogen stimulation: *In vitro* test of immune function that determines the proliferative response to a variety of stimulants (mitogens). This test is used to determine the effects of stress on cell-mediated immunity.

Lymphoid organs: These include the bone marrow, spleen, thymus, lymph nodes, tonsils and other clusters of lymphocyte-containing tissues.

Lymphokine: General term applied to all non-antibody immune messengers (e.g. interleukins, interferons) secreted by lymphocytes and which play a major role in regulating immune reactions.

Lysis: Disintegration of bacteria or of infected, cancerous or foreign cells by complement proteins or lysozymes.

Lysosome: A membrane-bound intracellular vesicle containing enzymes that digest bacteria, protein and some carbohydrates.

Lysozyme: An enzyme found in the saliva, sweat and tears, and within the lysomes of macrophages and neutrophils, that destroys the bacterial cell walls.

Macrophage: Any class of immune cells capable of engulfing and digesting foreign or toxic matter within tissues. Macrophages secret cytokines that function on immune cell activation. Besides their phagocytic properties, macrophages synthesize complement proteins. Macrophages also process and present antigens to T cells.

Major histocompatibility complex (MHC) proteins: Cell surface proteins coded by genes located in three regions of chromosome 6 in humans. Class I and II MHC proteins are integral to T-cell immune responses: a T cell will respond to an antigen only if it is presented in association with a MHC protein on the surface of another cell.

Mast cell: A cell found in connective tissue that contains intracellular particles or granules. These granules contain local hormones (such as histamine) that are released in response to tissue injury and thereby contribute to the inflammatory response.

Memory cell: A T or B lymphocyte that has developed as part of a primary immune response to a specific antigen, into a cell with a prolonged life that retains a memory of the stimulating antigen and circulates continuously between the blood and lymphoid organs. Upon re-exposure to that antigen, memory cells provide a secondary response that is more rapid and efficient than the primary response to the antigen.

Mitogen: A chemical derived from bacteria or plants (e.g. pokeweed) used to stimulate B- or T-lymphocyte proliferation *in vitro*. Different mitogens stimulate different subpopulations of lymphocytes.

Monocyte: A phagocyte that originates from bone marrow, enters the circulation and on returning to the tissues, matures into a macrophage.

Monokine: A molecule produced and secreted by monocytes and macrophages. Monokines are involved in the regulation of the immune response.

Natural killer (NK) cell: A white cell capable of killing tumour cells and virus-infected cells without previous exposure to an antigen. NK cells are thought to provide an important defence against cancer and viral infections.

Neutrophil: A white blood cell that performs phagocytic and degradative functions similar to the macrophages. Neutrophils are the first cells to appear at a site where an inflammatory response occurs.

Opsonization: A process in which complement proteins or antibodies coat a foreign substance or microorganism, thereby facilitating phagocytosis by a neutrophil or macrophage.

Phagocyte: A white blood cell capable of ingesting foreign particles and microorganisms. Phagocytes include monocytes, macrophages and neutrophils.

Phagocytosis: Process whereby phagocytes ingest and destroy bacteria, etc.

Phagosome: A vesicle that forms around a bacterium or other particles as it is ingested by a phagocyte in the process of phagocytosis.

Stem cell: A non-differentiated precursor cell that undergoes maturation to a variety of cell types. One type of stem cell gives rise to T cells, B cells, monocytes, neutrophil and red blood cells.

Stressor: External influence on the mind and body. Stressors have widespread, subtle and profound effects on the body, especially on the neuroendocrine and immune systems.

Suppressor T cell: See T lymphocyte.

Thymocyte: A cell that is derived from the bone marrow and migrates to the thymus, where it develops into an immunocompetent T cell.

T lymphocyte (or T cell): A type of lymphocyte that migrates from the bone marrow to the thymus, where it acquires the ability to recognize antigen via antigen-specific receptors. T cells leave the thymus and circulate in the blood or reside in other lymphoid organs. There are several types of T cells, including the following:

- Helper T cells, which respond to antigen by synthesizing and secreting lymphokines that stimulate protective functions of other immune system cells

- Cytotoxic T cells, which recognize foreign antigens on the surface of virus-infected cells or transplanted cells, and function to destroy these cells
- Suppressor T cells, which inhibit other immune responses such as antibody production by B cells, and thus help to prevent overreaction of the immune system
- Delayed-type hypersensitivity T cells, which react to antigens by producing lymphokines that induce localized inflammatory responses and attract macrophages and cytotoxic T cells to the area to assist in elimination of the antigen

Western blotting: Test in which viral antigens are separated on a gel, transferred to a blotting strip and exposed to a patient's serum. Uses include the detection of the presence of antibodies to HIV rather than the HIV antigen itself. Also called "immunoblot".

Index

Note: page numbers in *italics* refer to figures and tables

Index compiled by Jill Halliday